The Supreme Remedy

Reflections on applying natural healing arts
to the Bahá'í Fast

About the author

Deborah Walters is a Doctor of Naturopathy and runs a private practice welcoming clients from all over the globe. She specializes in spiritual, mental and physical healing. Deborah builds bridges between science and spiritual texts as well as blending approaches of modern medicine and natural healing methods. She lectures throughout the United States on topics of spiritual and physical well-being.

The Supreme Remedy

Reflections on applying natural healing arts
to the Bahá'í Fast

Deborah Walters

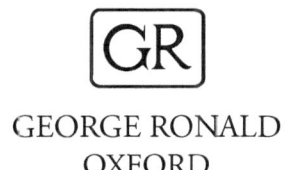

GEORGE RONALD
OXFORD

George Ronald, Publisher
Oxford
www.grbooks.com

© Deborah Walters 2014
All Rights Reserved
Reprinted 2016

*A catalogue record for this book is available
from the British Library*

ISBN 978–0–85398–567–9

Cover design: Steiner Graphics

CONTENTS

Introduction   vii

I	**A Call to Fast**	1
	1 Transformation and Renewal	3
	2 A Brief History of Fasting	9
	3 Prescription for Today's World	24
	4 The Human Experience	46
II	**The Human Temple**	67
	5 Fasting for the Body	69
	6 Preparing the Body for the Fast	79
	7 Recommendations for Fasting	101
III	**The Rational Faculty**	111
	8 Fasting for the Mind	113
	9 Preparing the Mind for the Fast	135
	10 Recommendations for the Fast	180
IV	**The Soul**	195
	11 Fasting for Spiritual Purposes	197
	12 Preparing the Soul for the Fast	220
	13 Recommendations for the Fast	272
V	**Where Do I Go From Here?**	283
	14 Alternatives for Those Who Cannot Fast	285
	15 Re-entry: Life after the Fast	293
	16 Recipes	304
	17 Prayers for the Fast	334

Annex 347
I   Reflections on the Badí' Calendar 347

Bibliography 351
References 355

INTRODUCTION

I have no objection to your interpretations and inferences so long as they are represented as your own personal observations and reflections.[8]

Individual interpretations based on a person's understanding of the teachings constitute the fruit of man's rational power and may well contribute to a more complete understanding of the Faith. Such views, however, lack authority. The believers are, therefore, free to accept or disregard them.[9]

Therefore, in the spirit of science, religion, and personal experience and interpretation, I offer the following pages with humility, in the hope that readers will find in them ideas to open their minds and hearts to new worlds and possibilities.

PART I

A CALL TO FAST

I

TRANSFORMATION AND RENEWAL

The more we search for ourselves, the less likely we are to find ourselves; and the more we search for God, and to serve our fellow-men, the more profoundly will we become acquainted with ourselves, and the more inwardly assured. This is one of the great spiritual laws of life.

Shoghi Effendi[1]

Transformation is directly linked to our actions. The universe provides a world that can transform both our inner and outer reality, and fasting is a very tangible path of change. Perhaps we eliminate sugar from our diet, or act kindly towards someone who challenges us. Small changes in habits create large internal shifts which give birth to new realities. We understand life on deeper levels.

Change is organic, whether it is individual or collective, and it is one of the only things we can rely on. All created beings evolve to reach a stage of maturity; for example, the maturity of a plant is to flower, the maturity of a tree is to give fruit, and maturity for a human being is to reach our capacity spiritually and attain the powers of our intellect. Humanity reflects a similar pattern to that shown in nature, tending toward ever greater levels of unity. Its highest level of attainment will be the unification of civilization, and one of the positive effects of the Fast will be to bring about such a transformation.

Humanity's current state of development can be compared to that of an adolescent. Any fair-minded person living today can readily recognize society's symptoms of rebellious teenager-like tendencies, desiring to strike out independently following its impulses and rejecting the standards of the past. The evidence of such a phase can be witnessed through economic unfairness and uncertainty, slack moral standards, lawlessness, terrorism, religious intolerance, prejudice of all kinds, the constant emphasis on vanity, riches and the pursuit of pleasure, the weakening of family and marital bonds, negligence in quality parental guidance, the spread of fear and paranoia and rampant excess of the tongue in speech and appetite.

Most influential theorists in the field of moral reasoning hold that moral development in childhood and adolescence rests on cognitive development – the shedding of egocentric thought and the growing ability to think abstractly. The perpetual round robin of 'Who am I?' plagues teenage minds and impinges on teenage choices. The quest to achieve certainty over self-consciousness and self-doubt marks this stage, which seeks to acquire the level of skills needed for success instead of inadequacy. Experience through crisis or a turning point often leads people to reevaluate their criteria for judging what is right and fair.

Like young adults, humanity as a whole is progressing toward expressing new virtues, new moral standards, and showing a capacity for self-discipline not only to survive but to thrive.

Habits and behaviours result in progress or stagnation or even regression. Unhealthy change in the individual takes place through acquiring negative habits – pursuing the impulses, the needs of self. Reflection on personal action and its results is the most important step to change, on both individual and collective levels. The transformation of human society is a result of a very complex set of interactions between profound changes that have to occur within the individual, and deliberate attempts to change the structure of society. The path of growth is not one of individual salvation alone; it implies constant efforts to create and strengthen new social institutions. The maturing of humanity requires individuals to collectively enter the stage of adulthood, to produce high-quality relationships, to responsibly attain a role in civilization through craftsmanship, arts or sciences, and to develop a high level of integrity. These themes are explored further by Paul Lample in his book *Revelation and Social Reality*.

In contemplating the verse by Bahá'u'lláh telling us about the 'innumerable effects and benefits' of the Fast[2] we can begin to see the widespread implications of transformation on an individual, community and global scale. This call for change challenges us to consider the benefits of spending a period of time every year focusing our efforts on cleansing ourselves, and refraining from self and passion. The challenge collectively, then, is to create a new mindset, a clearer lens with which to view the world, and optimal tools with which to respond.

What we perceive as reality is set by the limits of the mind. It's necessary to avoid the natural inclination to compartmentalize, dividing reality into categories and keeping them separate. We must be mindful to resist the ease of fragmenting life, which comes from several systems operating at once within an individual. Humans exist on many levels. The main categories include the 'human temple' – the body –, the rational faculty and the soul. While these 'expressions' communicate constantly with each other, we have not yet evolved enough to consciously administer these communications. The vastness of our reality requires us to break subjects down into smaller components in order to understand them. While each can be studied individually, they are indeed the very essence of one being and must be viewed in unity.

A fragmented approach creates opposing forces and an illusionary 'reality', and it is this that the individual must resist. While it is necessary to prioritize our time and resources with discernment, living in harmony requires that we see the interconnectedness of our lives. When we fail to see the whole, tension and anxiety arise from being pulled in so many directions. The result is confusion and reliance on old habits. Transformation can aid us to integrate ourselves internally. Beliefs such as 'If I want to advance in my career my family life will suffer,' or 'Serving my Faith pulls me away from my marriage,' are compartmentalized and not integrated. More integrated thinking might be, 'I can advance my career while engaging my family,' or 'Service helps enhance my marital relationship.' Some compartmentalize the spirit and intellect: 'Logic has no place with intuition.' A more integrated approach might be: 'Minds and hearts complement each other and are expressions of one reality.'

Bahá'u'lláh gave us the Fast, and we can seek and understand the benefits and stations laid within it. It is a bounty to humanity and a signpost to our approach to God. Just as humans have to obey the laws of nature such as gravity, they are also bound by the universal spiritual laws. God releases life-generating forces for the natural world, providing sustenance, assisting evolution. God also releases spiritual forces to develop the soul. The human body is subject to the laws of nature and involuntarily grows as dictated by nature. On the other hand, obeying the spiritual laws is purely voluntary. Following spiritual guidance in today's society is like arriving in a city we don't know and needing to find the hospital – we would obey and follow the street signs because we implicitly trust the authorities who have posted the signs.

Many symbols of the spiritual laws can be found in nature – for example, the sun, moon and stars. Just as these are essential to our lives, so Bahá'u'lláh characterizes the spiritual laws as the 'breath of life unto all created things', or 'the highest means for the maintenance of order in the world and the security of its peoples'.[3] He describes his Book of Laws, the Kitáb-i-Aqdas, thus : 'Blessed the palate that savoureth its sweetness, and the perceiving eye that recognizeth that which is treasured therein, and the understanding heart that comprehendeth its allusions and mysteries.'[4] Anyone who appreciates beauty can read the laws and understand their splendour. Bahá'u'lláh referred to His laws as a fortress, a mighty stronghold,[5] and also to the Fast as a fortress.[6] Following the laws, like following signs in a strange city, will lead us to the correct destination. In fact, Bahá'u'lláh testifies, 'By My life, were ye to discover what We have desired for you in revealing Our holy laws, ye would offer up your very souls for this sacred, this mighty, and most exalted Faith.'[7]

The laws given by every Manifestation of God have included fasting and prayer. Bahá'u'lláh says, 'Fasting and obligatory prayer are as two wings to man's life.'[8] Divinity anticipates humanity being plunged in the sea of self and illimitable pressures, and therefore offers devotional practices – prayer and fasting – to help human beings refocus on their true reality.

Physical aspects of fasting

The body and mind take in many substances and influences throughout the day, depending on the choices that surround us. As far as the body is concerned, when we experience ***deficiency*** (lack of nutrients), or ***congestion*** (excess of nutrition), imbalance and disease proliferate. Therefore, complete physical fasting always includes:

- refraining from impulses
- cleansing out toxins
- rebuild health with proper nourishment

Creation tells us about staying in balance. Nature in all its splendour reveals the mysteries latent in the universe. Investigating nature on any level, be it plants, clouds, solar systems or storms, exposes the following two truths: nature ingests and eliminates, and everything moves in cycles.

At present, whole populations in the rich industrialized countries are out of balance, ingesting more than eliminating. Simple daily living exposes us to toxins at an unprecedented rate in our history – polluted air and water, TV programmes that induce fear and melodrama, and inundation of information by junk mail, the Internet, and gossip. 'Abdu'l-Bahá points out that 'it is certainly the case that sins are a potent cause of physical ailments'.[9] Diseases have diversified rapidly as a result of affluence, addiction, nutritional deficiencies and excess. Although modern agriculture allows us to eat a greater quantity of food than at any time in history, we consume foods wrenched from soils overused and deficient in the micronutrients required for optimum health.

Renewal is a natural impulse found in nature. The body has a series of miraculous processes that automatically arise to heal when faced with a crisis. Like an army battling an invader, our immune system is stimulated and launches its defences the minute it senses an intruder; the body creates pus and mucus around foreign substances to protect the major organs and bloodstream from further contamination.

Though the body can handle natural detoxification, this process can break down gradually over time if unaided. Therefore, every spring, we have a chance for rebirth, renewal and transformation. For example, as the body ages the release of hydrochloric acid in the stomach gradually decreases, therefore decreasing the amount of flora and enzymes.

Detoxification is a beautifully complex series of systems intended to keep us healthy and in balance. Every day metabolic processes automatically accumulate toxic matter and eliminate it. When done properly, this process not only moves toxins out, but also helps renew and *rejuvenate* inner structures. This can include clearing congestion, fats and free radicals, and dealing with digestive and colon problems or problems in the respiratory system or the skin. A detoxified system works well, interpreting information more clearly than a congested system can. Bahá'u'lláh writes: 'To cleanse the body of its wastes is essential, but only in temperate seasons.'[10]

Because exposure to toxins is unavoidable, the best approach is to (1) lower your toxin intake as much as possible; (2) remove toxins from the mind and body; and (3) rebuild the health of your mind, body and soul during the Fast.

Many of my Bahá'í clients or fellow community members report the first week of the Fast as being the worst, because some of the old residue and waste products in the system are passing through the blood attempting to be eliminated. It's also a difficult week because of the change in eating habits, and the body has to adjust to mild dehydration and changing blood sugar levels. These same individuals experience the second week as better – once the body has adjusted and thrown out some of the initial waste, a lighter feeling can be experienced; there is more mental clarity and the senses can feel more acute, especially if they are eating clean healthy foods.

Rest is an essential factor in renewal, especially during the Fast. One cannot maintain the overscheduled lifestyle most of us live during this period without feeling the effects of the interrupted daily diet. Deliberately scheduling extra down time, pushing off errands that aren't essential, and prioritizing your time will help aid the body and mind to restore themselves. As you rest, get in tune with your body's 'thank you' and try to feel the vital force and nerves being restored.

Fasting is a sacred right of passage which strengthens this process. The Fast is a call to action and devotion, to arise and be aware of our choices and their consequences. It's a time for each one of us to bring our own selves into balance. It's a time to recognize that, as well as humanity as a whole, we as individuals need to be nourished and rejuvenated. The consequences of fasting are weighty. If one such new habit is integrated successfully, the more general habit of refraining from what is harmful and aligning with a higher purpose can stimulate new ways of thinking. What are the probable effects on an individual? A nation? The planet?

Studying the past helps shape future actions. The next chapter takes a look at the historical tradition of fasting, from both a healing and a religious perspective, in keeping with the spirit of harmony between science and religion.

2

A BRIEF HISTORY OF FASTING

> Prayer carries us half way to God, fasting brings us to the door of His palace, and alms-giving procures us admission.
>
> *Muslim proverb*[1]

Fasting is an integral part of transformation and healing, both of the individual and of society as a whole. By studying humanity's development throughout history, we come to have a stronger appreciation for fasting, recognizing that God asked the people who came before us to fast. Our global history is rich with the tradition of fasting. It is one of the oldest methods used for the improvement of health, and also most major religions in every era have prescribed it as a spiritual discipline. As history has unfolded, the purpose of fasting has remained surprisingly consistent.

The origin of fasting is unknown, but probably dates back to the time when present-day animals developed. Animals commonly fast when ill as an instinctive response rather than a planned healing response. Many factors regulate food intake for animals and humans, including hormones, appetite, social factors and activity levels. These factors regulate metabolism and homeostasis within the organism. In ancient days, fasting was an innate response to illness, or to not having access to food or water for a period of time, or sometimes a natural rhythm, as when penguins go without eating for several months every year. Human fasting has developed over the centuries through religious practice, medical experimentation, observation and study.

Some of the most brilliant scientific minds have contributed their knowledge to this healing method. One of the first records of human fasting is traced to early Greek and Eastern societies. Many well-known figures in history have used fasting and openly promoted its benefits. Spanning from Hippocrates, Aristotle, Galen, Paracelsus, Plato and Socrates to Gandhi and on to modern-day 'wellness centres', philosophers, scientists and physicians have used fasting as a method of cleansing, healing, balance, and working towards a goal or renewal.

A historical perspective

The benefits and purposes of fasting affect the body, mind and soul. Throughout history fasting has been used for material purposes, such as political agendas or to rid oneself of an evil presence. It is also seen in the advancement in medicine and the healing arts. Fasting also appears in disciplines of devotion and obedience, especially in the context of religion.

Table 2.1   Purposes of fasting

Body	For material goals, or for political or superstitious purposes
Mind	Creating a healing plan from knowledge available at that time in history
Soul	For obedience, cleansing and devotion

Most children are taught history only from their regional geopolitical point of view. But when we view humanity's various stages of development, considering spiritual influences, the purpose of life on earth is revealed. As the human mind developed from stage to stage, God sent messengers (divine educators, or Manifestations of God in Bahá'í terminology) reflective of the needs of that time. Parallels between the development of civilization, sciences and arts, and religious advancement begin to appear. In certain periods they were one and the same: the religious divines of that age were also the physicians who dominated the medical and political field. Over time there has been change, both progression and regression, and the variances between different parts of the world during each epoch have been vast.

One would expect that as civilization and the human mind evolved, so would the field of healing. In my perspective, however, the science of healing has not kept up with the pace of spiritual dynamics or the evolution of thought. One indication is the rapid spread of wasting conditions that plague society, and for which there are no cures. I believe that it is the divisions between rational thought, politics, domination and superstition that have caused this slower evolution. Despite this, the one consistent prescription in both religious practice and the science of healing is fasting.

The following sections give an overview of a time period, followed by a short discussion of the practices of medical, social and religious fasting during each epoch.

3000–1200 BC

Shamanic practices and herbs were used in all cultures. Many herbalists were considered to be 'gods' in their times. Chinese medicine was established around 3000 BC by Shen Nung, an emperor who was called the father of medicine. Evidence suggests that some cultures, such as the Egyptians in c.2000 BC, knew the effects of plant medicines on the body, as distinct from placebos or magic.

Fasting was only one of the numerous tools used by healers. For example, medicine combined magic, ointments, herbs and surgery. Everything was experimental at this point, whether casting out demons or relying heavily on plants, animals and minerals for healing. Medical practice in Mesopotamia relied strongly on astrology. As people and animals lived more closely together, medicine needed to become more formalized to deal with the new issues at hand. Often, village shamans yielded to specialists in sorcery and divination who worked with spirits. Illness was equated with the will of the gods.

The prophet Abraham is thought to have lived around 2000 BC. In the midst of superstition and idol worship, his core message to humanity was the reassurance of God's love and His oneness, and he was severely persecuted for teaching monotheism.

Abraham's Revelation had great influence on the Middle Eastern region, and created the stage for future Manifestations of God.

Fasting as religious practice

In another part of the world, Hinduism was flourishing. The most influential teachings in Hinduism are contained in the Avestas and the Maharabhata, of which the Bhagavad Gita is the best-known part. In the Sanskrit texts fasting is understood to mean 'to move near the Supreme'. Knowledge was represented by the three main gods, or forces: creativity (Brahma), preservation (Shiva), and destruction (Vishnu).

Reality is simply an expression of *the one* that is everything – Brahman. Food is really an aspect of Brahman, and is to be considered sacred. It is given to us by the gods and should be treated with respect. Eating was a sacrificial ritual, fulfilling an important role in social and ritual life.

For Hindus, the practice of fasting is personal and flexible, and there are some traditional fasting times. It is a spiritual practice, not simply a physical exercise: chanting, vows, meditation and silence accompany fasting. These times include the lunar schedules, festivals, or planetary influences. Sometimes fasting is defined by abstaining from certain foods or liquids. The objective is partly penitential, to purify the body and the mind and to honour one's personal gods. Fasting is vital to Hinduism and is considered one of the aids to spiritual growth. It is a sacred offering to the gods, sometimes done in order to accomplish something, or to seek an answer to a prayer. It is intertwined with meditation and obtaining 'yogic power'. Hindu wives often fast on behalf of their husbands.

1300–600 BC

Medicine now reached a higher standard, especially in Egypt. Although most doctors were general practitioners, they could specialize in various parts of the body and get specialist training. According to some experts, ayurvedic medicine also began at this time. Disease was often considered to be the 'wrath of God' and thus in some societies the clergy were 'in charge of' contagious diseases. Most events had superstitious explanations – nothing was in an individual's control. Forces of good and evil lurked. Fasting, diet, herbs, animals and casting out demons were some basic tools in medicine. Polygamy and superstition commonly pervaded societies.

The Revelation of Moses infused the region with a new religion that was ethically grand in comparison to what had existed before, and profoundly influenced the future Revelations to come. There were new inventions, such as the magnetic compass, the Phoenician alphabet, and in medicine. Literary works such as Homer's *Iliad* and *Odyssey* originated in this era.

In the Old Testament, God (Yahweh) is presented as both protective and quick to anger. This concept was both appealing and palatable to the developmental needs of the human mindset of the time. The traditional

Mesopotamian gods were capricious: one never knew what to expect in comparison with the God of the Hebrews. While the Mesopotamians believed that the gods preferred good to evil but did not demand ethical conduct, the followers of Moses knew they would be pleasing to God by living up to high moral standards and by worshipping Him, and that they would be collectively rewarded. The message was clear: like any good parent, God would not abandon them.

Fasting as religious practice

Hebrew scripture offers us two examples of fasting. The first is by Moses, who fasted for forty days and forty nights in remission of his people's sins and in preparation for his own mission. The other is by Elijah in the desert. A beautiful verse from Hosea says, 'It is love that I desire, and not sacrifice,'[2] which may indicate that fasting for love is more commendable in God's eyes than simply for sacrifice or obedience.

Traditionally, Jewish fasting is associated with dangerous conditions or periods of mourning. The major fast is Yom Kippur, or the Day of Atonement, when charitable giving, prayer and repentance are the major themes. This fast is the only one specifically prescribed in the Torah.[3] It is a day to 'afflict your soul'. The fast begins one hour before Yom Kippur until after nightfall on the second day, a total of 25 hours.

Most branches of Judaism acknowledge this fast, during which a *kittel* (shroud) is traditionally worn. Girls aged twelve and boys aged thirteen and older without health conditions are required to participate. Pregnant women and those who have recently given birth, or someone suffering from a life-threatening illness, are not required to observe the fast. No food or liquid is consumed. Sexual relations and bathing are forbidden during the fast.

For Jews, fasting provides reflection time on what the actions of their ancestors wrought, and similarly, on taking account of one's own personal actions and their implications in the present. The focus is on repentance for wrongdoing, leading to a change in behaviour and habits. It builds on the original relationship God had with the Jewish people. Physical fasting is thus an impetus for spiritual growth.

The Zoroastrian faith, on the other hand, does not value strict fasting, characterizing it as asceticism, an extreme measure. Everything should be done in moderation, even eating and drinking. It is a crime, an offence, to purposefully abstain from food. Zoroastrians focus on spiritual rather than physical fasting. One should fast one's whole life: fast with one's eyes to not see evil, fast with one's tongue to not speak evil, fast with one's hands to not do evil things. One should constantly be vigilant about surrounding forces, against evil, gluttony and deficiency. Fasting would diminish your ability to judge these forces, and weaken your ability to battle evil.

The Vendidad, the Zoroastrian Book of Law, states,

> The person who abstains from food, or takes insufficient food, has neither enough strength to practice active virtues, nor can he till the earth, nor beget children, nor is he able to withstand hardship and pain.[4]

There are, however, a few dietary traditions, such as not eating meat three days after a loved one has died. Another practice traditionally observed is to fast from eating meat throughout the month of *Bahman*. There are no other ceremonies, rituals or special prayers required during this month. Being vegetarian this month is considered to build spiritual discipline.

560–1 BC

The writings of Bahá'u'lláh describe the rise and fall of great civilizations:

> For every land We have prescribed a portion, for every occasion an allotted share, for every pronouncement an appointed time and for every situation an apt remark. Consider Greece. We made it a Seat of Wisdom for a prolonged period. However, when the appointed hour struck, its throne was subverted, its tongue ceased to speak, its light grew dim and its banner was hauled down. Thus do We bestow and withdraw.[5]

In this period there were leaps in technology across cultures. In India, the physician Susruta pioneered plastic surgery for the nose. Ayurvedic medicine was well developed by now and often used fasting to heal. In China, the first cast iron was set after developing a furnace to reach very high temperatures. The Chinese also discovered the hardening quality of lacquer, which is the sap from a tree. The philosophy of opposing forces, yin and yang, was introduced. Acupuncture meridian theory was also established at this time. In China, India and Greece, attempts were being made to classify plants and provide a taxonomy of medicinal herbs – what would in the next period be called 'materia medica' and would ultimately develop into modern pharmacology.

Hippocrates, the Greek physician who used fasting regularly, is considered the 'father of medicine' because he introduced a new method of thinking into the medical field. His philosophies were based in reason, rather than the supernatural; the causes of disease could be found and treated by close observation of the symptoms. He proposed moderation, 'nothing in excess'. His method was to not interfere with the natural healing powers of the body, and to treat the patient without focusing on a specific illness. Physicians would commonly start treatment with a seven-day fast. If symptoms were still present after the seven days, then medicinal herbs would be given.

Fasting as religious practice

Gautama Buddha grew up in the Hindu culture prevalent in the age. Like many in that society he practised asceticism, where self-denial is a principled way of life. He initially used very strict fasting practices, but starvation reduced his physical health to such an extent that he no longer had energy to meditate. The story says that his diet consisted of a grain of rice and a sesame seed each day. He could touch his spine by pressing on his stomach, and realized that *desire could not be overcome by force*. Upon breaking his fast, he became aware that the body should be honoured, that a well-balanced body enhances one's spiritual awakening. The Four Noble Truths and the Noble Eightfold Path resulted from this enlightenment. Although Gautama did not apply fasting as a core idea of His teachings, He emphasized that a 'middle path' was important.

Gautama suggested that monks should limit their diet after noontime. Fasting would help one to spiritually progress in rising above 'all desires', and to help focus on overcoming all cravings. Fasting always revolved around the middle path: desire is rooted in the mind, and should be transformed there, while fasting provides a means to subdue the body's desires and to transform the mind's desires into wisdom.

In the Buddhist traditions, monks have different rules from general believers for fasting. They practice 'dhutanga' (to shake up or invigorate). Meat is generally not consumed at this time. There are two meals a day, an early morning meal and one before noon, with abstinence thereafter. The remaining part of the day is open for meditation, which is better practised on an empty stomach. On festivals and at full and new moons, ordinary believers too practise this ritual. Fasting is considered to maintain purity in body and spirit and is often done to achieve a goal or wish.

After the Buddha passed away, the spiritual springtime of his divine revelation infused many parts of the world. It specifically aided India's 'golden era', enlightening this population with arts, sciences and advances in technology. In fact, historians place India's Gupta Dynasty alongside the Han Dynasty, Tang Dynasty and Roman Empire, as a model of a classical civilization.

1–600 AD

Modern medicine still uses many principles from Hippocrates, the 'father of medicine'. In the first centuries of the common era Greek and Roman medical knowledge spread widely, often influenced by the earlier Egyptian civilization. Aulus Cornelius Celsus, a Roman known for his medical encyclopedia, classified medicine into three categories: diet, pharmacy and surgery. He used fasting and dietary restrictions to treat infectious disease.

However, during this period shamanic medicine was often still preferred to 'rational' medicine. Whatever could not rationally be explained lent itself to 'magic'. Wild and domesticated animals became reservoirs for disease.

Fasting as religious practice

In this age of war and trade between nation states, Jesus came to renew the message of Moses and bring God's kingdom to earth with new understanding. He was raised under the laws of Moses, yet brought a revolutionary way of thinking to our planet. Jesus, like Moses, began his journey by fasting for forty days and forty nights in the desert. The union with his Father was the aim of this fast.

Jesus brought a new perspective on spirituality. Union with God in this age was something private – an intimate connection between oneself and God. This was especially true of fasting. Jesus encouraged those fasting to make it private between them and God:

> And whenever you fast, do not look dismal, like the hypocrites, for they disfigure their faces so as to show others that they are fasting. Truly I tell you, they have received their reward. But when you fast, put oil on your head and wash your face, so that your fasting may be seen not by others but by your father who is in secret; and your Father who sees in secret will reward you.[6]

There is no mention in the New Testament of how or when to fast, nor of Jesus and his disciples fasting. In contrast, one can read about them feasting. It was a day for recognizing the sacredness of breaking bread with one another, and the teaching that the meek shall inherit the earth.

Some people came and asked Jesus why He and the disciples were not fasting during the Jewish fast. Jesus replied, 'How can the guests of the bridegroom fast while he is with them? They cannot, so long as they have him with them. But the time will come when the bridegroom will be taken from them, and on that day they will fast.' He continued with a metaphor: 'No one pours new wine into old wineskins. If he does, the wine will burst the skins, and both the wine and the wineskins will be ruined. No, he pours new wine into new wineskins.'[7] There are numerous meanings here. We can envision the new revelation (the new wine) each prophet brings to each age of humanity (the new wineskin) and might understand how the prophets were from the same God (the wine maker). Therefore, Jesus brought a new message; the former traditions no longer applied.

There is a story in the Gospel of St. Mark of an afflicted child; the disciples tried but failed to cast out the spirit that tormented him. Jesus healed him, and when the disciples asked him why they had not been able to help the child, replied, 'This kind can come forth by nothing, but by prayer and fasting.'[8] This passage implies a working between spiritual health and physical health. It also indicates that fasting was a practice used to heal the body at the time.

After the establishment of the Church, early Christians linked fasting to penitence and purification. The earliest evidence of fasting during this era was in the second century when churches traditionally fasted prior to Easter. This fasting period turned into Lent. Originally, Christians fasted without food or water, a practice encouraged more in the early days. Later on, fasting was relegated to the most sacred times of the Christian year: eating less food during Advent, the four weeks prior to Christmas, and Lent, the forty days prior to Easter. Christians were encouraged to undertake their own fasts in order to become closer to God. Eventually, church policies evolved with cultural norms; today's practice differs according to the Christian denomination, but it is common to eat fish rather than meat on Fridays and to 'give up' something during Lent.

600–c.1750 AD

At the beginning of this period, shamanism had become a well-established science and healing art in the Americas. The shaman distinctly understood pharmacology and specific doses under certain conditions, but also employed standard rituals calling on the supernatural to induce healing. Using both forces, the sick person and the practitioner entered sacred space. Rituals became part of standard medicine, while fasting was a pillar of health and was used in vision questing. It was a perfect exchange, as the shaman was given credit for the healing, and the patient felt as though they played a part. This was a 'perfect blend' of science and religion.

But the Middle East was about to enter a revival infused by the Revelation of Muhammad. Islam affected not only the Arab world but also, and profoundly, the development of the West. Islamic medical knowledge and experience became far superior to that of Western medicine, enhancing Western knowledge of anatomy and pharmacology. Major advances in mathematics, philosophy and science ensued. The influence of Islam on the Middle East enabled it to flourish in technology, science and the arts. Islamic discoveries and inventions spread to Asia and Europe, setting the stage for the European Renaissance.

Greek and Roman medical knowledge had been faithfully preserved by the Byzantine scholars, and Islamic scientists now combined this with Hindu and Islamic practices. They continued the tradition of Hippocrates in medicine. Because this region was a path between Europe and the Orient, epidemics tended to break out and it was in fighting these illnesses that Islamic physicians developed a pharmacopoeia of

720 drugs which combined medicinal plants from the Greek, Hindu, and Persian traditions.

Around the 12th century, European scholars translated much of the work done in Persia and Arabia into Latin, focusing on anatomy and physiology, and the causes of illness. Huge contributions to pharmacology were made by experimenting with various substances. From the 16th century great advancements in medicine occurred again. Homeopathy, naturopathy and allopathy began. Fasting was widely practised and studied. Paracelsus, the famous Swiss physician, wrote, 'Fasting is the greatest remedy.' Across the globe during this time period, doctors were studying the effects of fasting on disease. Dr Von Seeland of Russia wrote, 'As a result of experiments I have come to the conclusion that fasting is not only a therapeutic of the highest degree possible but also deserves consideration educationally.' In Europe, Dr Adolph Mayer was studying fasting in practice and ascertained that 'fasting is the most efficient means of correcting any disease'.

Fasting as religious practice

Muhammad came to renew the message of the oneness of God and confirm the monotheistic faiths brought by Abraham, Moses and Jesus. He taught that one's life should be transformed into a form of worship, and that submitting to God's Will is an ultimate goal. Martyrdom was the highest station one could attain, and this included conforming one's actions to the laws of God and surrendering oneself entirely to God (Islam). Validating the past beliefs in the oneness of God and reaffirming the prophets of old, Muhammad intertwined faith and right action as inseparable practices. God was unknowable in His essence, but ever protective, loving and generous to His followers.

In Islam, Muhammad made fasting one of the five 'pillars', or religious obligations to God: 'O ye who believe! Fasting is prescribed to you as it was prescribed to those before you, that ye may (learn) self-restraint . . .'[9] One fasts for a month, the ninth month of the Islamic calendar. This is a celebratory time of energy, self-control, and inner reflection. In the Qur'án the specific spiritual passage is:

> Ramadhan is the (month) in which was sent down the Qur'an, as guide to mankind, also clear (Signs) for guidance and judgment. So

every one of you who is present (at his home) during that month should spend it in fasting, but if any one is ill, or on a journey, the prescribed period (should be made up) days later. God intends every facility for you; He does not want to put to difficulties. (He wants you) to complete the prescribed period, and to glorify Him in that He has guided you; and perchance ye shall be grateful.[10]

Elsewhere it is laid down that adults who are healthy can participate in the Fast from sunrise to sunset, abstaining from food, drink and sexual activity. The month of Ramadan enables one to reflect, express gratitude for God's guidance and blessings, practise generosity by giving to the poor and needy, and ask for forgiveness for past wrongdoings. It's a time to remember to be dependent upon God's Will. Families rise before sunrise to eat a meal sustaining them until the Fast is broken at sunset by a light meal. Special sweets are served at this time. Many go to the mosque to pray. The end of Ramadan, Id al-Fitr (Eid), is celebrated for three days with visits to family and friends and the exchanging of gifts. The last day of the Fast, called the Night of Power, is spiritually significant because it commemorates the time when the beginning of the Qur'án was revealed. Great rewards are promised for observing that night with prayer, fasting and reading the sacred Qur'án.

1750 AD–Present

There were extraordinary advances in Western medicine during this period, due to the rise of scientific research. Countless lives have been saved and many diseases eradicated or controlled. At the same time, these advances have led to a proliferation of specializations, so that today there is a sometimes confusing array of specialists and generalists as well as naturopaths, acupuncturists and homeopaths – not to mention many other valid fields of healing. Today, fasting is used frequently as medical doctors recommend it prior to certain tests and procedures, while natural medicine promotes short fasts to regain balance and recover from acute and chronic conditions. Outside the realm of medicine, many use fasting for political or personal solutions as well as in the spiritual traditions (Mahatma Gandhi was an example of fasting for political reasons). The Native American culture used fasting for healing, vision quests, and a rite of passage into adulthood.

Fasting in the medical field was being studied vigorously, especially in Russia, Germany, Switzerland and North America. The clinical research carried out in these countries alone has added to the world's body of knowledge on experimental fasting. The data gleaned from these studies has given us clear knowledge regarding the effects of fasting on the mind and body, and its precise phases and outcomes. We know much better how to fast, how the body reacts, when to fast and how to break a fast properly.

As we grow old, our metabolic rate slows down. Numerous studies conducted around the globe have confirmed that when animals and insects are forced to fast, their lifespan is greatly increased. Their cells return to a more youthful state. While these studies show more profound effect on lower forms of life, they also confirm a permanent increase in metabolic rates and assimilation powers in humans during fasting. During one of Gandhi's fasts in 1933, his physicians examined him when he was in the tenth day of fasting. One of them observed that 'despite his 64 years, from a physiological point of view the Indian leader was as healthy as a man of forty'.[11]

Fasting as religious practice

In 1844, when the Báb proclaimed His mission to Mullá Ḥusayn, who was searching for the Promised One, a new era began. The Báb revealed the Bayán as the set of laws for His short nineteen-year mission to prepare the world to recognize the Promised One of all ages. These laws included fasting as well, which was binding on those between the ages of eleven and forty-two.

> The substance of this gate is that before fasting thou must comprehend God's purpose thereof, regarding that which is the fruit of the fast...The purpose of fasting is to fast from anyone who is not godly...Guard thyself from drinking; eating; intercourse; contention, even in words; injustice, even to the slightest extent; and pronouncing judgment against God. Be especially careful with regard to the last three prohibitions inasmuch as, from the inception of the Revelation till the commencement of the next Revelation, whosoever pronounceth judgment against the Point hath pronounced judgment against God, which rendereth his fasting null.[12]

The Báb instructed His followers to search for 'Him Whom God shall make Manifest', the Promised One of all ages. This was Bahá'u'lláh (a title that means 'Glory of God'), who was born in Persia. Bahá'u'lláh claims to be the return and fulfilment of all the Messengers of the past, a fulfilment prophesied in all the holy books of scripture in all religions. His divine message is to unite all the peoples in one universal cause and establish unity on earth. His teachings will raise up a new race of men, enabling humanity to build this unity.

Bahá'u'lláh's central message is that 'the earth is but one country, and mankind its citizens'.[13] His teachings lay the foundations of a united global civilization. One could even read these prescriptions as the remedies for humanity today. Some of these basic tenets include:

- Abandonment of all forms of prejudice
- Men and women should be assured equality
- Elimination of extremes of poverty and wealth
- Economic problems have spiritual solutions
- Realization of universal education
- Each person is responsible to independently search for truth
- Establishment of a global commonwealth of nations
- Recognition that true religion is in harmony with reason and the pursuit of scientific knowledge
- Establishment of a universal auxiliary language

Bahá'u'lláh's teachings encourage daily prayer and communion with God, living a life dedicated to the service of humanity and consorting in fellowship with the followers of all religions. Spiritually, the highest station is no longer martyrdom, but teaching the Cause of God. The source of all wrongdoing is ignorance, and in overcoming ignorance teaching the Cause of God ranks above all. The purpose of God's Will on earth is the peace, tranquillity and advancement of its peoples. Bahá'u'lláh's teachings promote unity and concord, not only within an individual and between individuals, but for the whole of humankind as well. The only way to the peace and tranquillity of the world's peoples is through justice, fellowship and love.

Prayer and fasting are necessary to ensure the soul's development. As we have seen, Bahá'u'lláh likens them to the two wings of a bird which enable the bird to fly. Fasting and prayer offer a believer a devotional path and can be seen as symbolic in the context of the Bahá'í Faith. If we pull the lens back and view the Faith's destiny in this world, fasting can be seen as a symbol of purification and moving closer towards our Creator, putting us in touch with our duty and destiny here on Earth. The symbolism of fasting within the context of the Faith is further explored in the next chapter.

Bahá'ís fast from sunrise to sunset during the last month of the Bahá'í calendar. The Fast ends with the celebration of Naw-Rúz, the ancient Persian festival of New Year, on the Spring equinox.

The next chapter explains in detail Bahá'u'lláh's vision for the Fast, the laws pertaining to it, and the various practices associated with it. This chapter has shown that the importance of turning to God and devoting oneself to Him through fasting is a long-established practice and has been a requirement in every age during mankind's evolution. We can readily see its place amongst societies and its wisdom in reestablishing balance and progress for individuals.

3

PRESCRIPTION FOR TODAY

Know thou that religion is as heaven; and fasting and obligatory prayer are its sun and its moon.

Bahá'u'lláh[1]

God reveals laws in each age. Some laws benefit society as a whole – those listed in the previous chapter are among such laws revealed by Bahá'u'lláh. Other laws benefit the individual and develop their spiritual capacities such as forgiveness, purity and other virtues. Still other laws are given to guide mankind in its desire to draw nearer to God; among these are the laws of prayer and fasting. In the Kitáb-i-Aqdas Bahá'u'lláh characterizes His laws as the 'lamps of My loving providence', or 'the breath of life unto all created things'.[2] He encourages us to partake of these bounties. Often people find themselves doing things that are counterproductive to their spiritual growth; sometimes we find it difficult to follow Bahá'u'lláh's laws, not because the laws are difficult in themselves but because they usually differ from the habits of our culture and upbringing. For example, daily prayer and fasting can be challenging to integrate into our lives at first. But if we gradually practise them, the benefits become tangible as we form a new habit.

The Bahá'í Fast

The time during the Fast is potent with spiritual forces and bounty. Bahá'u'lláh states:

> Thou hast endowed every hour of these days with a special virtue, inscrutable to all except Thee, Whose knowledge embraceth all created things. Thou hast, also, assigned unto every soul a portion of this virtue in accordance with the Tablet of Thy decree and the

Scriptures of Thine irrevocable judgment. Every leaf of these Books and Scriptures Thou hast, moreover, allotted to each one of the peoples and kindreds of the earth.[3]

The ability to connect with these divine forces is reflected and is in direct proportion to the yearning and willingness to approach them. Because of the potency of the spiritual forces of the Fast, time to prepare the mind and body is required. Bahá'u'lláh has set aside some days prior to the Fast to prepare and to celebrate:

> to provide good cheer for themselves, their kindred and, beyond them, the poor and needy, and with joy and exultation to hail and glorify their Lord, to sing His praise and magnify His Name . . .[4]

These days are called Ayyám-i-Há, the 'Days of Há'. Baha'u'llah identifies these days with the Arabic letter 'Há', the days beyond the limitations of the year and its months. In Arabic, each letter is significant and has a numerological value. Words are created by arranging letters in a certain way – called the '*abjad*' system – to deliberately infuse the words with additional meaning. In the Bahá'í teachings the letter Há has been used as a symbol of the essence of God. Há has a numerical value of 5 in the *abjad* system. Accordingly, Ayyám-i-Há has a maximum of 5 days.

The significance of the Fast in the Bahá'í calendar

It was the Báb who introduced the new calendar which was later confirmed by Bahá'u'lláh and is used by Bahá'ís today. The calendar measures days from sunset to sunset. Each Bahá'í year consists of 19 months of 19 days with four or five extra days – the Days of Há. Each month is named after one of the attributes of God. The Báb determined the last month of the calendar, or 'Alá', to be the period of fasting and decreed the day of Naw-Rúz (New Year) to mark its end. Naw-Rúz is on the spring equinox in the northern hemisphere and marks the beginning of the Bahá'í New Year. (For further details about the calendar see the Annex.)

There is a special significance to the first month and the last month of the calendar. The first month is designated 'Bahá', in honour of Bahá'u'lláh, Him Whom God shall make manifest, and is the most excellent of all. In a prayer Bahá'u'lláh comments on the significance of the Fast being placed in the last month:

> All glory be to Thee, O my God, for Thou hast graciously enabled me to fast during this month which Thou hast related to Thy Name, the Most Exalted, and called 'Alá' (Loftiness). Thou hast commanded that Thy servants and Thy people should fast therein and seek thereby to draw nearer unto Thee. The days and months of the year have culminated with the Fast, even as the first month began with Thy Name, Bahá, that all might testify that Thou art the First and the Last, the Manifest and the Hidden, and be well assured that the glory of all names is conferred only through the glory of Thy Cause and the word expounded by Thy will and revealed through Thy purpose. Thou hast ordained that this month be a remembrance and honour from Thee, and a sign of Thy presence amongst them, that they may not forget Thy grandeur and Thy majesty, Thy sovereignty and Thy glory, and may be well assured that from time immemorial Thou hast ever been and wilt ever be Ruler over the entire creation.[5]

Innumerable effects of the Fast

The depths of this Revelation and the significance of its laws are limitless. In meditating on the Bahá'í calendar, we see the Fast placed in the last month to prepare for the new year. Bahá'u'lláh determines, 'There are various stages and stations for the Fast and innumerable effects and benefits are concealed therein. Well is it with those who have attained unto them.'[6] It's intriguing to imagine the stages, stations and innumerable effects and benefits of the fasting season. Through intention, the Fast can reveal individually and uniquely the various stages and the spiritual growth required. Every year the Fast will present various challenges and outcomes.

A metaphor for the various stages and stations for the Fast can perhaps be seen in nature, in the life of a caterpillar. Ayyám-i-Há is the time when the caterpillar prepares to cocoon. After it's well fed, it creates a cocoon for itself with the intention of transforming into a more brilliant, beautiful state of being. It tucks itself away from the elements of the world and allows metamorphosis to occur. This is called the pupa stage, or resting phase. It's an extremely vulnerable time for the insect, as it does not have any power to run away. In the cocoon, the caterpillar digests itself from the inside out, creating a soupy mixture. The biological process continues by using special reformative cells which remain hidden until the death of the caterpillar, when its power to rebuild itself is revealed. Once the transformation is complete, the tube-shaped caterpillar with a mouth on one end and an anus on the other is changed into a complex, perfectly sculptured adult insect. The butterfly must then struggle to be released from the cocoon, rushing the blood through its wings to give them the strength they need to fly.

The Fast reflects perfectly the pupa stage, and it can be a spiritually vulnerable time. It's a time of spiritual metamorphosis and transformation into a more complex vital being. It also can be a very messy time as, like the dead caterpillar, we shed our old habits and ways of being. With all our emotions and attachments, we sometimes feel like dissolving into a puddle on the floor! In the small deaths of sacrifice lie the hidden gifts and the mystery of sacrifice. Just as the caterpillar contains hidden jewels, so does the soul, and as the butterfly breaks out of the cocoon and reenters the world, Naw-Rúz takes us into the new year.

If we examine the prayer revealed by Bahá'u'lláh to be said during the Days of Há just before the Fast begins, we may find pearls hidden in its depths:

> My God, my Fire and my Light! The days which Thou hast named the Ayyám-i-Há (the Days of Há, Intercalary days) in Thy Book have begun, O Thou Who art the King of names, and the fast which Thy most exalted Pen hath enjoined unto all who are in the kingdom of Thy creation to observe is approaching. I entreat Thee, O my Lord, by these days and by all such as have during that period clung to the cord of Thy commandments, and laid hold on the handle of Thy precepts, to grant that unto every soul may be assigned a place within the precincts of Thy court, and a seat at the revelation of the splendors of the light of Thy countenance.
>
> These, O my Lord, are Thy servants whom no corrupt inclination hath kept back from what Thou didst send down in Thy Book. They have bowed themselves before Thy Cause, and received Thy Book with such resolve as is born of Thee, and observed what Thou hadst prescribed unto them, and chosen to follow that which had been sent down by Thee.

Thou seest, O my Lord, how they have recognized and confessed whatsoever Thou hast revealed in Thy Scriptures. Give them to drink, O my Lord, from the hands of Thy graciousness the waters of Thine eternity. Write down, then, for them the recompense ordained for him that hath immersed himself in the ocean of Thy presence, and attained unto the choice wine of Thy meeting.

I implore Thee, O Thou the King of kings and the Pitier of the downtrodden, to ordain for them the good of this world and of the world to come. Write down for them, moreover, what none of Thy creatures hath discovered, and number them with those who have circled round Thee, and who move about Thy throne in every world of Thy worlds.

Thou, truly, art the Almighty, the All-Knowing, the All-Informed.[7]

This beautiful prayer reflects the pure sentiments and encouragement for all to attain their capacity and transform themselves in approaching the divine. The ultimate goal in immersing ourselves in prayer and fasting is self-surrender to the will of God. This is the dying of the self, or caterpillar body. The object of our quest daily through prayer and yearly through fasting is to shake loose the shackles of our physical existence so as to become transformed into a more complex beautiful being, giving us spiritual wings to fly. Our vision becomes world-embracing rather than limited to ourselves. We enter prayer and fasting by regarding our desires as utter nothingness compared to God's purpose. With diligence, yearning and joy, we arise to fulfil these commandments of God. Daily practice in the surrender of one's will and merging with God's will helps us to become a clear channel for His purpose.

As a sacred practice, the Fast is essential for a healthy soul. Bahá'u'lláh states:

> O Pen of the Most High! Say: O people of the world! We have enjoined upon you fasting during a brief period, and at its close have designated for you Naw-Rúz as a feast. Thus hath the Day-Star of Utterance shone forth above the horizon of the Book as decreed by Him Who is the Lord of the beginning and the end.[8]

The station of absolute self-surrender transcendeth, and will ever remain exalted above, every other station.

> It behoveth thee to consecrate thyself to the Will of God. Whatsoever hath been revealed in His Tablets is but a reflection of His Will. So complete must be thy consecration, that every trace of worldly desire will be washed from thine heart. This is the meaning of true unity.[9]

Bahá'u'lláh's mission is unity, yet He states, 'No two men can be found who may be said to be outwardly and inwardly united.'[10] True unity will develop through studying what is revealed in His Tablets (the Will of God), and purifying our hearts from any worldly desire. This unity is reflected when God asks for action and we follow through in this earthly realm of existence with implicit obedience and radiant acquiescence. 'Abdu'l-Bahá wrote that

> every great Cause in this world of existence findeth a visible expression through three means; first, intention; second, confirmation; third, action. Today on this earth there are many souls who are the spreaders of peace and reconciliation and are longing for the realization of the oneness and unity of the world of man; but this intention needs a dynamic power, so that it may become manifest in the world of being.[11]

It's interesting to consider that God's Will searches for ways of being expressed in the material world. Our love and praise and prayers cleanse us to be an expression of this Will. Nature is a pure receptacle, as is reflected in Bahá'u'lláh's words, 'Nature is God's Will and is its expression in and through the contingent world.'[12] The Fast is a time to align our will with the Will of God and cleanse our intentions for the new year.

God is self-sufficient and we are dependent upon Him for aid and assistance. This can only be drawn to us as a magnet when we purify our intentions and put them into action. We see this most poignantly in this statement by Shoghi Effendi:

> The unseen legions, standing rank upon rank, and eager to pour forth from the Kingdom on high the full measure of their celestial strength on the individual participants of this incomparably glorious Crusade, are powerless unless and until each potential crusader decides for himself, perseveres in his determination, to rush into the

arena of service ready to sacrifice his all for the Cause he is called upon to champion.[13]

And,

> Thus, when a person is active, they are blessed by the Holy Spirit. When they are inactive, the Holy Spirit cannot find a repository in their being, and thus they are deprived of its healing and quickening rays.[14]

The Baháʼí Fast allows for true unity 'outwardly and inwardly', as Baháʼuʼlláh describes. Although physical benefits of detoxification are manifest during this time, the Fast has a higher purpose. Undertaken in the correct spirit, it brings potential spiritual and physical unity when our efforts are accepted by God. In fact, fasting during any time of the year will produce physiological results in the mind and body, but fasting during this sacred time benefits the relationship of the created to the Creator in the most potent way because it combines obedience, love and self-surrender. The Baháʼí Fast is about sacrifice, making our efforts sacred, and it has many benefits:

- ***It allows us to draw nearer to our Beloved.*** In our busy society, we often miss time to build our relationship to God. This is the soul's true longing – to draw nearer to God. The Fast is a time of quiet contemplation through prayer and meditation. We follow the Prophet's example in order to draw nearer to Him. Baháʼuʼlláh's sufferings were immense; they would have been insurmountable for any human. Through the Fast, and our slight experience of hunger, we can gain empathy for the sufferings of the destitute.
- ***It prepares us for the New Year through spiritual recuperation.*** This is a welcome opportunity to reflect where we've been in the last year, to let go of the old, and make intentions for the coming year: to plan personal and spiritual goals, to acquire spiritual attributes and awaken latent spiritual forces in our soul.
- ***It strengthens discipline and moderation.*** It's a time to overcome personal addictions and bad habits, to make adjustments

to our inner and outer lives, to practise and habituate the skill of overcoming our lower nature and insistent self. Resiliency and self-discipline are built during the Fast; these qualities are applicable to all aspects of life.
- ***It helps us regain balance and purifies us.*** The Fast is a time to focus on purifying and balancing body, mind and spirit.
- ***It cleanses our hearts of attachments.*** The Fast will reveal our attachments. It's a golden opportunity to work on releasing attachment and reattaching our hearts to the eternal.
- ***It preserves us from tests.*** Our spiritual work during the Fast causes spiritual progress and revitalization. How many times have we unconsciously made traps for ourselves in relationships or job choices because of our lack of clarity? Many tests in life result directly from the natural consequences of our free-will choices.

How the Fast works

The rest of this chapter addresses questions specifically answered in the sacred texts or by 'Abdu'l-Bahá, Shoghi Effendi or the Universal House of Justice. The remaining chapters of the book are simply my own observations and recommendations for optimal, safe fasting, and for exploring the innumerable potentials latent in the Fast.

How does the Fast work?

The Fast begins at sunrise on 1 March and lasts until sunset on 19 March when the upcoming equinox is on 20 March and begins on 2 March lasting until sunset on 20 March when the equinox is on 21 March. It is observed by abstaining from food or drink from sunrise to sunset each day. It's helpful to find a sunrise/sunset calculator to be accurate with the time in your particular city or region.

Who fasts?

All adults, from age 15 until they reach the age of 70.

How should the Fast be observed?

Fasting and prayer go hand in hand – like the sun and moon, where 'fasting is illumination, and prayer is light'. This is a spiritual and material fast, conducive to the spiritual transformation of each individual.

Under what circumstances is one not required to fast?

Baha'u'llah states, 'In clear cases of weakness, illness, or injury the law of the Fast is not binding . . . Well is it with them who act accordingly.'[15] If you have any doubts, please check with your doctor prior to participating in the Fast. The Universal House of Justice offers the following advice:

> Regarding the Fast, as you know, there is exemption for those who are ill. The answer to your question, therefore, should be determined on the basis of competent medical advice. Ultimately, the keeping of the Fast and saying of the obligatory prayers are left to the conscience of the individual.[16]

Fasting is not recommended 'in clear cases of weakness, illness or injury'. My understanding of this is that it is all right to fast when the body can handle detoxification, and has been properly nourished. If you are undernourished, it is not recommended to fast. (Some overweight people are undernourished because of their food choices and lack of vitamin and mineral content in their diet.) People who have degenerative diseases, weak hearts or heart failure, who have had surgery recently or will soon have surgery, who have low immunity, cancer or severe mental illness, should refrain from fasting unless under a doctor's supervision. If you cannot physically participate in the Fast, read Chapter 14 later in this book on options for those who cannot fast.

The Bahá'í teachings on exemptions from fasting have been summarized by Shoghi Effendi, Guardian of the Bahá'í Faith, and the Universal House of Justice:

5. Exemption from fasting is granted to:
   a. Travellers
      (i) Provided the journey exceeds 9 hours

      (ii) Those travelling on foot, provided the journey exceeds 2 hours.
      (iii) Those who break their journey for less than 19 days.
      (iv) Those who break their journey during the Fast at a place where they are to stay 19 days are exempt from fasting only for the first three days from their arrival.
      (v) Those who reach home during the Fast must commence fasting from the day of their arrival.
  b. Those who are ill.
  c. Those who are over 70.
  d. Women who are with child.
  e. Women who are nursing.
  f. Women in their courses [menstruating], provided they perform their ablutions and repeat a specifically revealed verse 95 times a day ['Glorified be God, the Lord of Splendour and Beauty'].
  g. Those who are engaged in heavy labour, who are advised to show respect for the law by using discretion and restraint when availing themselves of the exemption.
6. Vowing to fast (in a month other than the one prescribed for fasting) is permissible. Vows which profit mankind are however preferable in the sight of God.[17]

Can I smoke during the Fast?

In one of His Tablets 'Abdu'l-Bahá, after stating that fasting consists of abstinence from food and drink, categorically says that smoking is a form of 'drink'. In Arabic the verb 'drink' applies equally to smoking.

Is sexual intercourse permitted during the Fast?

Although the Báb in the Bayán appears to have proscribed intercourse during the Fast (see Chapter 2), there are no writings specific to this topic in the Bahá'í Writings pertaining to the Fast.

Notes for travellers

As stated above, travellers are exempt from fasting, but if they want to fast while they are travelling, they are free to do so. You are exempt the whole period of your travel, not just the hours you are in a train or car, etc.

What if I forget and accidently eat?

If one eats unconsciously during the fasting hours, this is not breaking the Fast as it is an accident.

If I'm over 70 can I fast?

The age limit when fasting is obligatory is 70 years, but if one desires to fast after this age limit is passed, and is strong enough, one is free to do so.

Fasting in high or low latitudes

It's difficult to fast by the sun if one lives in latitudes where the sunset and sunrise are in great disproportion from the rest of the world, and where some days the sun does not set at all. In this case, it's permissible to rely on clocks rather than relying on the rising and setting of the sun to determine fasting hours.

Is it permissible and acceptable to fast in a month other than the month of 'Alá' if pledged to do so?

> The ordinance of fasting is such as hath already been revealed. Should someone pledge himself, however, to offer up a fast to God, seeking in this way the fulfilment of a wish, or to realize some other aim, this is permissible, now as heretofore. Howbeit, it is God's wish, exalted be His glory, that vows and pledges be directed to such objectives as will profit mankind.[18]

Observance of the Fast during school

If a student lives at a boarding school or university and depends upon the school for meals, while it can present difficulties, the student should make every effort to obtain permission from school authorities to fast. If food is unavailable past sunset, food service departments may be willing to set aside a dinner or breakfast for individuals following religious practices. If the request is refused the only alternative would be to obey the administration.

* * *

The laws of fasting are simple and straightforward. Reading the writings about the Fast will help enhance our spiritual understanding of its sacredness. With these sacred laws in mind, further detail on ways to enhance our fasting capacities will allow us to enjoy the full benefit of this blessed undertaking.

The Bahá'í Sacred Writings on fasting

I would now like to share with you some Bahá'í Writings that relate to the Fast. As an introduction to them I offer you insights into what I see as some ways to get the most out of the Writings. Our understanding of the Writings on the Fast is equally important to our commitment to fast. Bahá'u'lláh asks us: 'Immerse yourselves in the ocean of My words, that ye may unravel its secrets, and discover all the pearls of wisdom that lie hid in its depths.'[19] And also:

> Meditate profoundly, that the secret of things unseen may be revealed unto you, that you may inhale the sweetness of a spiritual and imperishable fragrance, and that you may acknowledge the truth that from time immemorial even unto eternity the Almighty hath tried, and will continue to try, His servants, so that light may be distinguished from darkness, truth from falsehood, right from wrong, guidance from error, happiness from misery, and roses from thorns.[20]

When we read the Word of God only through the eyes of intellect or our emotions our understanding is bound to have limitations. For example, a person who treasures compassion above all will interpret the Writings differently from one who treasures justice above all. We can tend to see everything through the lens of our personal leanings rather than the whole. And we can also be limited by our understanding of what 'compassion' or 'justice' might mean.

While reading, it's helpful to keep in mind the capacity and limits of our own understanding. The nature of your life today will obviously change in a year. Where you stand at 'the ocean of His words' today will be a far different place from where you will stand in the future. Today you may have a sandy beach with calm waters, but next year you may find yourself on a rocky shore buffeted by torrential winds. All through our lives, the meanings we glean from the Writings will change, depending upon our vantage point on the ocean.

Bahá'u'lláh points out the three aspects of limitations on our understanding:

> The understanding of His words and the comprehension of the utterances of the Birds of Heaven are in no wise dependent upon human learning. They depend solely upon purity of heart, chastity of soul, and freedom of spirit. This is evidenced by those who, today, though without a single letter of the accepted standards of learning, are occupying the loftiest seats of knowledge; and the garden of their hearts is adorned, through the showers of divine grace, with the roses of wisdom and the tulips of understanding. Well is it with the sincere in heart for their share of the light of a mighty Day![21]

When sitting down before the Writings, it is good to do so in an attitude of humility and to feel great yearning in our heart, for God will cast the light of understanding in the hearts He chooses. Bahá'u'lláh assures us that those who desire knowledge and understanding will not be denied:

> Know thou moreover that thy letter reached Our presence and We perceived and perused its contents. We noted the questions thou hast asked and will readily answer thee. It behoveth everyone in this Day to ask God that which he desireth, and thy Lord will heed his petition with wondrous and undeniable verses.[22]

The Báb and Bahá'u'lláh explained that personal interpretations are based upon one's own spiritual capacity, station and upon the degree of spiritual discernment in each individual. These stations are numerous and varied; it would be hard to imagine all Bahá'ís adhering to a similar viewpoint where personal interpretation is involved. Bahá'u'lláh responded to the friends in a kindly manner concerning their personal interpretations, sometimes explaining how one could come to that point of view. This does not mean that Bahá'u'lláh was indicating that each point of view is equally valid, only that he made it clear that there can be a multiplicity of meanings, that the meaning of the Word of God 'can never be exhausted'.[23]

Personal interpretation is only condemned by Bahá'u'lláh when the obvious meaning is lost deliberately, or if its rightful outward meaning is interpreted away through discourse and vain imaginings. Bahá'u'lláh said this was the day of unity, where veils have been rent asunder. Each individual is capable of recognizing his Lord, and no one who seeks will be disbarred from the door of knowledge. Bahá'u'lláh encourages us to shed the waters of wisdom on the world!

It is important to view the Writings as a harmonious whole, being aware of both the symbolic and literal meanings, otherwise we run the risk of misinterpretation. The symbolic meaning and literal direction go hand in hand. The Fast is both literal and mystical, and the differences are obvious. For example, if through some kind of selfish motive we interpreted the Fast only metaphorically, we could reframe it to mean refraining from 'spiritual foods' from sun-up to sundown, rather than literally interpreting it correctly and not putting anything in the mouth from sunrise to sunset. When Bahá'u'lláh writes that we are to abstain from food, it is meant as a literal direction. And as we refrain physically, we are also growing spiritually.

We should resist the temptation to compartmentalize our understanding of these texts. When you read, try these thoughts from the perspective of unity – 'and' rather than 'or': 'The Fast is this and it is also . . .', 'It is also true that the Fast . . .' The Writings all flow from the same source and therefore are unified, though sometimes they appear to contradict each other. It's as though Bahá'u'lláh is describing a beautiful piece of art in various ways and from various perspectives. The children's parable *Seven Blind Mice* illustrates this point. Seven blind mice disagree on what is next to them. Each one of them has touched a different part of an elephant and describes only that one part – the ear, the leg, the tail. The last mouse runs up and down the elephant and puts all the pieces together to describe the entire beast.

As we move forward on our journey of understanding the Fast, the following prayer of 'Abdu'l-Bahá offers encouragement and support:

I pray for each and all that you may be as flames of love in the world, and that the brightness of your light and the warmth of your affection may reach the heart of every sad and sorrowing child of God.

May you be as shining stars, bright and luminous for ever in the Kingdom.

I counsel you that you study earnestly the teachings of Bahá'u'lláh, so that, God helping you, you may in deed and truth become Bahá'ís.[24]

Writings by Bahá'u'lláh

We, verily, have set forth all things in Our Book, as a token of grace unto those who have believed in God, the Almighty, the Protector, the Self-Subsisting. And We have ordained obligatory prayer and fasting so that all may by these means draw nigh unto God, the Most Powerful, the Well-Beloved. We have written down these two laws and expounded every irrevocable decree. We have forbidden men from following whatsoever might cause them to stray from the Truth, and have commanded them to observe that which will draw them nearer unto Him Who is the Almighty, the All-Loving. Say: Observe ye the commandments of God for love of His beauty, and be not of those who follow in the ways of the abject and foolish.[25]

All praise be unto God, Who hath revealed the law of obligatory prayer as a reminder to His servants, and enjoined on them the Fast that those possessed of means may become apprised of the woes and sufferings of the destitute.[26]

One who performeth neither good deeds nor acts of worship is like unto a tree which beareth no fruit, and an action which leaveth no trace. Whosoever experienceth the holy ecstasy of worship will refuse to barter such an act or any praise of God for all that existeth in the world. Fasting and obligatory prayer are as two wings to man's life. Blessed be the one who soareth with their aid in the heaven of the love of God, the Lord of all worlds.[27]

Cling firmly to obligatory prayer and fasting. Verily, the religion of God is like unto heaven; fasting is its sun, and obligatory prayer is its moon.

In truth, they are the pillars of religion whereby the righteous are distinguished from those who transgress His commandments. We entreat God, exalted and glorified be He, that he may graciously enable all to observe that which He hath revealed in His Ancient Book.[28]

Know thou that religion is as heaven; and fasting and obligatory prayer are its sun and its moon. We entreat God, exalted and glorified be He, to graciously aid everyone who acteth according to His will and good-pleasure.[29]

Be not neglectful of obligatory prayer and fasting. He who faileth to observe them hath not been nor will ever be acceptable in the sight of God. Follow ye wisdom under all conditions. He, verily, hath bidden all to observe that which hath been and will be of profit to them. He, in truth, is the All-Sufficing, the Most High.[30]

We beseech God to assist His people that they may observe the most great and exalted Fast, which is to protect one's eye from beholding whatever is forbidden and to withhold one's self from food, drink and whatever is not of Him. We pray God to confirm His loved ones that they may succeed in accomplishing that which they have been commanded in this Day.[31]

This is one of the nights of the Fast, and during it the Tongue of Grandeur and Glory proclaimed: There is no God beside Me, the Omnipotent Protector, the Self-Subsisting. We, verily, have commanded all to observe the Fast in these days as a bounty on Our part, but the people remain unaware, except for those who have attained unto the purpose of God as revealed in His laws and have comprehended His wisdom that pervadeth all things visible and invisible. Say: By God! His Law is a fortress unto you, could ye but understand. Verily, He hath no purpose therein save to benefit the souls of His servants, but, alas, the generality of mankind remain heedless thereof. Cling ye to the cord of God's laws, and follow not those who have turned away from the Book, for verily they have opposed God, the Mighty, the Beloved.[32]

These are the days of the Fast. Blessed is the one who through the heat generated by the Fast increaseth his love, and who, with joy and radiance, ariseth to perform worthy deeds. Verily, He guideth whomsoever He willeth to the straight path.[33]

Even though outwardly the Fast is difficult and toilsome, yet inwardly it is bounty and tranquillity. Purification and training are conditioned and dependent only on such rigorous exercises as are in accord with the Book of God and sanctioned by Divine law, not those which the deluded have inflicted upon the people. Whatsoever God hath revealed is beloved of the soul. We beseech Him that He may graciously assist us to do that which is pleasing and acceptable unto Him.[34]

Verily, I say, fasting is the supreme remedy and the most great healing for the disease of self and passion.[35]

All praise be to the one true God Who hath assisted His loved ones to observe the Fast and hath aided them to fulfil that which hath been decreed in the Book. In truth, ceaseless praise and gratitude are due unto Him for having graciously confirmed His loved ones to perform that which is the cause of the exaltation of His Word. If a man possessed ten thousand lives and offered them all to establish the truth of God's laws and commandments, he would still be beholden unto Him, since whatsoever proceedeth from His irresistible decree serveth solely to benefit His friends and loved ones.[36]

Moreover, in the traditions the terms 'sun' and 'moon' have been applied to prayer and fasting, even as it is said: 'Fasting is illumination, prayer is light.' One day, a well-known divine came to visit Us. While We were conversing with him, he referred to the above-quoted tradition. He said: 'Inasmuch as fasting causeth the heat of the body to increase, it hath therefore been likened unto the light of the sun; and as the prayer of the night-season refresheth man, it hath been compared unto the radiance of the moon.' Thereupon We realized that that poor man had not been favoured with a single drop of the ocean of true understanding, and had strayed far from the burning Bush of divine wisdom. We then politely observed to him saying: 'The interpretation your honour hath given to this tradition is the one current amongst the people. Could it not be interpreted differently?' He asked Us: 'What could it be?' We made reply: 'Muhammad, the Seal of the Prophets, and the most distinguished of God's chosen Ones, hath likened the Dispensation of the Qur'án unto heaven, by reason of its loftiness, its paramount influence, its majesty, and the fact that it comprehendeth all religions. And as the sun and moon constitute the brightest and most prominent luminaries in the heavens, similarly in the heaven of the religion of God two shining orbs have been ordained – fasting and prayer. "Islám is heaven; fasting is its sun, prayer, its moon." '37

Thou seest, O God of Mercy, Thou Whose power pervadeth all created things, these servants of Thine, Thy thralls, who, according to the good-pleasure of Thy Will, observe in the daytime the fast prescribed by Thee, who arise, at the earliest dawn of day, to make mention of Thy Name, and to celebrate Thy praise, in the hope of obtaining their share of the goodly things that are treasured up within the treasuries of Thy grace and bounty. I beseech Thee, O Thou that holdest in Thine hands the reins of the entire creation, in Whose grasp is the whole kingdom of Thy names and of Thine attributes, not to deprive, in Thy Day, Thy servants from the showers pouring from the clouds of Thy mercy, nor to hinder them from taking their portion of the ocean of Thy good-pleasure.38

There are various stages and stations for the Fast and innumerable effects and benefits are concealed therein. Well is it with those who have attained unto them.39

In clear cases of weakness, illness, or injury the law of the Fast is not binding. This injunction is in conformity with the precepts of God, eternal in the past, eternal in the future. Well is it with them who act accordingly.40

The law of the Fast is ordained for those who are sound and healthy; as to those who are ill or debilitated, this law hath never been nor is now applicable.41

Writings and Talks by 'Abdu'l-Bahá

Obligatory prayer and fasting are among the most great ordinances of this holy Dispensation.42

In the realm of worship, fasting and obligatory prayer constitute the two mightiest pillars of God's holy Law. Neglecting them is in no wise permitted, and falling short in their performance is of a certainty not acceptable. In the Tablet of Visitation He saith: 'I beseech God, by Thee and by them whose faces have been illumined with the splendors of the light of Thy countenance, and who, for love of Thee, have observed all whereunto they were bidden.' He declareth that observance of the commands of God deriveth from love for the beauty of the Best-Beloved. The seeker, when immersed in the ocean of the love of God, will be moved by intense longing and will arise to carry out the laws of God. Thus, it is impossible that a heart which containeth the fragrance of God's love should yet fail to worship Him, except under conditions when such an action would agitate the enemies and stir up dissension and mischief. Otherwise, a lover of the Abhá Beauty will assuredly and continually demonstrate perseverance in the worship of the Lord.[43]

Well is it with you, as you have followed the Law of God and arisen to observe the Fast during these blessed days, for this physical fast is a symbol of the spiritual fast. This Fast leadeth to the cleansing of the soul from all selfish desires, the acquisition of spiritual attributes, attraction to the breezes of the All-Merciful, and enkindlement with the fire of divine love.[44]

Fasting is the cause of the elevation of one's spiritual station.[45]

Fasting is a symbol. Fasting signifies abstinence from lust. Physical fasting is a symbol of that abstinence, and is a reminder; that is, just as a person abstains from physical appetites, he is to abstain from self-appetites and self-desires. But mere abstention from food has no effect on the spirit. It is only a symbol, a reminder. Otherwise it is of no importance. Fasting for this purpose does not mean entire abstinence from food. The golden rule as to food is, do not take too much or too little. Moderation is necessary. There is a sect in India who practise extreme abstinence, and gradually reduce their food until they exist on almost nothing. But their intelligence suffers. A man is not fit to do service for God with brain or body if he is weakened by lack of food. He cannot see clearly.[46]

Besides all this, prayer and fasting is the cause of awakening and mindfulness and conducive to protection and preservation from tests . . .[47]

There is but one power which heals – that is God. The state or condition through which the healing takes place is the confidence of the heart. By some this state is reached through pills, powders, and physicians. By others through hygiene, fasting, and prayer. By others through direct perception . . . All that we see around us is the work of mind. It is mind in the herb and in the mineral that acts on the human body, and changes its condition.[48]

Some people lay stress on fasting. They affirm that in augmenting the weakness of the body they develop a spiritual sensibility and thus they think to approach God.

Weakening one's self physically does not necessarily contribute to spiritual progress. Humility, kindness, resignation, and all these spiritual attributes emanating from great physical strength are acceptable to God. That an enfeebled man cannot fight is not accounted a virtue. Were physical weakness a virtue the dead would be perfect, for they can do nothing.

If a man be just, kind, humble and merciful and his qualities are acquired through the will-power – this is Godlike. A child cannot kill a man; but a Bonaparte can abstain from war, from shedding blood, from devastating countries. A dumb person will not speak ill of any one, a paralyzed hand cannot strike; but a strong arm can refrain from striking. Justice, love and kindness must be the instruments of strength, not of weakness.

Exaggerated fasting destroys the divine forces. God has created man in a way that cannot be surpassed; we must not try to change his creation. Strive to attain nearness to reality through the acquisition of strength of character, through morality, through good works and helping the poor, through being consumed with the fire of the love of God and in discovering each day new spiritual mysteries. This is the path of intimate approach. [49]

The nineteen-day fast is a duty to be observed by all. All should abstain from eating and drinking from sunrise to sunset. This fast is conducive to the spiritual development of the individual. The Greatest Name should be read every day.[50]

The Divine wisdom in fasting is manifold. Among them is this: As during those days (i.e. the period of fasting which the followers afterward observe) the Manifestation of the Sun of Reality, through Divine inspiration, is engaged in the descent [revealing] of Verses, the instituting of Divine Law and the arrangement of teachings, through excessive occupation and intensive attraction, there remains no condition or time for eating and drinking. For example, when His Holiness Moses went to Mount Tur (Sinai) and there engaged in instituting the Law of God, He fasted forty days. For the purpose of awakening and admonishing the people of Israel, fasting was enjoined upon them.

Likewise, His Holiness Christ, in the beginning of instituting the Spiritual Law, the systemizing of the teachings and the arrangement of counsels, for forty days abstained from eating and drinking. In the beginning the disciples and Christians fasted. Later the assemblages of the chief Christians changed fasting into lenten observances.

Likewise the Koran having descended in the month of Ramadan, fasting during that month became a duty.

In like manner his holiness the Supreme [the Báb], in the beginning of the Manifestation, through the excessive effect of descending Verses, passed days in which His nourishment was reduced to tea only.

Likewise, the Blessed Beauty [Bahá'u'lláh], when busy with instituting the Divine Teachings and during the days when the Verses [the Word of God] descended continuously, through the great effect of the Verses and the throbbing of the heart, took no food except the least amount.

The purpose is this: In order to follow the Divine Manifestation and for the purpose of admonition and the commemoration of their state, it became incumbent upon the people to fast during those days. For every sincere soul who has a beloved longs to experience that state in which his beloved is. If his beloved is in a state of sorrow, he desires sorrow; if in a state of joy, he desires joy; if in a state of rest, he desires rest; if in a state of trouble, he desires trouble.

Now, since in this Millennial Day, His Holiness the Supreme [the Báb] fasted many days, and the Blessed Beauty [Bahá'u'lláh] took but little food or drink, it becomes necessary that the friends should follow that example. For thus saith He in the Tablet of Visitation: 'They, the believers, have followed that which they were commanded, for love of Thee.'

This is one wisdom of the wisdoms of fasting.

The second wisdom is this: Fasting is the cause of awakening man. The heart becomes tender and the spirituality of man increases. This is produced by the fact that man's thoughts will be confined to the commemoration of God, and through this awakening and stimulation surely ideal advancements follow.

Third wisdom: Fasting is of two kinds, material and spiritual. The material fasting is abstaining from food or drink, that is, from the appetites of the body. But spiritual, ideal fasting is this, that man abstain from selfish passions, from negligence and from satanic animal traits. Therefore, material fasting ia a token of the spiritual fasting. That is: *'O God! as I am fasting from the appetites of the body and not occupied with eating and drinking, even so purify and make holy my heart and my life from aught else save Thy Love, and protect and preserve my soul from self-passions and animal traits. Thus may the spirit associate with the Fragrances of Holiness and fast from everything else save Thy mention.'*[51]

4

THE HUMAN EXPERIENCE

> The goal of fasting is inner unity . . . And when the faculties are empty, then the whole being listens. There is then a direct grasp of what is right there before you that can never be heard with the ear or understood with the mind. Fasting of the heart empties the faculties, frees you from limitation and from preoccupation. Fasting of the heart begets unity and freedom.
>
> *Confucius, as interpreted by Thomas Merton*

The thoughts in this chapter stem from my professional training and experience and my own personal understanding of the Writings of the Bahá'í Faith. I humbly offer these musings in the hope that the reader's understanding of our reality may be enriched.

The essential message of Bahá'u'lláh is the oneness of reality. While we shall study the body, mind and soul in different sections of this book, the overall goal is unity. Humans are complex beings with complex systems. Each component has its own systems and communications, and yet they are integrated to such a high level that one cannot separate them. They communicate constantly and are of one reality. Shoghi Effendi acknowledges that

> . . . we have three aspects of our humanness, so to speak, a body, a mind and an immortal identity – soul or spirit. We believe the mind forms a link between the soul and the body, and the two interact on each other.[1]

Bahá'u'lláh's Writings also elucidate this point:

> Say: Spirit, mind, soul, and the powers of sight and hearing are but one single reality which hath manifold expressions owing to the

diversity of its instruments. As thou dost observe, man's power to comprehend, move, speak, hear and see all derive from this sign of his Lord within him. It is single in its essence, yet manifold through the diversity of its instruments.[2]

Body, mind and soul united in one purpose

For the mind to manifest itself, the human body must be whole; and a sound mind cannot be but in a sound body, whereas the soul dependeth not upon the body. It is through the power of the soul that the mind comprehendeth, imagineth and exerteth its influence, whilst the soul is a power that is free.[3]

'Abdu'l-Bahá encourages us in the statement above to look to the end of things in the beginning. As the year dwindles out in March, we come to celebrate and anticipate thoughts of spring – a new beginning. As Samuel Coleridge wrote, 'And Winter slumbering in the open air, wears on his smiling face a dream of spring!' Every year the Fast, the last month in the calendar, gives us an opportunity to transform ourselves and be reborn into the new year. It's a time for reflection. What have I done with the time I've been given? What qualities have I developed? How have I served? What negative habits have I acquired? As we prepare for the Fast, how do we want to answer these questions at the end of next year?

Let's return to an example from Chapter 3. I have found that the lifecycle of a butterfly can be seen as a metaphor for the spiritual benefits of the Fast, reflecting both individual potentiality and participation. The caterpillar, or larva, is active; it eats leaves and grows tremendously. During the year, the soul takes in the Writings of Bahá'u'lláh to feed the spirit, pointing it in the right direction. The caterpillar also moults a few times – a process likened to when God challenges us in our attachments to this world through tests and difficulties. The mind is asked to shed old habits and beliefs throughout the year; to view reality in a new light. After each moulting, the caterpillar becomes larger, just as the soul's capacity to function in this world becomes stronger and the mind becomes clearer. The caterpillar then prepares to be transformed by eating sufficiently, then finding an appropriate, safe place to build its cocoon. This reflects the time we take in February to prepare the body, mind and soul for the upcoming Fast.

Bahá'u'lláh asks us to protect our eyes from beholding what is unseemly; creating a safe place is essential to **detoxification and reunion**. The tools used to construct our cocoon are:

- *Protection for the mind and body.* Sanctify the mind and heart from the elements of the world and dangerous predators such as junk food, television, advertising or gossip.
- *Yearning from the heart.* Seek God and His good pleasure, wishing to draw nearer.

Figure 4.1   *Pupa to butterfly*

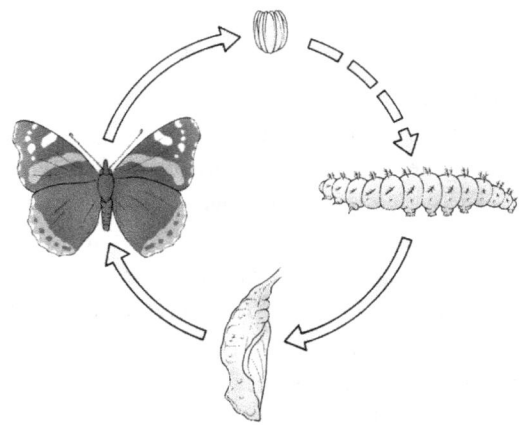

When the heart uses attraction to become a receptacle of love, it's as though the chrysalis is set, as shown in Figure 4.1. Once the cocoon is solidified, like the caterpillar in dormancy, the Fast begins by welcoming the mysterious 'forces released' – the catalyst to transformation. The pupa stage of the caterpillar, or resting phase, reflects its sensitive nature – especially to predators or influences and poisons from the outer world. People who fast develop susceptibilities to these influences. Within the caterpillar, latent cells begin to digest themselves from the inside out, creating a soupy, messy mixture. For fasting individuals, this is a time when emotions run higher than usual, and anything at all can potentially affect our drawing nearer to God. Some people experience the heightened awareness during the Fast as 'messy', being manifested as tears of joy or sorrow. Transformation can be painful if toxicity is high. The mysterious forces of the Fast, like the intent of the caterpillar's hidden cells, help to reconstruct us into more complex selves. Bahá'u'lláh assures us of the 'various stages and stations for the Fast and innumerable effects and benefits [that] are concealed therein'.[4]

At the apex, the newly constructed butterfly struggles to release itself from the cocoon. After the Fast the soul, recharged and drawn nearer to its Creator, is ready to emerge into the world. Therein lies great inner conflict, yet also an opportunity to consolidate discipline. A person's newly detoxified system struggles with animal impulses, longing to rush back into its physical delights and comforting habits – especially eating the things missed! For the butterfly, the struggle is necessary because the blood rushing through its wings gives it the necessary strength to fly. Similarly, if a person's mind is properly disciplined during the Fast, it can overcome the struggles faced on reentering the world when the Fast is over.

The material world reflects the spiritual world

'Abdu'l-Bahá clarified the similarity and reflection between the spiritual world and the world of creation.

> The spiritual world is like unto the phenomenal world. They are the exact counterpart of each other. Whatever objects appear in this world of existence are the outer pictures of the world of heaven.[5]

In creation, each object contains some aspect of Revelation and according to its own capacity expresses the knowledge of God. All things are 'a door leading into His knowledge, a sign of His sovereignty, a revelation of His names, a symbol of His majesty, a token of His power, a means of admittance into His straight Path',[6] so the physical and spiritual worlds have similar properties and counterparts in all the worlds of God. The laws and principles in the material world are equally applicable in the spiritual worlds. The spiritual world is a higher kingdom, and therefore possesses qualities not found in the lower human kingdom, but the laws and principles still exist and are applied at that higher level. If every created thing in the universe is a door that leads to God, then surely the human temple – the body – can reveal some of these mysteries.

Each world has its counterparts and yet they are interrelated. By studying the rational faculty, the nature of the soul, or the human temple, we can glimpse how each of the others functions. The seat of the soul is the human heart, but the soul does not reside there. The mind is connected to the brain, but is not found in the brain. It's no wonder that in the human temple, one cannot survive without a functioning brain or heart!

Fasting provides us with an opportunity to bring into balance these three existences. The qualities of purity, simplicity and sincerity shine through and enable us to discern our human as well as our spiritual needs. We need to purify our bodies from impediments and bad habits, purify our minds from maladies of the mind, and purify our hearts from selfish desires. Simplicity comes with a simple diet, simplifying what our minds are exposed to, and making simple what we are attracted to. Our society makes our diet overly complex, exposes us to too many influences and makes our hearts vulnerable to carnal desires and instant gratification. Bahá'u'lláh states:

> In this day the tastes of men have changed, and their power of perception hath altered. The contrary winds of the world, and its colours, have provoked a cold, and deprived men's nostrils of the sweet savours of Revelation.[7]

We are vulnerable to the winds of self and natural emotions which tempt us; purity can easily be lost. We can manifest selfish disorders, intellectual maladies, spiritual sicknesses.

Health and the systems of body, mind and soul

The following is my current understanding of the body, mind and soul, of my belief that optimal treatment lies in comprehending how they can work together, assuring constant progress.

The lack of an approach to healing through balancing and unifying the systems of body, mind and soul weighs heavily on our medical system. Medicine has evolved into specialists mastering one part of the body or system, giving prescriptions to patients. Healthcare experts often don't communicate with each other, and this can lead to long-term harm to patients. While specialization in science is vital to ingenuity and new understandings, and no one can deny the enlightening and useful information that emanates from these studies, yet most doctors are frank about their lack of true understanding of how the body's systems work together in their totality.

Each expression of our being has various qualities which can lead to health or imbalance. Most approaches to medicine segregate the various aspects of the human experience and compartmentalize disease. With the aim of eliminating the symptoms displayed, the disease is searched out and destroyed. But this focuses on only one aspect, disregarding the totality of a human being: we affect our reality and our reality affects us. The human is not an isolated being, nor is the sum of influences on it isolated. One individual may experience degrees of imbalance ranging from minor to severe, while another will seem unaffected by external influences or internal disturbances.

Numerous clients give me pages of symptoms, have already seen several specialists; although they look sick, feel sick and experience sickness, nothing can be found in the tissues so they are told there is no disease. Frustrated, disempowered and often feeling invalidated, they come to me for clarity: What do all these symptoms mean? How many times has a person out of balance, nervous, taking sleeping pills for years, gone uncured? In a few years or decades this person will become affected in the body and finally manifest a disease dictated by life circumstances and inherited genes, although this imbalance was present all along. The struggle our bodies experience can be affected by our genetics as well as strong infectious diseases in the past and how they were treated.

Bahá'u'lláh states,

> Know thou that the soul of man is exalted above, and is independent of all infirmities of body or mind. That a sick person showeth signs of weakness is due to the hindrances that interpose themselves between his soul and his body . . .[8]

This truth is reflected in homeopathy's view of disease, where the soul is the animating force of the body, and the spirit, or vital force, is the animating principle that flows through the body. The soul is not in the body, but associates with it, and is 'in tune' with it. If something interferes with the frequencies, the connection can become 'mistuned'. If you think of a radio receiving a station, the clearer the signal is, the better. The same is true for the health of the body. Many things can become a veil or obstruction when the body/mind is in receiving mode, causing the connection to become mistuned. So the soul is never ill; it is just the connection between it and the body that becomes impeded, and health begins to decline.

Regarding homeopathy, the following letter to an individual from the Universal House of Justice states:

> One of the friends in Persia wrote to Shoghi Effendi and asked this question: 'Is it true that 'Abdu'l-Bahá has said that biochemical homeopathy, which is a form of food medicine, is in conformity with the Bahá'í medical concept?' The beloved Guardian's reply to this question in a letter dated 25th November, 1944 was as follows: 'This statement is true, and the truth thereof will be revealed in the future.' (The question and answer are translated from the Persian.)
>
> The Universal House of Justice has also asked us to inform you that it does not wish the above statement to be circulated in isolation from the many and varied other texts in the Writings on medicine. However, you may share it with any of your friends who are interested.[9]

The most potent healing force is the Word of God or, as Bahá'u'lláh refers to it, the Divine Elixir that can transmute substances, transforming an individual. It is evident in the first line of the healing prayer, 'Thy name is my healing, O my God.' When we tune back into our source, this can realign the mistunement and whatever is impeding the association of the soul with the body. There are many ways of healing, and many things can help retune the connection, including diet, remedies and medicaments, prayer and meditation. Both physical and spiritual means should be used at the same time as they harness the spirit to the body and mind. Once the connection is retuned, then one can use self-regulating techniques such as diet, good habits, good psychology and spiritual practices to maintain health.

In his *Lectures on Homeopathic Philosophy* James Tyler Kent states:

> All that there is of the soul operates and exists within every part of the human body, and thus it is that simple substance acts as a vital force. The soul adapts the human body to all its purposes, the higher

purposes of its being . . . when it exists in the living human body [it] keeps that body animated, keeps it moving, perfects it uses, superintends all parts and at the same time keeps the operation of mind and will in order. Let any disturbance occur in the vital substance and we see how suddenly incoordination will come . . . We see also that this vital substance when in a natural state, when in contact with the human body, is constructive . . . and in its absence there is death and destruction.[10]

Humans can adapt extremely quickly to their environment. The spirit force within us can adapt to our individual susceptibilities, but it must arrange its 'home' (or body) in order to process the adaptation.

The human body, together with all its elements, has its own degree of intelligence and life substance ranging from the finest to the coarsest levels of being. Each tissue, each cell has within it its fair portion of this innate spirit, allowing each part of the body to have its own unique functioning. This hidden spirit flows through humans, giving off an aura or atmosphere. Everything in the universe has an energy surrounding it, including plants and animals. The body reflects this energy through the perceptible, dynamic personality. It is the internal activities of a person that create disorder. This lack of balance and harmony then results in the body and mind showing symptoms, evidence of the internal disturbance. An internal disease, or mistunement, pervades every cell. A person can sense this change and know there is something happening internally. This occurs long before there are visible changes in the tissues of the body.

If there wasn't an initial internal disturbance in the system or susceptibilities inherent in the person, we would experience total freedom. As you are sitting and reading this book you are probably unaware of your eyes moving, the feeling in your back, or your heart beating. In total freedom, one would have to stop to become aware of these sensations. When you have no consciousness of your body's movement it means the body is in freedom.

It's no wonder this perfect state of health is reflected in the Bahá'í teaching that the highest station is selflessness and servitude. We find that even the mind displays this truth. When the mind is free from inner disturbances or anxieties, when one has to consciously think about the noise in the head, it is freedom. When the heart is free from attachments, and we are in the midst of teaching or serving others, we are at our happiest, because we don't have consciousness of self. When we are interrupted by our thoughts, feelings or pain in the body, we are brought into the self by the phrase, 'I feel'. Everything comes from a cause, and the 'I feel' is directly originated from an invisible, internal disturbance.

Symptoms are really a language of nature, the body's reaction, in order to maintain homeostasis. Our inner intelligence creates this disturbance to fight off whatever invader or crisis we've encountered. When we are experiencing a particular symptom we can assume that our system has prevented something worse from appearing. Every unpleasant symptom we may be suffering can be attributed to our body's protection, guidance and assistance to health.

When disease is found in a specific organ and we heal the organ or remove it, the internal nature of what caused the illness still remains. In my approach, I look for *who* (the immaterial) is sick, and secondarily, *what* (the material) is sick, for the *what* reflects the *who*. The body reveals the entirety of a person, on all levels. True healing does not merely manage symptoms and make them disappear, but focuses on the whole person.

Each of us is, however, susceptible to certain diseases, as the homeopath George Vithoulkas[11] writes:

> When the system is exposed to disease agents our system responds to counteract it. We have inherited and acquired levels of susceptibility, or sensitivity to certain influences. When our system is weak it's more susceptible and causes a predisposition to disease. We could therefore conclude that one's system resonates with that particular susceptibility. We can be sensitive to not only pathogens like viruses or bacteria, but environmental factors, emotional shocks, or medicines. Throughout life we have a certain level of sensitivity or susceptibility. It can stay at a certain level, but can shift throughout our lives. This explains why one person can walk in a room of colds and not come down with it. If the body is in homeostasis and balanced, the system is strong, our level of susceptibility decreases.[12]

In a significant Tablet, 'Abdu'l-Bahá emphasizes the importance of balance, and of diet in healing:

The outer, physical causal factor in disease, however, is a disturbance in the balance, the proportionate equilibrium of all those elements of which the human body is composed. To illustrate: the body of man is a compound of many constituent substances, each component being present in a prescribed amount, contributing to the essential equilibrium of the whole. So long as these constituents remain in their due proportion, according to the natural balance of the whole – that is, no component suffereth a change in its natural proportionate degree and balance, no component being either augmented or decreased – there will be no physical cause for the incursion of disease . . .

This question requireth the most careful investigation. The Báb hath said that the people of Bahá must develop the science of medicine to such a high degree that they will heal illnesses by means of foods. The basic reason for this is that if, in some component substance of the human body, an imbalance should occur, altering its correct, relative proportion to the whole, this fact will inevitably result in the onset of disease. If, for example, the starch component should be unduly augmented, or the sugar component decreased, an illness will take control. It is the function of a skilled physician to determine which constituent of his patient's body hath suffered diminution, which hath been augmented. Once he hath discovered this, he must prescribe a food containing the diminished element in considerable amounts, to re-establish the body's essential equilibrium. The patient, once his constitution is again in balance, will be rid of his disease . . .

. . . When highly-skilled physicians shall fully examine this matter, thoroughly and perseveringly, it will be clearly seen that the incursion of disease is due to a disturbance in the relative amounts of the body's component substances, and that treatment consisteth in adjusting these relative amounts, and that this can be apprehended and made possible by means of foods.[13]

In all circumstances of healing, I prefer to strive for sustained long-term cures and continued preventative health measures where possible.

Ultimate health

We have at least until death to grow spiritually. In my practice, I see clients brought into balance through diet, movement, mind-balancing techniques, and various types of treatments including herbs or homeopathy. I see them live a fuller life, more free and able to make choices in difficult conflicts. Life always presents more challenges and conflicts. It enables us to know where our spiritual opportunities lie. How we handle the challenges depends upon our losing or gaining spiritual energies. When we use our spiritual energies wrongly, such as in working towards our own selfish ends, it will lead to layers of further disease. However, an intention to bring joy and not harm others takes great spiritual energy and can cause some deep conflicts within, as we confront past habits and selfish desires. The more advanced we become spiritually, the more energy it takes to keep moving up the mountain. As we resolve each challenge, there is a rush of spiritual energy, or confirmations, and we experience freedom as well as newly found health in mind and body.

A wrong application of ourselves in the world empties us of our virtues and attracts the negative weighted energies of the ego. As we empty ourselves of our spiritual energies we will experience a need for more energy or stimulation of the nervous system. Our choices then become attracted to stimulating forces like entertainment, coffee or other substances, and we have to work harder or face degeneration. Just as God does not interfere with free will, healing is clearly a human choice. No matter how many remedies I can give, they cannot touch human free will; sometimes I've encountered situations where there seems to be a force that is resisting healing efforts. Through our free will, our empowered choices, we can use the grace and spiritual energies offered to us either for healing or towards a state of disease.

When we sleep, the body rejuvenates while the soul travels without being bound by the ego, so that the consciousness can heal as well. During sleep we are united with universal energies; our dreams help us to process our day. We do not set up any hindrance between the soul and the universal healing energies. When we are awake, it is more difficult to set aside the ego in order to have God's energies or the Holy Spirit flow through us. When the limited ego takes over, our vastness, limitlessness and eternal perspective gets cut off. Therefore, ultimate health would require us to entirely let go of the ego in order to stay connected, all the time, to the ever-flowing energies. We would not be resisting the flow of the will of God. In this context, it's interesting to note that in the Bahá'í teachings selflessness is considered the highest state a soul can attain in this day.

Figure 4.2   Physical, mental and spiritual forces

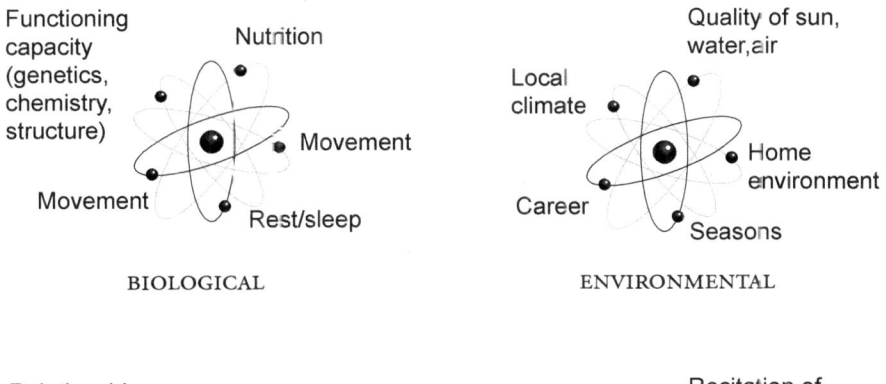

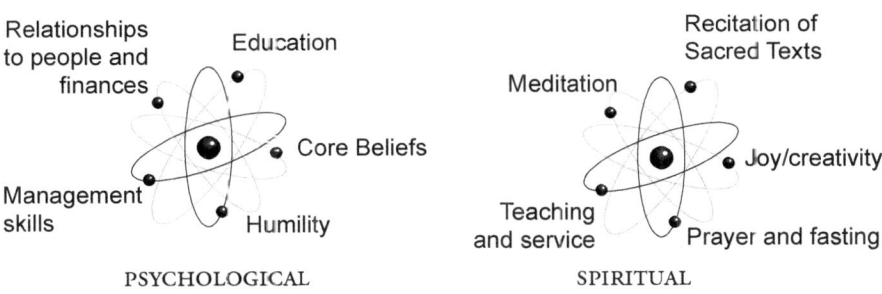

The forces that may act on a person can be summarized in Figure 4.2. A true approach to healing takes into consideration our connectedness to the influences shown in the figure. Like separate atoms, each influence has its own sphere of balance. Each unit, such as 'meditation' in the spiritual atom, has its external influence reflected in the electron, and its internal influences reflected in the neutrons and protons. Each human expression of mind, body and spirit has receptors which initiate a defence mechanism, regulating stimuli from the external and internal environment and trying to maintain equilibrium, to balance, find the 'middle way'. These influences are initially received by these receptors and result in varying effects, felt on all levels. However, the manifestation of disease or imbalance depends upon the predisposed weakness of the individual.

Figure 4.3 *The human experience*

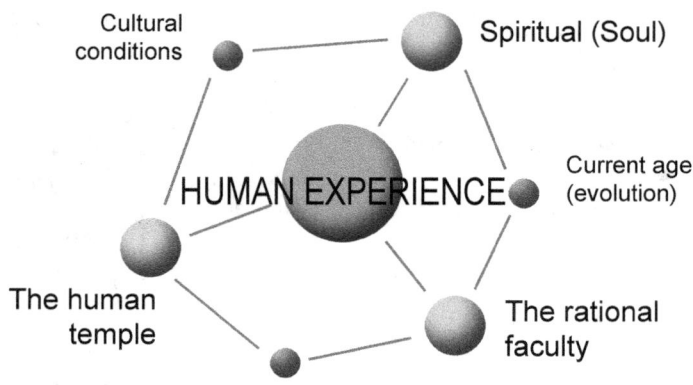

Just as science reflects how atoms join together by sharing electrons, creating molecules, the human experience reflects what is created when we put together the expressions of mind, body and soul, creating a unified vision, as shown in Figure 4.3. The figure reflects the interrelationship of these aspects, acknowledging that any effect on one affects the others. Conceptually they are separate, yet when connected they create a single pulsating, dynamic unit. The human body with its various components and systems is not linear. Researchers have explained this synchronicity by placing billions of molecules in a container. It was observed that while the movements of these molecules were initially random, after some time they became spontaneously synchronized, moving and vibrating together as a coordinated system. When synchronized, the molecules in the container created something more than the sum of its parts, an invisible unified essence – like the soul – which could not be found in any of the molecules, but was associated with each one. As in the human body, each level of experience constantly synchronizes in a fluid way through its essence or intelligence to maintain homeostasis while it responds to its surrounding environment.[14]

The human body has its own intelligence. It acts according to instinct, carnal cravings and desires, or subconscious programming. It can make order out of chaos and learn new information. However, when the mind has been exposed to non-material influences that cause it to become imbalanced, the intelligence of the body becomes mistuned. In nature, bears have been known to prefer the junk foods left at campsites over their natural choices. This tells us that animals are prone to cravings and tastes. Exposure to these tastes resets the palate, creating imbalance, then demanding more of that substance. 'Abdu'l-Bahá encouraged us to live and eat 'according to a natural, inborn equilibrium' and not by our lustful appetites.'[5] Humans have been given the rational faculty, or mind, enabling us to choose our destiny.

The body acts as a hologram of the mind. The images our eyes see create the vision of our future; memories of the past lead to wonderful imaginative adventures utilizing the power of the soul. The vibrations our ears hear translate syllables into melodies that we can replay in our minds at will. Symbolically we choose which part of life we want to listen to, which thoughts streaming forth we deem important, and whether or not we listen to the breezes of confirmation from the Holy Spirit. The sensitivity of the body to the elements, to soft or rough textures, reflects the soft or rough feelings of the heart or the coldness in a friend's comment. Hands and feet create action and inaction. They represent how love is shared or withheld, how thoughts are articulated or reflected upon.

Examining how the human body works, with its various systems and intelligence, can also reveal how the mind and soul operate. The body takes in nutrition and eliminates toxins. This is similar to the mind's ability to only receive information or to also transmit information – though we constantly try to do both at once. Listening skills are far more important for understanding than talking. Transmitting information effectively happens only after 'digesting' the information, or having some sort of reflection time. The Fast gives us an opportunity to retrain the mind to crave good information, and eliminate past baggage.

The soul parallels these systems by ingesting proper nutrition through sacred scripture. We can eat a spiritual breakfast by reading scripture, eat a hearty noon lunch with the Obligatory Prayer and have a light evening meal through more reading. The detoxification of the soul is done by finding out what the heart is attached to in the material world, detaching one's soul from it and reattaching it to the eternal. The soul is allowed to quicken through the mindful intention of reconnecting with God. The process of refraining from the cravings of body and mind allows the soul's cup to be filled.

Table 4.1 Processes of the body, reflected in the mind and soul

Processes	Body	Mind	Soul
Nutrition/ respiration	Foods, air, absorption through skin	Impressions from the five senses, experiences, imagination	Daily writings, prayer, music
Digestion	*Enzymes & flora required* Chewing, swallowing, breaking down nutrients into molecules	*Intelligence required* Comprehension through contemplation, writing a journal, or talking to a 'witness'.	*Yearning required* Reflection and meditation
Transformative processes	Assimilating nutrients or moving toxins into bloodstream; deep relaxation and rest	Assimilating events into memory; identifying negative thought patterns from the ego	Assimilating spiritual knowledge into understanding; recognizing attachments
Catalysts	Enzymes/ neuropeptides/ hormones	Will/submission/ acceptance	Desire/sacrifice/ faith
Elimination	Removal of bodily wastes	Removal of negative thoughts through forgiveness	Releasing of attachments to material world, Kingdom of Names
Movement	Aerobic exercise, flexibility, strength training	Expressing oneself, social interaction, learning a new skill	Servitude, teaching, actions aligned with God's will
Cleanliness	Washing/bathing	Purifying the mind and intentions/ motives	Purifying and cleansing the heart/ desires
Protection	Clothing, sunscreen & sunglasses, avoiding unhealthy foods . . . moderation	Obedience to His Laws, avoiding influences of ego, seeking the Middle Way	Avoiding the 'ungodly' and things that spark passion and desires of the self; contentment
Resistance	Illness/exhaustion	Stubbornness/ disobedience/ contention	Apathy/estrangement/ heedlessness

For further examination, Table 4.1 displays the main processes of the body: *intake of nutrition, digestion, transformation of digested products and elimination*, and *movement* and how their counterparts are reflected in the mind and soul. This checklist will help assess toxicity levels and health in each area. 'Ageing' represents the breakdown of the cells in the body, including brain cells. Loss of intelligence breaks down the mind, just as lack of strong spiritual infusion brings a soul to darkness.

True healing

One of the greatest questions is, 'How do the mind, body and soul interact and/or relate to each other?' My personal experience led me to look at God's relationship to mankind in order to find some clues. Bahá'u'lláh explained how the Prophet, or Manifestation of God, mediates between God and man, bringing God's message to earth and sharing it with its inhabitants. God allows all humans the ability to recognize the Manifestations of God, but He also gives us free will to do so. Without the Manifestations, man could not know God; He is the Hidden Mystery we can never comprehend except through them. By seeing how a Manifestation of God conducts himself, by recognizing his teachings and their fruits, we can know God on a very limited scale. The Holy Spirit is the force which moves through the three to connect them.

On an individual level, the soul, mind and body relate in a similar manner. The spirit, 'Abdu'l-Bahá explains, is the energy or light that emanates from the soul. True healing involves unity within this relationship. 'Abdu'l-Bahá teaches us:

> There are two ways of healing sickness, material means and spiritual means. The first is by the treatment of physicians; the second consisteth in prayers offered by the spiritual ones to God and in turning to Him. Both means should be used and practised.
>
> Illnesses which occur by reason of physical causes should be treated by doctors with medical remedies; those which are due to spiritual causes disappear through spiritual means. Thus an illness caused by affliction, fear, nervous impressions, will be healed more effectively by spiritual rather than physical treatment. Hence both kinds of treatment should be followed; they are not contradictory.[16]

And Shoghi Effendi comments:

> Physical ailments should be treated by skilled physicians through remedies. Spiritual disease results from grief, fear or nervousness and should be treated through prayer. Both means of healing are not contraindicated, and should work together. In fact, the spirit and the body meet at the sympathetic nerve. The nervous system is neither wholly physical nor spiritual and works well when both conditions are normal.[17]

'Abdu'l-Baha is reported to have said:

> There is one power that heals – God. The state or condition through which the healing takes place is the confidence of the heart. By some this state is reached through pills, powders, and physicians. By others through hygiene, fasting, and prayer, by others through direct perception . . . All that we see around us is the work of mind. It is mind in the herb and mineral that acts on the human body, and changes its condition.[18]

We may, then, conclude that it's the mind that will determine the quality of healing. The mind will also determine the ability to fast. If it believes fasting is hard, impossible, or wonderful, it will be so. The mind determines reality. 'Abdu'l-Bahá said:

> It is the mind that is the all-unifying agency that so uniteth all the component parts one with the other that each dischargeth its specific function in perfect order, and thereby cooperation and reaction are made possible.[19]

One of the goals in the Bahá'í Fast is to attain inner harmony and unity with God's will. The Fast and its inherent challenges – eating and drinking before sunrise and after sunset with the effect on blood sugar levels and dehydration – can wreak havoc on the body and mind. However, I've found that there is a way to eat and drink in a way that will ease the discomfort of the day, to ease the stress on the mind and to build the spiritual strength and gain the rejuvenation intended in the Fast. We shall go into this in more detail in Part II.

The Fast helps detoxify the body, mind and soul so that the spirit can flow freely. Medicine in most oriental traditions is in fact based upon regulating the 'chi' flowing – not too much or too little. The Bahá'í teachings talk about the heat generated by the Fast. Bahá'u'lláh specifically asserts, 'Blessed is the one who through the heat generated by the Fast increaseth his love.'[20]

The Bahá'í writings define the purpose of the Fast as to:

- protect one's eye from beholding whatever is forbidden;
- withhold one's self from food and drink; and
- withhold one's self from whatever is not of Him.

The physical fast is simply a symbol of an inner fast, the true fast. 'Abdu'l-Bahá tells us that

> this physical fast is a symbol of the spiritual fast. This Fast leadeth to the cleansing of the soul from all selfish desires, the acquisition of spiritual attributes, attraction to the breezes of the All-Merciful, and enkindlement with the fire of divine love . . .[21]

and that

> physical fasting is a symbol of . . . abstinence, and is a reminder; that is, just as a person abstains from physical appetites, he is to abstain from self-appetites and self-desires. But mere abstention from food has no effect on the spirit. It is only a symbol, a reminder. Otherwise it is of no importance.[22]

In this way, those who cannot physically fast can still participate in the spirit of the Fast! And analysing the physical fast reveals the inner fast.

Protecting one's eye from beholding what is forbidden involves vigilance and awareness in the present moment as to our thoughts, actions and intentions. This acute awareness of thoughts creates discipline to withhold from food and drink and whatever is not permissible according to the Bahá'í teachings. Table 4.2 gives a glimpse into how we fast:

Table 4.2 How we fast

Processes	Body	Mind	Soul
Cleanse	Toxic matter	Negative patterns and impressions	Attachments
Enhance nutrition	Purifying the body through eating fresh, organic, whole foods; taking supplements and herbs to rebuild cellular health	Eliminating junk food for the mind from TV, Internet, video games, gossip, magazines, and advertising; 'consuming' nutritional information and nurturing relationships	Eliminating earthly attachments to objects and people; 'consuming' the sacred texts, praying and meditation; immersing oneself in nature
Recreate and repair	Moving the body, deep breathing, rest and relaxation	Taking time to process unfinished business from the past	*Feeling* the vibration of love and joy while praying and invoking the Greatest Name
Continue good habits formed during the Fast	Continuing healthy patterns to serve God	Continuing to reorient the mind to the spiritual world – as in consulting a GPS to find directions	Continuing to follow the teachings of God

Reflection, consultation and action

When we build a home, we would be unwise to start by visiting the wood yard and buying materials straight away. Instead, we consult an architect or an engineer who prepares the blueprints and plans that must exist prior to construction taking place. I wonder if the same applies to our intentions in the Fast. Our architect is Bahá'u'lláh; it is His teachings that have laid out the vision. The chapters ahead may be thought of as tools and equipment. They lay out in detail how one might fully participate in the *innumerable effects and benefits* of the Fast.

The next parts of this book look in more detail at the 'three aspects of our humanness': the body (The Human Temple), the mind (The Rational Faculty), and the soul (The Soul). Each part is made up of three chapters: an introduction, a chapter on preparing for the Fast, and a chapter of recommendations for the Fast. The primary idea is to first present the theory – general information on health in the broadest sense. Following this, you can then plunge into the art of applying these theories during the Fast to explore the innumerable benefits and bounties contained in it. The interaction of these two; theory and application, creates a knowledge base and refinement of the principles every year. It is important to reiterate here that, although based on my understanding of the Bahá'í Writings, these ideas do not themselves form part of Bahá'í teaching – they are simply my personal understanding.

In general, it's a good idea to give time for reflection on the Fast before it actually begins. What is happening in the external world, and in my internal world? What qualities and attributes would I like to polish for next year? What negative habits can I release? How can I best utilize this time of transformation? I suggest you reflect on these matters, and then consult with family members, and with professionals if necessary, to create a plan. Here are some suggestions, based on my own experience of the Fast:

If you like, choose a theme or dedication. Each Fast I choose a theme to study, such as radiant acquiescence, detachment, etc. In preparation, I find as many sources on these themes as possible, creating a wealth of information to have on hand. This deepening carries me into the next year, allowing my soul to practise these themes through tests and difficulties, applying the Writings in each instance by looking at the world through the lenses of that teaching. Sometimes I've chosen a specific book for the Fast, or a period in the Faith's history. Is there a particular book or topic you've always wanted to deepen on? Perhaps try using the Long Obligatory Prayer every day to integrate a new habit? I've even dedicated days or entire Fasts to certain individuals. If you are truly trusting and courageous, you can pray for tests to integrate your learning and draw you nearer to God.

Identify acquired negative habits. 'Abdu'l-Bahá eloquently laid out the differences between character and personality. One is born with a God-given personality and capacity. This is easily seen in children from the time they are born, with their various talents and behaviour tendencies. Character, on the other hand, is based upon acquired habits and knowledge. It's usually seen in how we respond to situations. One can overcome personality deficiencies through education and discipline of the mind. For that reason alone, identifying habits that plague our thought patterns and beliefs are critical to transformation.

Write yearly goals. Refraining from the outer world allows time to reflect upon various aspects of daily life such as relationships, children, our role as a parent, profession, finances, spiritual growth, and service. Where would I like to be a year from now? What are some tangible goals? Where do I need to bring balance?

1. Write your goals in positive statements. Sometimes it's easier for the mind to determine what it doesn't want, and that's OK, too. Start with writing what you don't want in order to clarify for yourself what you do.
2. Write statements in the present tense as though they already exist. When 'Abdu'l-Bahá laid the cornerstone of the Mother Temple of the West, He said, 'The Temple is already built.'
3. Check your goals weekly to maintain a course of action. Be flexible when needing to reshape your goals. Remain detached from any outcomes and have faith and confidence.

Above all, remember that human beings respond well to gentleness and mercy when eliminating bad habits. Allow a transitional period to solidify new habits, depending upon your age and volition. This is why goals are important. They give us a broader picture of core issues within us, and help us to deal fairly with ourselves.

> O God! as my body has become purified and cleansed from physical impurities, in the same way purify and sanctify my spirit from the impurities of the world of nature, which are not worthy of the Threshold of Thy Unity![23]

PART II

THE HUMAN TEMPLE

5

FASTING FOR THE BODY

The spirit, or human soul, is the rider; and the body is only the steed.
'Abdu'l-Bahá[1]

The soul acts in the physical world with the help of the body.
'Abdu'l-Bahá[2]

This chapter is based on ideas that have emerged in my work and studies from various emerging scientific fields, in the light of teachings of the Bahá'í Faith. I hope it will elicit awe and a deeper respect for this 'wondrous creation' that is the human body.

The purpose of the Fast is to draw closer to God, to eliminate bad habits and acquire spiritual attributes. Yet the relationship the soul has with the body is vital to our quality of life, as it's the animating force of the body. Taking good care of the body during the Fast will help enable us to take the time to meditate and reflect upon our lives. Having a deficient body in pain can be such a distraction to the mind as to make it near impossible to focus on what we truly desire.

The body as the gate

The soul requires a noble steed to take action in this world. Shoghi Effendi uses this metaphor, explaining that the body 'is like a horse which carries the personality and spirit, and as such should be well cared for so it can do its work!'[3] Good riders will guide their horses by feeling as one with them, directing them through intentions in the mind. Reins are a good metaphor to imagine what tool directs the horse – the rational mind. These three expressions – the rider, the horse, and the ego which vies for the reins of the horse, that is, soul, body and mind – all have their own consciousness. Just as untrained horses are free to do as they please and follow their desires, so if the body is addicted to a substance, it demands it. Just as a horse always wants to go to the pasture, the body also sends us unhealthy cravings if we are out of balance. Both the horse and the rider – the body and the soul – are to be respected, for they reflect one another in this lifetime. The Báb writes:

> As this physical frame is the throne of the inner temple, whatever occurs to the former is felt by the latter. In reality that which takes delight in joy or is saddened by pain is the inner temple of the body, not the body itself. Since this physical body is the throne whereon the inner temple is established, God hath ordained that the body be preserved to the extent possible, so that nothing that causeth repugnance may be experienced. The inner temple beholdeth its physical frame, which is its throne. Thus, if the latter is accorded respect, it is as if the former is the recipient. The converse is likewise true.[4]

The Writings of the Báb are rich in metaphor and symbolism. He alludes to the various parts of the body and their relationship to the mystical realm, revealing spiritual truths. The body's processes are symbolic and act as a metaphor to show us how to connect spiritually and draw nearer to God. Our body takes in food, and our spirit also needs to take in 'food'. The respiratory system allows us to inhale fragrances and oxygen for delight and sustenance. Spiritual sustenance and intoxication are drawn in through the Writings, or 'Breath of the All-Merciful', symbolized in the body by the nose. The Bab states, 'It behooveth the faithful to inhale the fragrance of sweet savours, for verily, that is the food ordained by God for it.'[5] During the Fast many find their sense of smell and taste heightened. One becomes hungrier for more wholesome foods and their fragrances. In parallel, the Fast offers a time for the heart to become hungry for the Word of God and we can better inhale its sweet fragrances during this heightening.

The Báb also uses the analogy of the body and food to demonstrate the hierarchy and the diversity of spiritual levels.

> For verily I have demonstrated this truth to thee through thine outward body, whereby that which is partaken by the ear cannot be enjoyed by

the eye. Thus, it is incumbent upon thee to comprehend, in a similar way, such manifestations, that each station hath its own food. That which delighteth the eye is not the same thing that delighteth the ear, inasmuch as the ear beholdeth not and the eye heareth not.[6]

If we had not experienced having a nose, breathing, exhaling, speaking, partaking of food, we could not understand these symbols in the Writings. If we did not speak and hear the Word of God with the ears and see the words on a page, we could not understand the various spiritual 'foods'. God speaks to us in a language we can relate to and understand.

The body prepares the soul for the next life. It is the prime instrument which creates the opportunity to develop the latent spiritual skills after the human temple is destroyed. 'Abdu'l-Bahá likened it to a mirror that reflects the soul into this world. It's essential to keep this temple healthy so that the soul may gain maturity.

The body endures many conditions in this world, and these are all opportunities to progress spiritually. All the Prophets have this human element as well, for it's something we can relate to. Shoghi Effendi is reported to have said: 'The human element in the Prophets is human, but the power working through their atoms is from God, is stronger than in other humans. The soul works through our bodies . . . the Spirit of God through Theirs.'[7]

The human temple is laden with secrets. It reflects the possible unity of the world, its members consulting and acting with one common purpose. It also reflects the truths of the greater universe:

> . . . this limitless universe is like the human body, all the members of which are connected and linked with one another with the greatest strength. How much the organs, the members and the parts of the body of man are intermingled and connected for mutual aid and help, and how much they influence one another! In the same way, the parts of this infinite universe have their members and elements connected with one another, and influence one another spiritually and materially.[8]

Some thoughts on the expressions of the soul in the body

It's easy to perceive the connection between stress, mental and emotional attitudes and physiology and health. The latest scientific research has brought compelling evidence of how anger or fear increase the rate of heart disease, for example. These are states of mind that are not trained and prevent the spirit from flowing through the body. A disciplined ego and trained mind leads to coherence in thought and these rhythms are plainly seen in physiological changes and benefits. Shifting our emotions to care, love or appreciation changes the body's destructive stress response. It allows the spirit to flow through the body and create positive feeling states, increasing the synchronization of body systems and their efficiency, emotional stability and mental acuity, not to mention improvements in behaviour. We may conclude then the importance of the emphasis in the Bahá'í teachings of the expression of virtues, even simply in relation to our physical health without taking into consideration the wider issue of the impact of virtues on society. Science is continually finding out more on how our thoughts and emotions change our biochemistry and physiology.

The body itself has its own 'thinking' capabilities, or intelligence, processing billions of chemical messages per minute. Instead of sinking into chaos, it evaluates new data and creates various responses.

We perceive the world through our senses, our instincts, our intellect and our intuition. Even at the cellular level, we are interpreting the world around us, making choices, adjustments and reactions. Our bodies take information from our environment, the foods we eat, the emotions we experience and others, and interpret that information on many levels. For example, in a balanced system the kidneys are responsible for maintaining a certain level of body fluids, but in instant consultation with the whole body. While the body is made up of many different systems, there is an underlying message that water is needed everywhere. The body then asks for water. Therefore, the entire body is always listening, communicating and reacting to its environment. Complications arise when there is a mis-tuning, a misalignment, between the spirit and body, disrupting the unity or the consultation and wisdom required to maintain balance within.

Body systems: A city

The soul expresses itself through all the systems of the human temple. Maintaining the human temple requires many systems working together in harmony with their wisdom. Eleven organ systems create and maintain homeostasis in the body. These systems are rather like a city. Cities need clear ways to transport goods, clean up wastes, protect its inhabitants and provide structure. Regulation occurs by delivering goods, sending aid or taking out various elements. Cohesion is achieved through one central point maintaining good clear communication with all involved.

A city contains individuals, families and neighbourhoods. In a multicellular organism the levels of organization include cells, tissues, organs and organ systems. Each group works together towards a collective function. Tissues are groups of cells that perform a single function, and organs are groups of tissues that synthesize together. Organ systems include groups of organs working for a purpose. The interrelationships of these systems create unity.

Communication and sharing data augments unity in a diverse environment, whether in a city or in the human body. It's the key to success. Cells usually do not respond independently, but coordinate efforts based upon a commonality such as organs, or the immune system. Each cell within that system must *acquiesce in giving control* to the informed decision of the whole. Every cell has receptors that allow the various systems to talk to each other. The nervous, immune, neural and digestive systems coordinate and control systems in the body, responding directly to internal and external information and communicating with all the body systems.

Cities need to provide their inhabitants with services and proper fuel. In the body, digestion provides the ultimate fuel for all its energy requirements. The circulation supports this process by flow and distribution, like a large city moving goods and refuse around. The muscular and skeletal systems provide protection for the internal organs, store minerals, and support the body with structure and movement.

While good communication is vital to health, regulation maintains order. The body's regulators, or city officials, protect, send aid and remove harmful agents. The immune system supplies an army when we have too much toxicity, and fights off unwanted agents. It defines the boundaries of the organism, distinguishing between what is community and what is not. The excretory system, like the refuse service, uses the kidneys as a filter to remove waste products, maintain blood pH and regulate the water content in the blood. (In fact, the kidneys maintain balance of the blood.) The skin is the largest organ in the body and also provides the largest source of elimination.

Microcosm reflects macrocosm: The cell

On a larger scale, the body's health is dependent upon the health of the cell. The three processes required to sustain life are visible in cellular life: (1) nourishment; (2) transformative processes; and (3) elimination. Cells have internal regulators as well as external regulators. In the process of disease, alterations in the cell membrane function are the main factor. Cells may lose the ability to hold water, vital nutrients and electrolytes, or to communicate with each other. They can become subject to regulating hormones and insulin.

Cellular membranes change when too toxic or undernourished. Fats are the primary fuel for the body and critical to cellular structures, especially hormone precursors and regulators of the metabolism. Essential fatty acids enable healthy cells, while saturated fat results in membranes holding lower levels of fluids. Without the correct oils in the system, detoxification is difficult to achieve. The pH level in a cell's fluid can also determine its health. The cell maintains homeostasis if the pH level is kept between 6.5 and 7.5; lower or higher levels will affect the chemical reactions. (Further discussion on how to maintain pH levels is provided in Chapter 6. There are body controls, however, which buffer large shifts in pH levels.) Another health factor resides in cellular respiration, which depends upon proper amounts of oxygen. Oxygen and water help break down food to release energy, creating carbon dioxide.

Digestion is the master key to maintaining the body and providing fuel energy for cellular health. Fifty per cent of the immune and detoxification system resides in the gut, so it's difficult to heal any disease until the gut is healthy. Digestion also uses the three processes listed above: (1) proper nourishment; (2) transformative processes; and (3) elimination. Digestion begins with smell. The smell of food triggers the brain to release chemicals in the mouth to process the food. The digestion of carbohydrates begins primarily in the mouth. If carbohydrates are not fully masticated, there is a tendency towards flatulence and indigestion after eating them. The foods are moved to the 'blender' or stomach. The right acids, flora and enzymes enable chemical transformations of the food into nutrition. The blender churns foods until the more liquid on top blends and spins into the more solidified base; the food then enters the small intestine for distribution. Enzymes help cells regulate chemical pathways, make materials our cells need, and transfer information. The end products of digestion are then moved into the holding tank, or large intestine, where there is a last attempt to extract salts and water. The bowel then eliminates the waste.

Stress and chronic fatigue have a detrimental effect on the digestive track. Anger burns the liver[9] and negative emotions diminish healthy enzymes in the gut.

Healing by means of foods

One of the great contributions of Hippocrates, considered the father of medicine, came from his experience and observation of fasting. Given an inability to understand what was going on in the interior of the body, or the action of medicinal plants, or the nature of a disease, he adopted fasting on a moderate diet as a universal method of healing. Hippocratic medical knowledge developed around this simple process. He understood that when someone fasted, the body could release encumbrances within four to seven days, at which point the person experienced a healing crisis, usually in mucus discharges. At that time the physician could see the dynamic of the disease clearly, based upon the types of discharge.

Fasting on a moderate diet until the body is able to detoxify itself is a broad-based cure that can cross cultural differences, regardless of the person's constitution or disease. I see clients from all over the world, which presents an immense challenge in prescribing diet, understanding what foods a person has had access to, and what they eat in their culture. There are so many varied food habits throughout the world that it seems impossible to find an 'ideal diet': some parts of the world favour a protein-based diet, others subsist on a corn-based diet, and yet others carbohydrates such as rice or potatoes. How can one reconcile this? However, when examining cultures that do not have high levels of heart disease or cancer, we find they have something in common: no processed foods. Regardless of the local foods people rely on, as long as processed foods are not part of the picture there is health. The body has not developed cravings, and the tongue and brain have not been distorted.

The body can regain balance through fasting and proper food choices. Bad fuels will greatly affect a city: not only do they create pollution, but the machines used for construction will not run efficiently. In the body, the Western diet in particular has a tendency to provide 'bad fuel': it is acidic and mucus-forming through its dependence on heavily refined, high-sugar, salty foods which are often fried, laden with non-healthy fats, dairy and animal products.

'Abdu'l-Bahá explains that

> the cause of the entrance of disease into the human body is either a physical one or is the effect of excitement of the nerves.
>
> But the principal causes of disease are physical, for the human body is composed of numerous elements, but in the measure of an especial equilibrium. As long as this equilibrium is maintained, man is preserved from disease; but if this essential balance, which is the pivot of the constitution, is disturbed, the constitution is disordered, and disease will supervene.
>
> . . . When by remedies and treatments the equilibrium is reestablished, the disease is banished . . . if one of the constituents which compose the body of man diminishes, and he partakes of foods in which there is much of that diminished constituent, then the equilibrium will be established, and a cure will be obtained. So long as the aim is the readjustment of the constituents of the body, it can be effected either by medicine or by food.
>
> . . . When the science of medicine reaches perfection, treatment will be given by foods, aliments, fragrant fruits and vegetables, and by various waters, hot and cold in temperature.[10]

The founder of homeopathy Samuel Hahnemann, who lived in Germany in the nineteenth century, discovered laws and principles in healing through clinical experience, resulting in the science of homeopathy. 'Abdu'l-Bahá's statements confirm Hahnemann's findings that

> the only way the medical-art practitioner can remove such morbid mistunements (the diseases) from the dynamis is by the spirit-like

tenement-altering energies of the serviceable medicines acting upon our spirit-like life force. These energies are perceived through the ubiquitous feeling-sense of the nerves in the organism.[11]

Modern bacteriology has established that both the microbe and constitutional susceptibility can initiate disease, as 'Abdu'l-Baha explained disease in the quotation above. Ultimately,

> There is but one power which heals – that is God. The state or condition through which the healing takes place is the confidence of the heart. By some this state is reached through pills, powders, and physicians. By others through hygiene, fasting, and prayer. By others through direct perception . . . All that we see around us is the work of mind. It is mind in the herb and in the mineral that acts on the human body, and changes its condition.[12]

Bahá'u'lláh advises:

> Treat disease first of all through diet, and refrain from medicine. If you can find what you need for healing in a single herb do not use a compound medicine. Leave off medicine when the health is good, and use it in case of necessity.[13]

Changing the diet at the time of the Fast is to be recommended. Most naturopaths will advise a cleansing fast in the spring and in the fall – to maintain equilibrium during the change of seasons. Bahá'u'lláh, in the Tablet to a Physician in Arabic, mentions that cleansing the bowels during temperate seasons is beneficial, a pillar of health. Spring is the perfect time to fast, as the winter diet is especially conducive to eating heavy foods. Fasting in the spring prepares the body for the lightness of the summer diet. Colds and flu are a natural way for the body to burn off and cleanse the impurities stored in the body from the winter diet. Refraining from eating allows the body space to decompose tissues that are damaged, diseased or unneeded, and to purge them.

The Fast also allows us to 'reset the palate'. If the body is addicted to sugar, the Fast gives an opportunity to refrain from sugars. Refraining from a substance we crave for a little over two weeks is enough time to change the tongue's taste. After that, even fruits will taste like a heavenly dessert! Tongues and taste buds grow accustomed to the foods regularly eaten, so fasting allows time to change many habits and addictions. 'Abdu'l-Bahá wrote:

> At whatever time highly-skilled physicians shall have developed the healing of illnesses by means of foods, and shall make provision for simple foods, and shall prohibit humankind from living as slaves to their lustful appetites, it is certain that the incidence of chronic and diversified illnesses will abate, and the general health of all mankind will be much improved.[14]

When we don't fuel the body with food, unneeded tissues and wastes are transformed into fuel. This is the perfect recycling system! Fasting enables us to clean out unwanted trash in our bodies, providing our systems with better clarity for communication. In this we attain unity. Fasting helps create new and healthier habits in food choices, eating styles, and treating the body well. It's a time to bring peace to the city.

6

PREPARING THE BODY FOR THE FAST

> No specific school of nutrition or medicine has been associated with the Bahá'í teachings. What we have are certain guidelines, indications and principles which will be carefully studied by experts and will, in the years ahead, undoubtedly prove to be invaluable sources of guidance and inspiration in the development of these medical sciences. Moreover, in this connection the Guardian's secretary has stated on his behalf that 'It is premature to try and elaborate on the few general references to health and medicine made in our Holy Scriptures.' The believers must guard against seizing upon any particular text which may appeal to them and which they may only partially or even incorrectly understand . . . In matters of diet, as medicine, the Universal House of Justice feels that the believers should be aware that a huge body of scientific knowledge has been accumulated as a guide to our habits and practices.
>
> *The Universal House of Justice*[1]

The following pages are based upon my experience in working towards the best results, as well as personal reflections on some of the Bahá'í teachings and how they relate to healthy living.

Before the Fast begins, it is good to become mindful of one's daily lifestyle. Notice how the body might be out of balance. What routines and habits need changing? Make some mental notes on the following:

Nutrition: What you are eating, how often and when?
Movement: How often do you move your body? Are you raising your heart rate to an aerobic level at least 4 times per week? 30 minutes per day?
Waste management: Am I eliminating at least 2 times per day? Is my skin healthy? Am I hydrated? Do I breathe deeply?

Rebuilding: How long do I sleep? Do I feel rested and relaxed?

Take one week prior to the Fast to gradually eliminate harmful foods so as to prevent sickness during the first 3–5 days of the Fast. Elimination of caffeine, sugar, nicotine, alcohol, red meats and other animal products will help the side effects of fasting to be less intense. Increase your intake of water, fresh salads, organic vegetables, fruits and their juices, and green drinks (e.g. barley greens, chlorella, spirulina, wheatgrass) to promote the elimination of waste. Reduce carbohydrates. Start walking regularly – a brisk 25 minutes per day – if you don't already have an exercise programme. Some find it helpful to take a gentle herbal laxative such as liquorice, slippery elm or psyllium husks, to stimulate the colon the night before the first day of the Fast.

In your kitchen, clear out all those fatty, sugar-laden comfort foods you subconsciously reach for when you are hungry or stressed. Refill your pantry and refrigerator with the healing foods described below and in Chapter 16 on recipes. Buy all the supplements, herbs or equipment you need, such as a juicer. Keep these on the kitchen counter so that they are readily accessible.

For cleaning supplies, replace poisonous cleaning solutions with more natural, environmentally friendly ones. Ensure the bathroom is mould-free and toxin-free. Replace personal care items with more environmentally friendly non-toxic items. Buy a fresh loofah made of natural fibres. A skin brush will be an essential tool as well. Replace perfumes with 100% pure essential oils – choose with your nose, rather than by the name.

Our living and working environments should as far as possible encompass the virtues of cleanliness and orderliness. (Doing this ahead of time will eliminate the potential distraction of wanting to clean while fasting.) Prepare your bedroom with clean natural sheets, and provide an extra blanket in case the weather is chilly.

Some people set themselves goals for the physical fast to eliminate addictions like certain over-the counter drugs, smoking, sugar or coffee; to change eating habits such as becoming vegetarian/vegan, or simply to acquire a taste for healthier foods.

Components of physical health

Specific food choices will be based on individual needs. As we have seen, 'Abdu'l-Bahá states that health is a result of the constituents of the body being in balance:

> ... if, in some component substance of the human body, an imbalance should occur, altering its correct, relative proportion to the whole, this fact will inevitably result in the onset of disease.'[2]

The body has various processes and systems to maintain homeostasis. The following table is extracted from Table 4.1 (Processes for body, mind and soul), on p. 61:

Table 6.1   Processes for the body

Processes	*Body*
Nutrition/ respiration	Foods, air, absorption through skin
Digestion	*Enzymes & flora required* Chewing, swallowing, breaking down nutrients into molecules
Transformative processes	Assimilate nutrients or moving toxins into bloodstream; deep relaxation and rest
Catalysts	Enzymes/neuropeptides/hormones
Elimination	Removal of bodily wastes
Movement	Aerobic exercise, flexibility, strength training
Cleanliness	Washing/bathing
Protection	Clothing, sunscreen & sunglasses, avoiding unhealthy foods ... moderation
Resistance	Illness/exhaustion

Nutrition

Diets should reflect nature as much as possible – especially during a cleansing period. Eat living, fresh, organic, whole foods with unrefined and whole fibre, complex carbohydrates and essential fats. Fibre, fruits, vegetables, whole grains, nuts and essential fatty acids provide the best fuel. Some basic recommendations include the elimination and/or minimizing of caffeine, nicotine, meats, milk products (except yogurt and kefir), baked goods, refined flours, fried foods, sweets and fatty foods. The Master teaches us, 'The golden rule as to food is, do not take too much or too little. Moderation is necessary.'[3]

Living foods are full of light. Vegetables once digested metabolize into carbon dioxide (CO_2) and water (H_2O). The body extracts these elements, but the light (EM wave) stored in the plant from the sun and photosynthesis ends up being stored in the body. The body stores light waves through the energy of photons and scatters the frequencies throughout the spectrum of EM frequencies in the body.[4]

Our eating habits can affect the physical well-being of the planet. Environmentally, the best tips are to eat more plants and fewer animals, cook home-made meals, eat foods that are the least processed and packaged, grow and harvest your own foods where possible, and compost and recycle. Recent research is available on many websites, such as that of the Brighter Planet organization.[5] Emission outputs were examined in three distinct dietary choices with the same number of calories: an omnivorous diet, a vegetarian diet (no meat) and a vegan diet (no animal products). The average omnivore diet was responsible for emissions of 4.3 grams of CO2 per calorie consumed, while a vegetarian diet was 79 per cent of that average, and a vegan diet just 68 per cent. And most vegetarians or vegans do not eat the same amount of calories as an average American diet! Not only does livestock greatly add to the carbon dioxide output, but transportation, fertilizers and packaging the foods add to the problem. The greatest impact on global warming comes from the transportation of foods, but the second greatest is the nitrous oxide and methane used to tend livestock, with the largest amounts of emissions from red meats, then fish, dairy products, and lastly poultry. And greenhouse gases are produced even after the meal is over. Food scraps and waste decompose in landfills, adding to methane gases. Composting, recycling and cutting down on packaging can greatly contribute to our individual carbon footprint.

In his book *The End of Overeating*, David Kessler clearly portrays how the food industry promotes foods with the optimal combination of fats, sugars and salt to access the pleasure centre of the brain, creating a desire for these foods again and again. Not only do such foods usually come in heavy packaging, but the combination of ingredients is such that we find it difficult to stop eating. These foods access part of the addiction centre of the brain. Our biology is designed to maintain balance, yet that can easily be upset through easy access to a variety of foods high in sugar and fats. Foods that offer rewards, especially connected to emotional eating, can rewire our brain. As we anticipate the rewards and pleasure of eating these foods, and the synapses of our brain rewire repeatedly, it becomes harder to control our responses because our *biology* has been changed by these highly palatable foods habitually ingested. Once behaviour becomes a habit, the stimulus driving it becomes stronger. It becomes so routine that we act before we are conscious of the stimulus. In fact, researchers have measured intention by brain activity prior to the subject's awareness of their movement.[5] We have to take this into consideration as we begin the Fast. Many of us are in the hyper-eater camp, and our body and mind will react to fasting from these foods.

Eating is very personal; everyone's tastes vary depending upon culture, family traditions and personal preference. The key with nutrition is that it should be consistent. If you eat vegan one day, and another day fried foods and sugars, your body will become overworked. Your nutrition should be assessed on a weekly basis to ensure you are properly nourishing your body. Living in a fast-paced society makes it more difficult to track nutrients on a daily basis.

In the northern hemisphere, the Fast occurs right before spring, when the diet naturally turns to more natural, fresh foods. Greens are optimal foods filled with chlorophyll, while sprouts symbolize new growth. As the seasons change, the body craves different foods. In spring, it also desires to move, come alive, to create and to eat less amounts of food. A more simplified diet in the spring can help identify food allergies. The following list can apply to every season, but the types of foods our bodies crave will alter.

During the Fast, you will want to eat foods in these categories:
- natural, local and in season
- varied and rotational

- alkaline/acid balance
- proper proportions
- proper food combining
- proper oils
- with moderation

Natural food

Foods should be as close to nature as possible because these foods are the most vibrant and vitamin-filled. When foods are cooked their vitamin content drops. Foods are best when they are grown locally and in season. Our bodies have natural biorhythms that respond to local climate and seasons, so that foods in season fuel the body for the needs of the environment. Foods are also more nutrient-packed if eaten close to the time they have been picked. Rancid, old foods become poisonous, especially rancid oils, nuts, seeds and dairy products. (Even packaged foods are best shortly after packaging.) Organic foods are the best, but if you can't find organic, simply peel the skins or remove the outer leaves. There are also products you can buy to wash fruits and vegetables, or use an additive-free soap to soak them in.

Cooking your foods as gently as possible is recommended. The higher the heat and the longer food is cooked, the more nutrients and enzymes are cooked out (not to mention the taste). One can lightly steam or stir-fry vegetables. Baking or roasting squash and root vegetables are other fine alternatives. Fresh salads (without fruit) are a wonderful choice.

Currently, foods with the lowest amounts of pesticides are onions, avocados, corn, pineapples, mangoes, asparagus, sweet peas, kiwi fruits, cabbages, eggplants, papayas, watermelons, broccoli, tomatoes and sweet potatoes. Foods with the most pesticides are peaches, apples, bell peppers, celery, nectarines, strawberries, cherries, kale, lettuce, imported grapes, carrots and pears. (Keep checking with online groups such as the Environmental Working Group for updates.)

Check your intake of simple carbohydrates compared to complex carbohydrates. Simple carbohydrates are those that are digested quickly, like candy, white flour products, processed foods, boxed foods, crackers, pastas, milk, fruit juices and baked goods. Complex carbohydrates can be found in more 'natural' food' like multi-grains, whole grains, vegetables, wild rice, oatmeal, rye, whole barley, fruits and soy milk.

Varied and rotational

Eating the same foods every day, every week, can lead to imbalanced nutrition. Eating different foods weekly also prevents us from becoming sensitive or even allergic to a particular food. Just as we get a calloused finger when we rub it too many times, the biochemistry in the body produces antibodies which cause an immune response to eating the same food repeatedly. A varied and rotational diet also ensures that one of the constituents in the body will not become imbalanced.

The phytochemicals in plants have powerful effects on the body. Micronutrients such as vitamins and minerals, or phytonutrients, are naturally occurring substances that are powerful health promoters. There are also non-vitamin, non-mineral components of foods that have significant health benefits. Some help facilitate the ability of cells to communicate, have anti-inflammatory qualities or prevent cellular mutations.

Choosing a variety of colours in fruits and vegetables is the best remedy. Go to the grocery store and examine the varying shades and colours – the phytonutrients are one of the elements responsible for the intense colours. Whether you are shopping for raspberries or bananas, buy the one with the deepest, most vibrant colour. The deeper the shade, the more micronutrients and the higher the levels of antioxidants. (Even dark chocolate is better for you!) Various coloured foods also affect certain organs.

All naturally coloured food contains an antioxidant, but of the top twenty, seven are coloured red. Red pigments are protective, cancer fighters. Orange/yellow produce helps heart health, comfort and hypertension. Green can help eyesight and is the most life-giving colour. Purple/blue colours promote brain health and stress reduction and reduce free radicals. Ringing the colour changes will ensure a full vitamin spectrum. Next time you shop, take children to have an 'orange colour' day and explore which fruits and vegetables fall within that hue. They can have fun adventures finding the different colours in the store and trying different things.

Besides variety in colour, consider a variety of tastes. Chinese and ayurvedic medicine is based on various tastes – sour, bitter, sweet, spicy, pungent and salty. These are matched with various elements and conditions. A well-balanced diet keeps rotating various colours, tastes and types of food throughout the week.

Alkaline/acid balance

Alkaline foods heal more than acid foods; an acidic body manifests more diseases than an alkaline system. As stated in Chapter 5, pH levels in the cell should be kept between 6.5 and 7.5 to maintain health. Eat more alkaline foods in order to rebalance body chemistry. Acidic foods can contain high amounts of phosphorus, sulphur, chlorine and iodine and create acidic residues within the body, robbing tissues and bones of vital calcium. The Western diet is highly acidic, which creates degenerative disease and chronic conditions of inflammation, congestion, allergies and infections. Alkaline foods contain calcium, magnesium, potassium and sodium and are generally higher in water content.

When we feel irritable, or are aware of noises in joints and muscles, fatigue, flushed face or coated tongue, the problem is often acidosis. Table 6.2 will help you choose appropriate foods.

Proportions

In Western society, proportions are simply too large. Eating the proper proportions at mealtimes – not too much or too little – is essential to nutrition. Overeating makes illness more severe, as Bahá'u'lláh confirms in the Tablet to a Physician. It's easy when breaking the Fast to fall into temptation to overeat. The stomach tends to shrink after many days of fasting, and to eat with moderation and only until full is the key to building energy and good health during the Fast. Overeating causes stress on the digestive tract. Serve food on smaller dishes like a salad plate. You will be impressed by the results and feel satisfied after a small serving. We have a tendency to fill the plate, whatever size we are holding.

Food combining

Proper food combination when eating leads to optimal digestion. 'If two diametrically opposite foods are put on the table', writes Bahá'u'lláh, 'do not mix them. Be content with one of them.' And further: 'Take first the liquid food before partaking of solid food. The taking of food before that which you have already eaten is digested is dangerous . . .'[7]

Table 6.2 Food choices

Alkaline	Slightly alkaline	Neutral	Slightly acidic	Acidic
Apples Alfalfa sprouts Apricots Avocados Asparagus Bananas Beets Bell peppers Broccoli Cabbage Cantaloupe Cauliflower Cayenne Celery Dates Figs Garlic Ginger Grapefruit Grapes Green beans Guavas Kelp Kiwi fruits Lemons, Limes Leafy green herbs & lettuce Mango Melons Nectarine Oranges Papaya Passion fruit Parsley Peaches Pears Peas Pineapple Potatoes Pumpkin Raisins Raspberries Strawberries Squash Sweet corn Turnips Vinegar (apple cider) Watercress Watermelon	Almonds Artichokes Brussel sprouts Cherries Chestnuts Coconut (fresh) Cucumbers Eggplant Goat's milk Honey (raw) Leeks Mushrooms Okra Olives Olive oil Onions Pickles Radishes Sesame seeds (whole) Soy Sprouted Grains Tomatoes Vinegar (rice)	Butter (unsalted) Cow's milk (raw) Oils (not olive) Plain yogurt	Barley Blueberries Bran Butter Cereals (unrefined) Cheeses Crackers (unrefined) Cranberries Beans: Mung, adzuki, pinto, kidney, garbanzo dried Dry coconut Eggs (hardboiled) Milk (homogenized) Honey (pasteurized) Ketchup Maple syrup Molasses (unsulfured) Most nuts Mustard Oats Pasta (whole grain) Pastry (whole grain) Plums Potatoes Prunes Rice (basmati and brown) Pumpkin seeds Sunflower seeds	Artificial sweeteners Beef Beer Breads Brown sugar Cereals (refined) Venison Fish Flour (white/wheat) Molasses (sulphured) Pasta (white) Pastries (white flour) Pickles Pork Poultry Seafood Sugar (white) Soda Table salt Tea (black) White bread White vinegar Whole wheat Wine Yogurt (sweet)

Here are some simple rules to follow:
1. **Drink water properly.** Water is best on an empty stomach. You can sip up to 4 ounces during or after meals at room temperature, but any more than that amount can push the meal through too quickly and dilute digestive enzymes. It's best to drink water 30 minutes prior to eating. Ice water will kill digestive enzymes prior to a meal!
2. **Fruits alone.** Fruits should be eaten on an empty stomach or with other fruits. They pass through the stomach quickly, unlike other foods such as starches, proteins and fats, which linger up to two hours. When you eat fruit with these types of foods, it can cause fermentation in the stomach. Eat fruits raw, except apples. You can eat those baked. Other fruits baked are simply sugar.
3. **Proteins and starches alone.** Proteins, whether animal or vegetable based, require hydrochloric acid production, while starches require an alkaline atmosphere to digest. These two are contraindicated and produce a confused message to the stomach when ingested together – the stomach has difficulty processing them together, so that they generally pass through mildly digested and their nutrients are not utilized. This can lead to indigestion, bloating, gas or other discomforts. Proteins include animal proteins, dairy and nuts. Starches include simple and complex carbohydrates. It is best to choose only one per meal and mix them with vegetables. Therefore, breakfast could be a protein and vegetable meal, while dinner would be starch and vegetables.
4. **Eat simply**. 'Abdu'l Baha writes,

> If humankind . . . lived according to a natural, inborn equilibrium, without following wherever their passions led, it is undeniable that diseases would no longer take the ascendant, nor diversify with such intensity.
>
> But man hath perversely continued to serve his lustful appetites, and he would not content himself with simple foods. Rather, he prepared for himself food that was compounded of many ingredients, of substances differing one from the other . . . The result was the engendering of diseases both violent and diverse.[8]

Try to eat simply during the Fast and not mix too many different foods together. I would recommend up to seven ingredients per sitting. Choose from fats, vegetables, fruits, carbohydrates, proteins and dairy.

Proper oils

Fats are connected to inflammation and all types of body imbalances. Essential fatty acids are ones the body cannot make itself and must obtain from foods. But trans-fatty acids, so common in our Western diet, displace the good oils in the cells, specifically in the mitochondrial membrane. The result is an impossibility to lose weight and a constant feeling of sluggishness. Soybean oil, hydrogenated oils, margarine and shortening are some of these. The hydrogenation used to make these products creates trans-fatty acids and triggers free radicals. This is why detoxification requires omega-3, 6 and 9 in order to balance body chemistry.

We need omega-3 and omega-6 fatty acids daily in the correct ratio. Omega-3 is more difficult to obtain than omega-6. It comes from green leafy vegetables, walnuts, flax seed, canola oil, primrose oil and borage oil. Salmon, sardines and herring have amounts of omega 3 in them as well. As for cooking oils, ensure they are cold-pressed, because heat will damage the essential fatty acids. Olive oil is recommended for salads and cooler cooking temperatures. Higher cooking temperatures do better with canola oil or coconut oil. Cell health depends upon proper oil intake, so add omega-3 foods.

Some special notes on foods

Blood types. Many have found wonderful benefits from Peter J. D'Adamo's book, *Eat Right for your Type: Complete Blood Type Encyclopedia*. It's an excellent study on blood types and how they respond to various foods. You can also simply buy the guidebook for your own blood type and take it to the grocery store.

Ageing. If you are concerned about ageing, you can choose foods from an anti-inflammatory diet which includes many of the food recommendations already given. Minimize meats, especially 'deli' meats and red meat. Choose vegetable proteins: soy, legumes, beans, lentils, whole grains, seeds and nuts. Choose fish with the least amount of toxic contaminants.

Juices. Freshly squeezed, or put through a juicer are best. There are some pure alternatives in the health food stores. The best tasting and healing juices can be made from the following fruits: apples, pears, grapes, pineapples, lemons and other citrus fruits. Healing vegetables include spinach, kale, carrots, celery, garlic, beet greens and beets, and wheatgrass. Juices should be made from organic produce and washed well. If you cannot obtain organic produce, peel the skins prior to juicing. As for juicers, juice compressors are the best and highly recommended, but they are expensive. The next best choice is the rotary-blade juicers. They are efficient with pulp and are moderately priced.

Nuts and seeds. Nuts and seeds can easily turn rancid. They should be bought shelled, and stored in an airtight container in the refrigerator or freezer, where they will keep for 6–12 months, but only 2–3 months if in the shell and stored in a cool dark place.

Legumes. Properly cooked beans will not cause flatulence. Simply soak them overnight in water in the refrigerator to prevent fermentation. Skim off any of the skins that have floated to the surface, drain and rinse with clean water. Bring to a gentle boil with minimal stirring for a little over an hour. Don't add anything salty or acidic to the beans until they are fully cooked. To retain the B vitamins, use the cooking water for the entrée. Eat complex carbohydrates in proportion to how much energy you expend.

Vegetables. Fresh vegetables are the highest in nutrient value, fibre and carotenes. Frozen vegetables are preferred to canned. If you cook vegetables, steam or stir-fry them. Boil vegetables only if you are making soup.

Meat and fish. If you choose to eat meat during the Fast, eat only an amount the size of your palm. Avoid well done, cured or charbroiled meats. Try to eat fish instead of meat as a protein source. Research the best caught fish, without heavy metals or from poisonous waters.

Sweeteners. Try stevia, agave, maple syrup, or blackstrap molasses. Eat honey raw, not cooked. Artificial sweeteners cause weight gain and are called excitotoxins. They overstimulate brain cells until they die.

Foods to avoid. Caffeine, nicotine, meats, milk products (except yogurt and kefir), baked goods, refined flours, fried foods, sweets and fatty foods, mixing many types of foods at once, or large portions in one sitting.

Digestion

Chewing. Make sure you chew food thoroughly when you eat. A large part of digesting carbohydrates takes place in the mouth through enzymes in the saliva. Bahá'u'lláh wrote,

> Do not swallow until you have thoroughly masticated your food . . . That which is difficult to masticate is forbidden by the wise. Thus the Supreme Pen commands you.[9]

Enzymes. Enzymes are the catalyst to digesting food, and without them food remains undigested in the gut, causing heartburn, gas, colitis, indigestion, bad breath, yeast infection and many other problems. The small intestine has a difficult job assimilating nutrients and keeping toxins from passing into the bloodstream. You can take enzyme supplements with food: purchase a full spectrum enzyme that covers fats, carbohydrates and proteins. Enzymes are further discussed below in the following section 'Catalysts'.

Flora and bacteria. Flora and friendly bacteria are usually eliminated by the use of antibiotics and long-term high stress and anger. As a body ages, it's essential to replace these flora and bacteria. Probiotics clean out the gut and work on any 'crud' stuck on the walls; they also strengthen the immune system, aid in the treatment of allergies and skin problems, get rid of viruses, increase the availability of certain vitamins, and aid cell development and detoxification by breaking down foods into their smallest elements. It's best to take probiotics in the morning on an empty stomach.

Catalysts

Enzymes help the process of digestion because they are biological catalysts. Catalysts help speed up a chemical reaction. A catalyst is any substance, even if it's a very small proportion, that reacts chemically with another substance, affecting that substance without being changed or consumed itself. One molecule may transform several million reactant molecules a minute. Catalysts may be gaseous, liquid or solid; they may be inorganic compounds, organic compounds or complex combinations. They tend to be highly specific because they react with only one substance, or with a small number of select substances.

There are three types of enzymes: enzymes found in raw foods, the digestive enzyme, and metabolic enzymes. They are proteins that increase or decrease the rate of particular biochemical reactions. Most metabolic pathways are controlled by enzymes – in fact, all chemical reactions in the body necessary to sustain life are mediated by them, especially the digestive process. Three molecules make up all food consumed: fats, proteins and carbohydrates. Without enzymes, the body is unable to adequately digest food; the enzymes break down foods into their essential forms and nutrients, sending them into the circulation to be distributed and assimilated by the cells of the body. Enzymes are also catalysts in intestinal health, collecting wastes such as dead tissues, chemicals and toxins and helping them to be eliminated. They break down the foods and determine what is to be nutrition and what is to be eliminated in the gut, as well as in the cells of the body.

If digestive enzymes are absorbed into the bloodstream along with the other things, this can be very beneficial. Enzymes travel through the bloodstream, selectively latching onto any waste or toxins that may be accumulating there. They help relieve the burden on the liver and immune system. For example, if something wants to pass through the intestinal wall, it is analysed prior to passing through. If detected as harmful, fighting antibodies are called up and it's attacked. These cells take the antigens back to the intestinal mucosa where they are gobbled up and destroyed by macrophages. Therefore, enzymes help immunity by breaking down the foods in the gut and preventing them from going into the bloodstream.

Enzymes are thus essential to our health and body processes. They discern between nutrition to be integrated into the body, and waste to be eliminated. Some human bodies have more enzymatic content than others. The general populace has sufficient digestive enzymes if they eat proper amounts of raw foods until their thirties. Digestive enzymes can die with normal absorption into the circulation, through stress, heat or certain medicines. During the Fast, taking digestive enzyme supplements and replenishing the amounts will help bring balance to the gut.

The body has other catalysts besides enzymes. In a number of non-enzymatic examples, a reactant or product can act as a catalyst as well. Vitamins can function as catalysts in the body, so are also included in the recommendations given in Chapter 7.

Respiration and absorption

Air

Consider leaving a bedroom window open throughout the night; even if the weather is cold, try cracking it open to welcome fresh air in. If you live in a polluted area, consider a room air ionizer system to keep the air fresh and cleansed. Spend time outdoors – connecting with nature helps the connection to the spirit:

> 'Abdu'l-Bahá likened the country to the soul and the city to the body of man, saying, 'The body without the soul cannot live. It is good,' he remarked, 'to live under the sky, in the sunshine and fresh air.'[10]

Water

How many of us consider how toxic a shower can be? The vapour from the hot water inhaled can contain ingredients harmful to the body. Consider installing a charcoal filter to your water system, or consult an expert on attaining the best water possible.

Ingesting animals through air or water is natural, as 'Abdu'l-Bahá writes:

> Whensoever thou dost examine, though a microscope, the water man drinketh, the air he doth breathe, thou wilt see that with every breath of air, man taketh in an abundance of animal life, and with every draught of water, he also swalloweth down a great variety of animals. How could it ever be possible to put a stop to this process? For all creatures are eaters and eaten, and the very fabric of life is reared upon this fact. Were it not so, the ties that interlace all created things within the universe would be unravelled.[11]

However, the quality of our water is critical to good health. A human is composed of 70% water. Water, like the proper oils, lubricates cells and helps by flushing them. It regulates body temperature, boosts energy, carries nutrients, and creates 'space' in the brain. Distilled water, spring water and artesian well water are the best choices. Filtered water instead of tap water will suffice.

A Persian pioneer used to say, 'In the Name of God, the Most Pure, the Most Pure' five times before cooking or drinking water. This invocation comes from Bahá'u'lláh's Kitáb-i-Aqdas for use when no water is available for ablutions.[12]

Chemicals

Household cleaning products, perfumes, hairspray, soaps or emollients such as creams or lotions that soften the skin can all cause toxicity. Such toxins are absorbed through the skin and from inhalation. Replace cleaning solutions with natural less toxic ones. Reduce your use of plastics and microwaving. For scents, use products that are made of 100% essential oils. Avoid the following ingredients in your products: mineral oil, dioxane, 'fragrances', parabens (methyl, propyl, butyl, and ethyl), alcohols (ethanol, ethyl alcohol, methanol, benzyl alcohol and isopropyl), petroleum jelly, talcum powder, colouring agents and sodium lauryl sulfates.

Movement

In the Tablet to a Physician, Bahá'u'lláh advises:

> Exercise is good when the stomach is empty; it strengthens the muscles. When the stomach is full it is very harmful . . . When you have eaten walk a little, that the food may settle.[13]

Regular aerobic exercise

Regular exercise significantly contributes to a non-toxic body. While long periods of hard-core workouts are not recommended during the Fast, keeping the body moving *is* highly recommended and essential to the detoxification process. Moving the body to the point of perspiration helps expel toxins through the skin – the body's largest elimination system. It helps the metabolic processes, stimulates the circulatory and lymphatic systems. Exercise helps increase the oxygen levels and endorphin rush into the brain – a key to boosting energy, peaceful moods, happiness and relaxation. Increasing muscle mass helps to prevent back pain, makes your body more efficient at using oxygen, promotes relaxation and aids sleep. The metabolic rate is raised when moving the body and circulation improves.

Flexibility

Movement also includes building *flexibility* through simple stretches and graceful slow movements such as dance and yoga. In addition, stretching muscles helps release toxins, allowing the acidity stored in the muscles to be released. A series of deep stretching helps the nerve bundles release nervous energy or built-up emotions alongside the spine. (Massaging these areas gently in long strokes helps, too.) Toning activity or building muscles would not be an appropriate activity during the Fast.

Strength building

As we age we lose muscle mass. Strength building should be an integral part of one's health and well-being, and takes place through resistance. It increases bone density. Although strength training would not be recommended during the Fast, it is worth mentioning for inclusion in your maintenance programme for the rest of the year. During the Fast, mental and spiritual strength building is more appropriate for your mind and soul's nearness to God.

During the Fast, exercise is really up to the individual. If the body feels it needs to move, then move; otherwise, be restful. Be mindful to exercise only on an empty stomach – never exercise on a full stomach! During the first week of the Fast the body will be adjusting to the new routine. I recommend walking and simple body stretching for 15–20 minutes. When you feel the body has adjusted to the Fast, low-impact aerobic exercise such as gentle walking, biking, swimming, tai chi and yoga are all excellent choices.

Cleanliness

A skin brush will be an essential tool during the Fast. Brush the skin for three minutes, only when it's dry and stroking towards the heart. (When brushing the legs, stroke upward.) The white powder coming off the skin is uric acid and other waste products. Never expose the brush to water. Then, use a fresh loofah made of natural fibres while bathing. Use 100% pure essential oils or fragrant herbs while bathing – choose with your nose, rather than by the name. Epsom salts help in detoxification and oatmeal sooths dry, irritated or inflamed skin. Avoid using regular soaps with detergents that strip the skin of its natural/protective oils. Use herbal hair rinses that clean the hair, rather than the harsh chemicals in commercial shampoos. Don't bathe right after eating.

Washing the body is reflective of the act of cleansing the spirit and mind. In the New Testament, Christ washed the feet of a 'sinner' with His own hair. In the Kitáb-i-Aqdas, 'the believers are exhorted . . . to bathe regularly, to wear clean clothes and generally to be the essence of cleanliness and refinement.'[14] Baha'u'llah asks us to wash before praying, but also to keep clean in our appearance internally and externally. 'Abdu'l-Baha confirms this when he speaks of children:

> A child that is cleanly, agreeable, of good character, well-behaved – even though he be ignorant – is preferable to a child that is rude, unwashed, ill-natured, and yet becoming deeply versed in all the sciences and arts.[15]

And in the following passage 'Abdu'l-Bahá suggests how a clean environment and cleanliness can connect one to the Kingdom:

> Arise and wash thy body, wear a pure gown, and, directing thyself to the Kingdom of God, supplicate and pray to Him. Sleep in a clean, well prepared and ventilated place, and ask for appearance (or display) in the world of vision. Thou wilt have visions which will cause the doors of doubts to be closed, which will give you new joy, wonderful dilation, brilliant glory. Thou wilt comprehend realities and meanings.[16]

Elimination

Of all the bodily processes, elimination is one of the most important ingredients to balance. When the bowel is underactive, the potential for absorption of toxic substances greatly increases through the bowel wall and directly into the bloodstream, circulating and depositing toxins into body tissue. A healthy bowel requires sufficient hydration, proper nerve and muscle tone, and the right balance of biochemical nutrients. Clean blood is directly related to a clean bowel. Our colon is sensitive to our emotions; in ancient times it was called 'the seat of the emotions'. Anxiety, nervous tension and stress can enable the colon to become tense, responding with diarrhea or constipation. All functional bowel disorders have a definite mental counterpart.

Relaxation is conducive to the best bowel movements. A body in balance eliminates after each meal. While all bodies are different, most individuals eliminate once a day, but 2–3 times is ideal. An ideal bowel movement should not float or sink, and should be shaped like a thin banana.

Don't worry too much about constipation during the Fast – it's a normal response of the body to less roughage in the system. Some suggestions for overcoming constipation are given in Chapter 7.

Transformative processes

Deep sleep

Most people need between 7 and 9 hours sleep, with deep sleep at some point. Take time to sit and relax prior to bedtime. Many with sleep problems find it helpful to create a bedtime routine so that their body knows it's time for sleep. Try sitting under dim lights for an hour before bed to prepare the brain for sleep. Complete darkness is required for the brain to produce melatonin for proper sleep; any amount of light can disrupt this, so if you wake up at night, try to keep the lights off. Use the bed for rest only, as this sends a message to the body about the purpose of the bed; so avoid doing work in bed. The bedroom is a place to recharge, so ensure it is clutter-free, with light, fresh air and a peaceful environment.

Heat therapy

Overheating the body with herbs in China, the saunas of Scandinavia and the sweat lodges of the Native Americans helped medicine for centuries. This healing method can help heal simple colds and flus, as well as degenerative diseases such as cancer, arthritis and AIDS. The heat allows the body's blood vessels to dilate and allow more blood to flow to the surface, allowing toxins to flow out through the skin. A true 'detox bath' is 104 degrees Fahrenheit, or 40 degrees Centigrade. Start at 10–20 minute periods at lower temperatures and build up the heat gradually.

Bathe daily during the Fast to stimulate the cleansing process. If you'd like to include heat therapy, do it at least 2 hours after eating. If possible, empty the bladder and colon first. Using a soft dry brush with strokes in an upward motion over the body, as described above, prior to treatment will help remove toxins from the skin. If you'd like to take a detox bath, ingredients to add to the hot water could be 5–6 drops of aromatherapy oils (chamomile or lavender), or ½ cup of sea salt, or ½ cup of baking soda, or herbs and seaweed, or Epsom salts, or 1 cup of cider vinegar.

In addition to heat therapy, you can interchange hot and cold hydrotherapy. In this situation, you alternate hot and cold water in the shower to improve circulation and relax muscles. Change the water temperature every couple of minutes for about three cycles.

Caution: **Don't use heat therapy during the day while fasting, or with certain physical illnesses.** If you start to feel dizziness, nausea, fast heart rate, irregular heart rate, headache, shortness of breath, or muscle cramps, stop the treatment. If the nervous system has been damaged, there may be a problem in sweating or a lack of toleration high temperatures. Those with chemical sensitivities, those taking certain medications such as for seizure, or those with metal parts in the body, chronic fatigue, MS or fibromyalgia, heart conditions, within 48 hours of an acute injury, or swelling on the body, or those who are pregnant, should be cautious about heat therapy.

Massage therapy

Massage can be used to treat the body to better metabolic processes, relaxation and to help pain control. The most helpful techniques are Swedish, deep tissue, or lymphatic massage. Hand and foot massages such as reflexology stimulate points connected to the organs of the body. Warm water soaks before massage help to stimulate immunity and to relax and soothe the sympathetic nervous system. If you wish to use aromatherapy in your massage, use your nose to choose the essential oil, not your knowledge. Make sure to use a carrier oil such as jojoba or olive oil, with 1–2 drops of essential oil. For healthy feet, simply rub the pads of your fingers and thumbs over your feet to find tender points. When found, gently press on the tender point to help eliminate waste products. These are felt like granular deposits which need to break down and move out.

Deep breathing

In order to support the physiological processes during the Fast, deep breathing will help not only clarify the mind, but bring about deep relaxation for the body. Regular daily practice of deep breathing throughout the Fast can produce a generalization of relaxation to the rest of your life. It prevents stress from becoming accumulative, as unabated stress builds up over time. Even sleep cannot break the cumulative stress cycle unless you've intentionally allowed yourself to deeply relax while awake. Sitting and unwinding in front of the television, or bathing, cannot bring about *deep relaxation*, which usually includes breathing exercises, progressive muscle relaxation, or visualization and meditation.

In the past 20 years research has shown the numerous benefits of deep breathing. It leads to increased energy levels and productivity, and to decreases in heart and respiration rate, blood pressure, skeletal muscle tension and metabolic rate. It also improves concentration and memory, reduces insomnia and fatigue, and prevents or reduces psychosomatic disorders such as headaches and various types of chronic pain. It also leads to an increased availability of feelings.

Studies show that those who are more anxious tend to breathe shallow from their chest, while those who are more relaxed breathe more slowly from their abdomens. It's easy to retrain your breathing patterns. Here is a simple abdominal deep breathing method which combines breathing with meditation; you can make it a practice for 20 minutes per day:

1. Sit in a relaxed position with the spine erect. Place your hand on your abdomen, below your belly button.
2. Inhale slowly and deeply through your nose sending the air as low as you can. Your hand should rise as you inhale.
3. Pause for a moment, and then slowly exhale through your nose or mouth fully. Allow your whole body to let go as you exhale.

4. Do ten full abdominal breaths. Keep breathing smooth and regular. It's helpful to count to 4 on the inhale and 4 on the exhale. Pause after 10 breaths and breathe normally for 2 breaths.
5. Repeat this for three sets of ten.

After about 10 minutes, you will notice the affects of this deep breathing on your body. Continue breathing normally and gently, and begin your meditation practice, which will be discussed further in the chapters on the soul.

7

RECOMMENDATIONS FOR FASTING

There are no set traditions or specified ways of eating during the Fast in the Baháʼí teachings. However you eat during the Fast will be all right – if you like to break the Fast with coffee, fine; if you like to eat oatmeal in the mornings for your Fast, great! The following recommendations are not designed to treat anything specific, but are simply general suggestions aimed at enhancing a fairly balanced system and to ease the body's discomfort during the Fast. The intention is to give you another way of looking at the Fast and a potential path to try out for yourself.

Cleansing and balancing the body

Before sunrise

'A light meal in the morning is as a light to the body,' says Baháʼuʼlláh.[1] We may be tempted to eat as much as possible in the morning, but overeating is the most harmful activity. To give the body ample time to adjust after waking, eat properly and slowly.

Dehydration is a challenge during the Fast. Therefore, upon waking, drink 1–2 cups of water. Fruits and their juices should be taken next. Allow enough time – at least 20–30 minutes – for the fruits to be fully digested before eating a light meal. You may wish to incorporate some fish oil supplements or flax oil, because fats help you feel satisfied longer. We eat proteins in the morning because they take longer to digest and give the most energy. Studies have found that white bread, white rice and carbohydrates tend to move through the digestive tract quicker, making you hungry faster. This is why the evening meal will include complex carbohydrates.

- ♦ Prepare morning foods the night before. Do any cutting or

- measuring of ingredients and set aside.
- Try playing soft, uplifting, meditative music while preparing food. Slowly enter the day with lightness and joy.
- Chew food thoroughly before swallowing.
- Remember to eat on an empty stomach, as foods imposed on a digesting stomach are harmful.
- After breakfast perform ablutions, washing of the face and hands, and move right into dawn prayers. It's such a joy to watch the sun rise as you turn east to connect with your Beloved, reciting and intoning His words.
- Once prayers are said, dry brushing the skin and bathing are a viable next step. Do some deep breathing to attain deep relaxation and welcome the day.

Here are some sample plans for morning meals during the Fast. Further options can be found in the recipes in Chapter 16.

Time	*Amount*	*Example*	*Notes*
Upon waking	1–2 cups	Spring water, or lemon in warm water	Some use master cleanser here.
		Probiotics, aloe juice	Take on empty stomach with morning water.
After 10 minutes	4 oz. or 100g	Fresh fruit/vegetable juice	See Table 6.2: Food choices.
	½ – 1 piece	Whole, fresh fruit	
After 30 minutes		Dates, dried fruits	Take digestive enzymes before the meal!
Breakfast 1	1–2 bowls	Wholegrain cereal	Oatmeal, oat bran, cream of wheat.
Breakfast 2	Protein and vegetable	1 egg and veggies	Salad plate portion.
Breakfast 3	Smoothie	Soy yogurt, flax, bananas, lecithin granules, soy protein powder, raw honey	
Just before sunrise	½ cup	Tea	Green, dandelion.
Time for meditation/prayer	15 minutes	Fasting prayer	'Turn towards the sun'.

During the day

The mouth can taste unpleasant the first week. This is normal. Some will use breath fresheners, rinsing the mouth out with mouthwash, or brushing the teeth frequently during the day if dealing at close quarters with clients/patients. More purist thinkers will allow nothing in the mouth until after sunset; however, Bahá'u'lláh also encouraged us to be refined, clean and fragrant.

At regular eating times, I would suggest taking a 'spiritual snack' by reading the sacred Writings, prayers or other inspirational writings, enabling the mind to refocus. This is the most precious opportunity to reflect and meditate on your journey. Practise seeing yourself as wrestling with desires and mastering your cravings.

What do I do when I feel spacey and tired in the afternoon?

Remedies for low energy	Notes
Take a nap	Limit your sleep to 20 minutes and you'll feel refreshed.
Take a brisk walk. Move the body, stretch.	Getting oxygen throughout the body will awaken your senses.
Get some fresh air. Connect with nature.	Fresh air will awaken the brain. A famous writer used to go out into New York city and watch ants if he wasn't in the country, and his writer's block would be removed.
Meditation. Deep breathing.	If you can't escape, sit quietly, set a timer for 10 minutes. Close your eyes, sit erect but comfortable, and repeat a mantra or the Greatest Name.

The daytime is a great time to incorporate some other healing methods, such as massage therapy (the best time is right before you break the Fast so you can drink water afterwards). Take time during the regular lunch hour to get fresh air, do some walking or stretching, to your personal ability. Be mindful of deep breathing, to really promote relaxation and well-being.

Breaking the Fast at sunset

The Fast does not end when the sun sets! The body will not starve or die within the next 30 minutes. This time period can become the greatest test through eating too fast and too much, but it is the opportunity to really train the body's urges. Breaking the Fast should be done slowly, so as not to create sickness or nausea. The sun does not instantly come out in its midday splendour; it rises gradually and allows us to adjust to its heat and light. We need to remember that our digestive tract has rested all day.

Breaking the Fast with some water will help prepare the digestive tract for food and help prevent dehydration. After approximately 10 minutes, fresh fruit/vegetable juice will stimulate the secretion of our digestive enzymes, prepare for more solid food and give us an instant 'vitamin rush'. This method also retrains the tongue to more natural tastes – when you are really hungry, whatever you eat tastes wonderful and the body remembers that taste as being satisfying.

- Do not break the Fast with any animal products, fried foods, refined foods, nuts or seeds.
- Resist the urge to snack, gorge or eat too fast.
- Begin eating by mention of God, and end by remembering your Lord.
- When you sit down to your meal, serve your portion on a salad plate.
- Chew your food thoroughly – at least 15 times per bite (22 times is recommended!). Fifteen chews may seem like an eternity, but realizing that mastication needs more work is a great observation. Taste and savour your food, give thanks!
- The first 9 days of the Fast can really benefit your body if you incorporate shredded vegetable salads as your first food to break the Fast. Shredded beets, cabbage, carrots, turnips, or broccoli slaw with a little avocado are great examples. They act like a 'street sweeper' for your intestines. Use citrus juices and olive oil (or flax oil) as a dressing. You can also spray amino acids on salad (see the recipes in Chapter 16).
- After the first 9 days, I recommend soups and liquid meals to keep bodily fluids flowing and to help hydration. Incorporate oils to make you feel more satisfied. Eat liquid or soft foods

- first, and then more solid foods at the end.
- Once your salad plate is finished, sit for 5 minutes. **If** you still feel hungry, take a helping the size of your palm. Remember you can snack in a couple of hours.
- Shortly after the meal and clean-up, take a stroll to stimulate digestion and get fresh air.
- About one-and-a-half hours after eating, drink more liquids such as water, hot water with lemon, or freshly squeezed fruit and vegetable juices. Drink tea throughout the evening for more hydration. Herbal teas specific to your personal detox programme can help (see below on supplements).

Before bed

Snack only after the stomach fully digests the previous meal. If proteins were eaten, this could take up to 2 hours; 2.5 hours with red meat. It's harmful to mix new foods into a stomach that is moving a meal into the small intestine.

Ensure that eating stops 2 hours before sleep. Drinking hot tea within an hour of sleep is all right, provided it is free of stimulants. Take herbal cleansers and drink a cup of tea: camomile, valerian root, ginger or peppermint are nice choices.

A potential healing crisis

What to do with the uncomfortable side-effects of detoxification

Remember the saying: 'It's darkest right before the dawn.' The healing crisis is recognized in most systems of natural healing. Whenever we begin healing, we come to a place where it gets worse before it gets better: it's when old toxins are being freed from their usual places of residence and affecting us with their full capacity. Many chemicals from pollution or medicines are stored deeply within our tissues. As accumulated wastes are taken out of the body, we may experience body odours, headaches or other symptoms. At such times we may panic or interpret them as a new problem.

A healing crisis is unpredictable as to when it will appear, but we know it doesn't last more than two days if it's a true healing crisis.

Some suggestions (see the recipes in Chapter 16 for more options):

Time	Amount	Example	Notes
Sunset	1–2 cups	Distilled/ spring water	Add lemon, or a master cleanse recipe, or 1–2 teaspoons of apple cider vinegar
10 minutes later	4–8 oz. (100–200g)	Fresh fruit/vegetable juices	See Table 6.2: Food choices
Before meal			Take supplements requiring an empty stomach, digestive enzymes.
20 minutes later	Salad plate portion		Carbohydrates and vegetables. If you ate carbohydrates for breakfast, choose protein and vegetables for dinner (and vice versa). Prepare small shredded veggie salads. Eat before cooked meal.
Dinner option 1		Herb-coated tofu with steamed vegetables, baked yam	
Dinner option 2		Steamed peppers stuffed with brown rice and tofu with diced tomato. Choice of cooked vegetable	
Dinner option 3		Stir-fried vegetables with brown rice	
Dinner option 4		Steamed greens with diced tomatoes and lots of garlic lightly cooked in olive oil and herbs. 1–2 slices whole grain bread	
During meal			Take any supplements required with food. Sip warm water if needed.
After dinner clean-up	15 minutes	Light movement	Walk, stretch, play with children.
Snacks	After 2 hours	Handful of nuts/seeds Air-popped popcorn and seasoned herbs if desired Organic apple slices	
Hydrate!			

If it lasts more than three days, you can generally consider it a new symptom. Sometimes we release toxins too quickly and become sick. In this case, it's recommended to increase your liquid intake and eat only vegetables and fruits until you feel better.

The following symptoms are signs of toxicity and their release: dizziness, nausea, aches or light-headedness in the first 3 to 5 days. Headaches and hunger pains are very common during the first three days of your fast. Changes in your skin, tongue, breath, urine and stools are common. Less common side-effects can include indigestion, joint pains, sinus congestion, flatulence or constipation. If you have restlessness and anxiety that you didn't have before the Fast, a food addiction may be presenting itself. Generally, the body can take care of itself; take time to physically and mentally rest. If there is any doubt, contact your doctor.

The colour of our tongue indicates how well we've cleansed. While fasting, the tongue can become coated with white, yellow or grey film; this represents detoxification. When the process is complete, the tongue will appear clear. These signs are not infallible, but are a general guide to the cleansing process.

Here are some recommendations to relieve some side-effects of detoxification without having to break your fast:

Remedies for side-effects	*Notes*
Headaches	Place 2 drops of peppermint or lavender essential oil on your fingertips. Rub your fingers together, then on the temples or the back of the neck. Be careful not to get the oil near your eyes. Press the acupressure points where the skull meets the neck for 60 seconds with gradual pressure. Have a friend give you a scalp massage, or massage the ears.
Gas pains, abdominal discomfort, indigestion, heartburn	Place 3 drops of peppermint essential oil in a tablespoon of carrier oil such as jojoba or olive. Rub together in your palms and rub gently over the abdomen.
Coldness in extremities, shivers	Dress in layers, ensuring you have an extra sweater.
Joint pains, sinus congestion	Bathe with 3 drops of eucalyptus oil, or place 2 drops in a tablespoon of carrier oil such as jojoba or olive, rub together between the palms of your hands and spread over affected areas.

Rebuilding physical health with supplements

Food supplements can help purification and rebuild cells. Although over-use of supplements is not recommended, in my experience they can be helpful during the Fast. Also, 'some vitamins can be hazardous to your health', as an article in the *Wall Street Journal* reveals:

> Most people are not aware that many of the synthetic vitamins, including some of the highly advertised 'name brands', are processed in a laboratory at high temperatures (which destroy the nutrient content), and contain petroleum derived chemical solvents, such as ethyl cellulose, coal tar, hydrochloric acid, acetonitrole with ammonia, methanol, benzene, formaldehyde, cobalamins reacted with cyanide and acetone and are coated with methylene chloride, a carcinogenic material.[2]

When shopping for supplements, therefore, it's best to find a source made from fresh organic whole foods grown from non-genetically modified crops. Powders or capsules are the best forms to purchase.

Vitamin C is a great example of a supplement usually sold in synthetic form, usually in the form of ascorbic acid. But ascorbic acid is only one of eight components of vitamin C, and does not fully create vitamin C in its whole form. Foods contain all eight: rutin, bioflavanoids, factor K, factor J, factor P, tyrosinase, asorbinogen and ascorbic acid.

When you are fasting, the body becomes sensitive to influences, whether natural or pharmaceutical. Always pay attention to how your body is responding and check with your healthcare practitioner. Consider giving your normal vitamins a break.

Here are some of my recommendations for supplements prior to and during the Fast:

Two weeks before the Fast: Essential fatty acids (EFAs); vitamin C: 2,000–4,000mg per day, taken in 500mg tablets throughout the day; glutathione: 400–800mg per day; L glutamine; echinacea: twice a day; selenium. Laxative if needed: aloe juice: 4 oz per day, and liquorice root.
During the Fast: Probiotics (take on an empty stomach), digestive enzymes (take with food), EFAs (take with food), dandelion root, spirulina.

A word of caution: *The right remedy will do very little if the foods ingested are contraindicative. Food choices and attitude in the mind will ultimately determine the success of the cleansing process.*

General purpose supplements for the Fast

The following supplements can help the body during the Fast:

Gentle herbal laxatives: Aloe juice works very well and is soothing to the digestive tract. Liquorice root and slippery elm also work. Try 1 teaspoon of blackstrap molasses in hot water. Don't worry too much about constipation during the Fast – it's a normal body response to less roughage in the system. Psyllium husks taken 1 hour after eating can stimulate bowel movements.

Essential fatty acids (EFAs): Flax oil, primrose oil, borage oil or fish oil. Some favour 1 teaspoon of cod liver oil (mercury free) daily, plus DHA (docosahexaenoic acid, which is an omega-3 fatty acid and a primary structural component of the brain, sperm and retina.)

Probiotics: Replenish your healthy flora and friendly bacteria. Take on an empty stomach in the morning.

Digestive enzymes: Use enzymes to fully digest your food. Choose full spectrum enzymes that use a balanced approach for lipids, proteins and carbohydrates.

Blood cleansers: Garlic, red clover, sarsaparilla root, goldenseal root, dandelion root, burdock root. Some of these make great teas.

Specific conditions

The following supplements will help with the specific conditions listed here. Choose 2–3 supplements. Start 2 weeks prior to the Fast and then stop taking these supplements when the Fast begins.

Sugar elimination:

Supplements to help withdrawal: B vitamins (take with food), vitamin C, zinc, amino acid L-glutamine, calcium/magnesium (take in the evening). Lipoic acid helps reduce sugar cravings.

Nutrition (replacing sugar snacks): Increasing protein can limit sugar cravings. Fruit slices, mixed nuts, vegetables, almonds, sunflower seeds, granola, protein smoothies.

Caffeine elimination: Drip and percolated coffee contain the most caffeine, while black and green teas have almost 1/3 the amount of caffeine.
Supplements: Vitamin C, potassium, calcium/magnesium (take in the evening), zinc and B1, B2, B6 (take with food). For headaches, use white willow bark herb.
Nutrition (replacing coffee): Allow yourself one cup per day. It's best taken in the mid- to late afternoon, fitting our biorhythmic clocks. You can replace the rest with green tea. If you feel that you need the energy, ginseng root can provide energy without the jitters!

Liver aid: Lethargy, cellulite, depression, poor digestion, headaches, bags under eyes.
Supplements: Dandelion root and leaf tea, milk thistle, digestive enzymes, chlorophyll-rich foods.
Nutrition: Fresh lemon squeezed in water upon waking and before going to bed. Keep fats low, as the liver needs rejuvenation. Beets, artichokes, radishes produce bile flow.

Allergies:
Supplements: CoQ10 30 mg; Quercetin: up to 2,000 mg daily with bromelain; Ester C up to 3,000 mg; digestive enzyme support with meals; echinacea, Siberian ginseng, goldenseal, dandelion.
Nutrition: Eat organic foods and cultured foods such as yogurt, miso and tofu. Drink cranberry, grapefruit and pineapple juices.

Anxiety/stress aid:
Supplements: Probiotics, electrolytes, antioxidants, and digestive enzymes with meals; Bach Rescue Remedy, calcium/magnesium (take in the evening).
Nutrition: Lemon water upon rising. Fresh green leafy vegetables, chlorophyll, high fibre foods. Avoid fats, sugars, sodas and stimulants. Focus on EFAs from primrose oil or flax oil. Eat alkalizing foods.
Aromatherapy: Camomile, lavender, ylang ylang.

PART III

THE RATIONAL FACULTY

8

FASTING FOR THE MIND

> There is, however, a faculty in man which unfolds to his vision the secrets of existence. It leads man on and on to the luminous station of divine sublimity and frees him from all the fetters of self, causing him to ascend to the pure heaven of sanctity . . . This is the power of the mind . . .
>
> 'Abdu'l-Bahá¹

While Part II has reviewed the material, the physical, body, Part III explores the rational faculty, which is the interior aspect of man – will and intellect. Part IV will address the immaterial, the soul or spirit that uses the mind and body to express itself.

This chapter combines my own professional experience with the latest scientific understanding of the mind, in particular how the mind reflects and moves in the body. It also reflects on some of the teachings of the Bahá'í Faith, and of Buddhism, that provide insights into the complex nature of the mind and its enormous potential.

What is the mind? Humans experience an internal dialogue, revealing an existence other than the body. When we say 'I'm hungry', the 'I' is the *body, the stomach*. But when we say 'I experienced', who is this 'I'? There is clearly another part of us than our body. When we contemplate and think, 'I wonder what I should do,' with whom are we consulting? The mind is an ethereal form that is connected with the body, as 'Abdu'l-Bahá explains:

> The mind which is in man, the existence of which is recognized – where is it in him? If you examine the body with the eye, the ear or the other senses, you will not find it; nevertheless, it exists. Therefore, the mind has no place, but it is connected with the brain.[2]

The mind makes scientific discoveries, explores mysteries and reveals beauty and art. In the Bahá'í teachings, various words are used to refer to it. Bahá'u'lláh often uses the term 'rational faculty', while you can also find the words 'intelligence', 'will', and 'thought'. The mind is a 'sign of the Revelation of Him', a 'mystery which cannot be comprehended,' a 'gift from God'.

In expounding this theme, Bahá'u'lláh quotes from the Qur'án: 'We will surely show them Our signs in the world and within themselves . . . He hath known God who hath known himself.'[3] This reference to self is the identity of the individual created by God, and not the self we mostly identify with, which is our stream of consciousness, the freeway continually humming.

Shoghi Effendi said that very little is known about the mind and its workings. Even the best minds cannot attain a true understanding of the mind, even if human beings have pondered its existence and tried to solve its mysteries for centuries. Bahá'u'lláh writes:

> Wert thou to ponder in thine heart, from now until the end that hath no end, and with all the concentrated intelligence and understanding which the greatest minds have attained in the past or will attain in the future, this divinely ordained and subtle Reality, this sign of the revelation of the All-Abiding, All-Glorious God, thou wilt fail to comprehend its mystery or to appraise its virtue. Having recognized thy powerlessness to attain to an adequate understanding of that Reality which abideth within thee, thou wilt readily admit the futility of such efforts as may be attempted by thee, or by any of the created things, to fathom the mystery of the Living God, the Day Star of unfading glory, the Ancient of everlasting days. This confession of helplessness which mature contemplation must eventually impel every mind to make is in itself the acme of human understanding, and marketh the culmination of man's development.[4]

Yet although the mind in its totality is mysterious and unknowable, science has made remarkable progress in the last century and disclosed some of this mystery. Understanding it according to our individual and collective capacity helps us to work with it. For example, we currently understand that we have a conscious and a subconscious mind.

The subconscious mind: Habits and experiences

The subconscious mind is the totality of our life experiences and acquired habits. It allows the conscious mind to focus on the present moment – as when you're driving a car and thinking about your day. The subconscious mind's programming lets your arms and legs and eyes avoid accidents while you think of other things. It's our autopilot programme. How many times have you driven somewhere and cannot remember the drive?

The subconscious mind also helps to run and regulate bodily processes such as heart rate, breathing, and immune responses. It is programmed according to past experiences including traumas, and often stores overwhelming emotion in the body. It's always in the present moment, so it can relive any memory just as it is happening in the now, in 'real time'. The subconscious mind filters billions of data bits, allowing us to focus on what the conscious mind determines to be important and to understand the world around us. I have found in my practice that the more interesting bits of data are the ones our consciousness rejects and the subconscious mind receives and may or may not process. All our belief systems reside in the subconscious, or what we believed at one point in our life and often didn't let go and evolve. It contains the lower impulses or lower self-programming and is a source of why we can't progress or move forward, heal. Our blocks often stem from a limited belief system found in the subconscious.

The conscious mind: Our creative force

The creative force behind our life lies in the conscious mind. Through focusing, the conscious mind can also to a certain extent determine breathing, heart rate and bodily systems.

We share up to 99 per cent of our genes with the animal kingdom. What differentiates us is the pre-frontal cortex in the brain, which enables humans to learn to control their emotions and impulses, to act unselfishly, and be self-aware. It allows us to dream, plan and make choices instead of relying on our impulses and subconscious reactions. God differentiated us from animals, and intellect is His gift to us. It enables us to find creative solutions to difficult problems, and indeed to recognize the existence of our Creator. Thus, the conscious mind is where we plan, make goals and choose our reaction to our reality, rather than relying on programming. The conscious mind can also cause inner conflict when its messages conflict with our subconscious programming. The conscious mind also has ability to express empathy and 'resonate' with another person. We usually protect this aspect of ourselves. Properly utilized and trained powerfully, the conscious mind directs our life and free will.

Curiously, other parts of the brain are also accessed in decision making. Using brain scans, researchers have found that most decisions come from the ventral pallidum area, sometimes called the reptilian part of the brain (well below the conscious part of the brain.) This draws attention to the fact that it is our genetics, together with our experiences, or core beliefs, that are responsible first for weighing decisions. This may explain why the conscious mind has subtle influence, and why it's more difficult to overcome habits that are from the subconscious or instinctual part of the brain.

Researchers do not yet understand why unconscious habits may suddenly become conscious or in what circumstances people are able to override subconscious programming by force of will. What we do understand is that the conscious mind and the focused power of it, used over time, produces amazing results.

In my professional practice I have found that the mind is the most crucial aspect of the health of the individual.

I know my clients are in optimal health when their mind shows clarity, rationality with logical succession, coherence, creativity and selflessness. Creativity is the primary force promoting an individual's happiness and purpose in the world. Freedom from selfishness, and the desire to create, are essential to balance. An individual in a balanced state of mind, not enslaved by his or her passions, is free to channel divine mysteries and divine beauty. Selfishness, desires and passions are the primary factors that mistune the mind. (Passions of the higher self, such as passion for serving one's fellow human beings, passion for teaching the Faith, passion for excelling in your work, are of course commendable!)

The key to optimal health is self-regulation. George Vithoulkas writes in his book *The Science of Homeopathy*:

> ... when there arise selfish tendencies and acquisitive desires, a state of pain is experienced. The selfish person is one who is diseased in

the deepest strata of being, in proportion to the intensity of the egotism . . . health on the mental plane is freedom from selfishness, having as a state complete unification of the person with the divine, or with truth, and whose actions are dedicated to creative service . . . health is freedom from pain in the physical body, having attained a state of well being; freedom from passion on the emotional level, having as a result a dynamic state of serenity and calm; and freedom from selfishness in the mental sphere as a result from unification of Truth.[5]

Freedom from self and desire helps to unify us, both internally and with divinity. Turning to the insights of the Bahá'í Revelation, we see that Bahá'u'lláh teaches us, 'The candle of thine heart is lighted by the hand of My power, quench it not with the contrary winds of self and passion.'[6] Our rational faculty allows us to attain higher states of consciousness and evolution, reflected in our actions through a dedication to creative service of humanity. It gives our lives meaning and texture. Through the power of the mind, even a physically debilitated person can live a happy and productive life full of service. 'Abdu'l-Bahá is reported to have said:

> Today the confirmations of the Kingdom of Abhá are with those who renounce themselves, forget their own opinions, cast aside personalities and are thinking of the welfare of others. Whosoever has lost himself has found the universe and the inhabitants thereof. Whosoever is occupied with himself is wandering in the desert of heedlessness and regret. *The 'master-key' to self-mastery is self-forgetting.* The road to the palace of life is through the path of renunciation.[7] [emphasis added]

The mind connects the body with the soul

Health in the mind requires connection to the body and the body's purpose, as well as knowledge of the soul and its purpose. The rational faculty is the pivotal point in the battle between the forces of our lower and higher nature. 'Abdu'l-Bahá states that the mental faculties 'are in truth of the inherent properties of the soul, even as the radiation of light is the essential property of the sun'.[8] He uses the metaphor of a lamp to explain: the lamp itself is the body, the light within the lamp is the soul, and the rays of the light are the mind. The power of the soul allows the mind to comprehend, imagine and influence. Bahá'u'lláh explains that every faculty in man, whether physical or spiritual, is a manifestation of the soul and emanates from the worlds of God. In the physical world the soul is signified by the mind; Shoghi Effendi confirms this in a letter written on his behalf: 'the rational faculty is a manifestation of the power of the soul'.[9]

The mind is an emanation of the soul, but not the same. The mind is the unifying agency that unites *all* component parts – body, soul, senses, powers, perceptions, memory, imagination . . . Everything is coordinated through the mind. Regardless of the source of knowledge – whether through the intellect or through inspiration of the heart – the mind processes it all. In fact, once the soul and body sever their ties, the intermediary between them will also cease to exist. Our mind has to process whatever we experience, and is able to process phenomena through the intellect, to help unravel mysteries. The soul on its own cannot solve mysteries or manifest the invisible. Bahá'u'lláh explains it thus:

> Consider the rational faculty with which God hath endowed the essence of man. Examine thine own self, and behold how thy motion and stillness, thy will and purpose, thy sight and hearing, thy sense of smell and power of speech, and whatever else is related to, or transcendeth, thy physical senses or spiritual perceptions, all proceed from, and owe their existence to, this same faculty... It is indubitably clear and evident that *each of these aforementioned instruments has depended, and will ever continue to depend, for its proper functioning on this rational faculty*, which should be regarded as a sign of the revelation of Him Who is the sovereign Lord of all.[10] [emphasis added]

Horse and rider, thoughts and emotions

In my observations, I find that every action is the outcome of free will, while simultaneously determined by divine influence. Since the mind is the intermediary between the soul and the body, it reflects the chasm between the spiritual and the physical, and therefore spiritual progress relies upon this faculty. 'Abdu'l-Bahá is reported to have said:

> As long as man is a captive of habit, pursuing the dictates of self and desire, he is vanquished and defeated. This passionate personal ego takes the reins from his hands, crowds out the qualities of the divine ego and changes him into an animal, a creature unable to judge good from evil, or to distinguish light from darkness. He becomes blind to divine attributes, for this acquired individuality, the result of an evil routine of thought, becomes the dominant note of his life.[11]

If the soul represents the rider, the body represents the horse. We can observe that the horse obeys the natural laws of the animal kingdom, while the rider obeys spiritual laws. If the horse is undisciplined and untrained, it will dominate and jeopardize the rider; and the experience of riding will be fearful and unpredictable. In this case the horse's mind will obey its animal impulses, moving in self-centred directions; it will be subject to the herd mentality of dominance, competition and getting its needs met. But when the horse's mind submits to, trusts, and unifies with the rider, horse and rider can together experience amazing feats. The mind is the power of the soul over the body.

In the case of human beings, God cannot force the 'horse' to advance towards Him; this is left up to the free will – its desires, what it pays attention to. God does not interfere with free will, as we see in Bahá'u'lláh's statement that one stroke of His pen would enable all on earth to recognize Him and follow His Teachings, but God forbade Him to do so because of free will. God's love and bounty is like the sun that shines on all creation: it does not distinguish between who will receive light and who will not. Our existence depends upon the sun, and it is our choice whether to receive its warmth and light. The sun will shine on us regardless of what we do. In the same way, God loves and helps us no matter what choices we make

During meditation, we observe how the mind connects with our emotions, with its properties of motion and stillness. The mind can focus on or still thoughts, while other thoughts pass by like clouds in the sky. In the midst of this motion and stillness, emotional responses will arise and then be released.

I imagine thoughts in the mind to be like waves on the ocean continually moving towards the shore, with an emotional quality attached to each thought. In his book *Quantum Healing*, Deepak Chopra draws on microbiology to explain thoughts and emotions as the horse and rider. The brain and body communicate through short amino acid chains called neuropeptides and cell receptors. Previously only known in the brain, scientists have now found them throughout the whole body. Thoughts are like the horse and come into existence as molecules of neuropeptides or interleukins.* The invisible rider represents the emotion and information attached to the thought molecule. The molecules are like horses; they gallop throughout the body communicating information. When these 'horses' interact with cells, the invisible riders share information and can drastically change the life of the cell. This throws light on how we can become enslaved by our emotions and consumed by them.

Shoghi Effendi also wrote about 'wayward thoughts':

> Of course many wayward thoughts come involuntarily to the mind and these are merely a result of weakness and are not blameworthy *unless they become fixed* or even worse, *are expressed in improper acts.*[12] [emphasis added]

Reading Shoghi Effendi's explanation, we may feel a sense of freedom, recognizing that we all have intrusive thoughts that float through the mind. Many of my clients are ashamed of their thoughts, and it is good to remember that unless we become fixated on those thoughts or act on them, they are not blameworthy. We can conclude that an individual in a serene state of mind channels creative energy, but a person ensnared by their passions experiences anxiety and resistance. Snared emotions prevent proper functioning and connection to the spiritual realms. Our goal is to attain freedom to experience a full range of spiritual and animal emotions without being enslaved by them from moment to moment. We live in a *dynamic* state of serenity – of movement and stillness.

Mind moves through molecules and light

I've found that if we understand the physiological influence of our thoughts and emotions, healing is more rapid and better results are

---

* Neuropeptides are small protein-like molecules released by neurons to communicate; interleukins act like neuropeptides but are secreted by the immune system, communicating with and affecting its behaviour.

obtained. We now find some cardiologists routinely asking their patients about forgiveness, for example. The horse and rider analogy in Deepak Chopra's book cited above, together with recent cutting-edge scientific research on the question of how molecular data is shared and affects cell function, has helped deepen my understanding of the relationship between mind and body. One very basic example that anyone can observe is that when we feel the emotion of fear, our heart rate increases.

An example of research in the field of the links between emotions and molecules is that carried out by Candace Pert, a Professor in the Department of Physiology and Biophysics at Georgetown University Medical Center where she conducts research on HIV/AIDS. In her book *Molecules of Emotions*, she explains how cells have receptors located on the surface of the cellular wall connecting deep within to the nucleus of the cell. These receptors sense and scan passing molecules, called peptides. Some molecules, she asserts, carry invisible information such as emotions or instructions. Each receptor vibrates constantly while it scans, binding to any peptide that matches it like a key fitting into a specific lock. When a receptor binds with a passing molecule, the information contained in the molecule enters deep into the cell, creating a response affecting cell division, manufacturing proteins, opening or closing ion channels, and changing the behaviour, physical activity or moods of the person as a whole.

According to Pert, the quality of life for the cell depends on which receptors are occupied. For example, the same receptor which hosts the molecule of the rhino virus (common cold) also hosts the molecule of happiness. If you are happy, it's unlikely you will come down with a cold, because that receptor site is occupied with a happy molecule. This may also explain why when you come down with a cold, you first become irritable.

Cellular memory is also a subject of much experimental research at present and as such controversial. Basically, it goes like this: our habits are physiologically ingrained at a cellular level. The cells habitually rely on certain active receptors and keep them active, requiring the nourishment and programming they give the cell. Sometimes, receptors rely so heavily on certain peptides that they become addictions, whether they are emotional peptides or peptides from drugs.

Cells continually release signalling molecules, as was also discovered by Fritz-Albert Popp in 1970. He called it photon exchange, that molecules exchanged information through light frequencies. He found that wave resonance was used for communication inside the body, and also between living beings. Beings exchange photons, which could explain flocking, and how we can easily pick up on other's moods.

Signalling molecules test out the environment and respond to external stimuli. This explains how one person can walk into a room and change the mood immediately – for good or ill – or how a swindler can identify which person to approach in a crowd. This phenomenon is 'resonance', in the same way that a resting violin string vibrates to another violin being played. Emotional resonance happens when we feel what others are feeling. Neuropsychology has acknowledged that the brain is hard-wired for compassion and empathy – that like mirrors, brains reflect the moods and emotions of others quite easily. Many of us have developed protective responses through fear and the unpleasant experience of pain.

The mind/body connection is easy to observe in the digestive system. Emotions can really affect elimination. The oesophagus through to the large intestine is lined with nerve cells. Digestive irritation often causes irritable feelings, whereas anger and fear create indigestion. The gastrointestinal tract is sometimes called our 'second brain'; it produces most of our neurotransmitters – for example, 95% of our serotonin is produced in the gut, as compared to 5% in the brain. Depression and anxiety are often felt in the gut.

Stepping out of the realm of science and looking at the Baháʼí teachings, we find that in the Tablet to a Physician Baháʼu'lláh states:

> The most great thing is contentment under all circumstances, preserving one from morbid conditions and from lassitude. Yield not to grief and sorrow, they cause the greatest misery. Jealousy consumeth the body and anger burneth the liver; avoid these two as you would a lion.[13]

Allowing yourself to lose your temper or your body to be consumed with jealousy can be like a first cigarette. Poisons pour into the bloodstream from the adrenal glands in an outburst of anger. Anger can sometimes be beneficial, but only when it's a justifiable response. In this case, you can consider it a call to action and use the energy anger has spawned within you to accomplish the feat ahead. Anger followed by action in an unjust or unfair situation causes feelings of optimism and empowerment.[14]

Research points out that stress influences our food choices. The processed foods we eat today have been engineered by the food industry to access the pleasure and reward centre of our brains. (No wonder we can't just eat a handful of chips!) The very sight of the food or thought of it creates the anticipation of pleasure, ultimately inducing us to eat it. It's also been found that video games can access the same addiction centre.

When a habit becomes imprinted on the brain, the behaviour becomes so routine that we respond before we are aware. Researchers can measure movement prior to the knowledge of one's movement – they can see the brain's impulse to reach for the cup of coffee prior to the hand lifting up to reach for it.[15] The circuits in the brain have been 'hard-wired'. Even after years of the body being free of these chemicals, the 'mind' or memory still contains the addiction, as in alcoholism. Post-traumatic stress disorder (PTSD) can arise decades later than the trauma too.

Microbiologists believe that the mind is actually the flow and storage of information as it moves through the body, and that this flow of information determines the organism's behaviour. Their view of health is a system in *balance*, where information sharing is rapid and unimpeded.

Contentment, in my experience, can preserve and protect the body at a cellular level from becoming addicted to any substance. Contentment is something we strive towards. From a perspective of wholeness, at any one time there are things we can be content with and things we can be dissatisfied with. As long as we try to get to the core issue of our stress, we can strive to be more content. For example, if you outgrow your shoes and they fit too tightly, you are in a lot of pain daily. You may not know you can buy new shoes (ignorance), or you may believe you can't afford new shoes, or even that you are not worthy of new shoes (illusion). Each day you force your feet into those shoes an inner conflict grows stronger, eventually leading to bitter contention and resentment. Eventually the mind would question the very compassion of God.

In such a situation where there is an unresolved problem, it will be more challenging to find contentment than to remain in pain out of illusion or ignorance. But I believe the teachings of Bahá'u'lláh are never unreasonable. They provide learning, growth and healing, but we must realize that there is a process that is sacred and has to be carried out correctly if we are to evolve. We can't just expect ourselves to be content without some real self-discipline and exploration.

Mind as a state of probability

Musing on all this, I have come to the hypothesis that the soul works in the body through atoms and that our mind influences this relationship. We know the soul is limitless, and yet the mind has both qualities of limitation and limitlessness. The conscious mind can determine reality (limitlessness) or we can live passively on autopilot by the subconscious mind (limited perspective and old belief systems). In the first verse of the Dhammapada, the Buddha states: 'All things are preceded by the mind, led by the mind, created by the mind.' And Bahá'u'lláh eloquently testifies, 'As to thy question whether the physical world is subject to any limitations, know thou that the comprehension of this matter dependeth upon the observer himself. In one sense it is limited; in another, it is exalted beyond all limitations.'[16]

These quotations remind me that studies have shown that when an electron comes into contact with another, it will retain a connection to that electron regardless of its global positioning. Research has demonstrated that once quantum particles make contact, they retain a connection even when separated so that the actions of one always influence the other.[17] Electrons constantly appear and disappear out of scientific measurement – and when they disappear, we have no way of tracing them. We might consider that this is a type of 'information sharing' with a different realm of existence. Since memory is not stored in the body, I wonder if it may be in this realm that it is stored.

From all this we may conclude that our conscious mind and its focus determines our perceptions and success. 'Abdu'l-Bahá writes that it is 'necessary to focus one's thinking on a single point so that it will become an effective force'.[18]

Purpose of the mind: Gaining victory over self

If optimal health lies in self-regulation, it would be reasonable to conclude that self-mastery is the key to victory. The first step is to know the self. If we search for God, the self will become apparent. 'True loss is for him whose days have been spent in utter ignorance of his self,' Bahá'u'lláh tells us.[19]

The ego is described in the Bahá'í teachings as the 'insistent self' or 'the prison of self'. Shoghi Effendi writes:

> . . . self has really two meanings, or is used in two senses, in the Bahá'í writings; one is self, the identity of the individual created by God. This is the self mentioned in such passages as 'he hath known God who hath known himself', etc. The other self is the ego, the dark, animalistic heritage each one of us has, the lower nature that can develop into a monster of selfishness, brutality, lust and so on. It is this self we must struggle against, or this side of our natures, in order to strengthen and free the spirit within us and help it to attain perfection.[20]

The two selves are explained in the Hidden Words:

> Thou art even as a finely tempered sword concealed in the darkness of its sheath and its value hidden from the artificer's knowledge. Wherefore come forth from the sheath of self and desire that thy worth may be made resplendent and manifest unto all the world.[21]

It is our struggle through daily living to take the reins away from the personal ego and redirect the mind to give the reins to the soul, so that we manifest our true selves. This is done by forgoing our lower impulses and desires. In the Bahá'í teachings the ego's desires are labelled 'vain imaginings' or 'satanic fancies'. Bahá'u'lláh likens them to worshipping idols. He encourages us:

> Arise, O people, and, by the power of God's might, resolve to gain the victory over your own selves, that haply the whole earth may be freed and sanctified from its servitude to the gods of its idle fancies – gods that have inflicted such loss upon, and are responsible for the misery of, their wretched worshippers. These idols form the obstacle that impedeth man in his efforts to advance in the path of perfection.[22]

> Even as the swiftness of lightning ye have passed by the Beloved One, and have set your hearts on satanic fancies. Ye bow the knee

before your vain imagining, and call it truth. Ye turn your eyes towards the thorn, and name it a flower.'[23]

Shoghi Effendi told the Bahá'ís, 'Ultimately all the battle of life is within the individual,'[24] and that

> Life is a constant struggle, not only against forces around us, but above all against our own 'ego'. We can never afford to rest on our oars, for if we do, we soon see ourselves carried down stream again. Many of those who drift away from the Cause do so for the reason that they had ceased to go on developing.[25]

The Bahá'í teachings tell us that God is an unknowable essence. We can't know God, but through further knowing and understanding the higher self we may get a glimpse of God's attributes. I see our spirits manifest through things that inspire us, that we love, that bring us joy. Anything we truly love is part of our higher self. But on our path to God we also quickly encounter the lower self, as it presents blockades. Therefore, the lower self, or ego, provides us with contrast. The human brain learns through contrast; in order to understand spirit, an ego needs to exist. The ego itself needs training and to be tamed. There is purpose in all of God's creation, and there is no evil inherently in anything in creation, but what our free will chooses to do with it can be used for selfish purposes. What the ego doesn't understand, it violates and misuses. I believe, therefore, that the ego has a great purpose: it provides us with the contrast we need for further understanding and for our spiritual progress. Without joy, we could not know sorrow. Without cold, we could not understand hot.

Most of my clients identify their egotistical tendencies only in pride and conceit. However, egotism also resides in the opposite polarity, in unworthiness and self-denigration. This is also egotistical because it focuses on the self: 'I'm no good, I'm not worthy.' It is genuine self-centredness in the other extreme, and as we see in the Bahá'í teachings, Bahá'u'lláh persuades us not to censure the self, but to arise to our noble station. The Hidden Words contains the clear direction: 'Noble I made thee, wherewith dost thou abase thyself?' 'Hear no evil, and see no evil, *abase not thyself*, neither sigh and weep.'[26] [emphasis added]

The qualities of the ego are similar in everyone, yet the ego expresses itself in diverse ways. From studying the Bahá'í and Buddhist texts, I have put together the following summary for my own work:

1. It's defensive and fearful.
2. Its driving power to acquire more never ceases.
3. It always wants its way.
4. It always has to be right, or to be superior.
5. It always wants something different from what it has.
6. It wants attention.
7. It's always attached to an outcome or expectation.
8. Its voice sounds urgent and judgemental.
9. It creates unworthiness and emptiness.

The ego's intention is ultimately to protect us, but it creates 'us vs. them' separateness. These walls unfortunately become our prisons. It's interesting to find that the 'prison of self' is a concept portrayed in the Bahá'í teachings, while the Buddha said, 'Your worst enemy cannot harm you as much as your unguarded thoughts.'

In healing, separateness is a vital concept. Every time we experienced trauma or did not receive what we needed as a child we experienced separateness in our consciousness. The separateness confuses us, we feel unsafe; it causes us to feel unloved, unprotected, not whole. In the science of psychology, this is how it's viewed. On a spiritual level, in my experience separateness is a source of suffering. It's hard to let go of it because it gives the illusion of safety, of protection. 'If I don't have that person or that situation in my life then I'll be fine' is usually the story of the ego. However, because of the principle or oneness or interconnectedness presented in the Bahá'í teachings, this cannot be so. I see that the moment people become aware of and comprehend the separateness inside themselves or with others, their misery is dissipated. When our perceptions are inaccurate, this gives the situation more energy and power than it really has; separateness can then become a fixed state and thus suffering, and the lower self, or ego will express itself.

In the Bahá'í teachings the pull of the ego is likened to gravity, as in this statement by 'Abdu'l-Bahá:

> Just as the earth attracts everything to the center of gravity, and every object thrown upward into space will come down, so also material

ideas and worldly thoughts attract man to the center of self. Anger, passion, ignorance, prejudice, greed, envy, covetousness, jealousy and suspicion prevent man from ascending to the realms of holiness, imprisoning him in the claws of self and the cage of egotism. The physical man, unassisted by the divine power, trying to escape from one of these invisible enemies, will unconsciously fall into the hands of another. No sooner does he attempt to soar upward than the density of the love of self, like the power of gravity, draws him to the earth. The only power that is capable of delivering man from this captivity is the power of the breaths of the Holy Spirit.[27]

We can receive the breaths of the Holy Spirit by reading the sacred text, and through prayer, meditation and serving God. The mind has the power to redirect us to receive the light of the soul, releasing us from the prison of self. One of the purposes of the Divine Messengers is to reorient our minds to remember our eternal selves.

Accurate perception and proportionate action

The battle within is contained within a broad spectrum of perception and action. We can work within this paradigm when we discern between the things we can change and those we cannot. The rational faculty expresses itself well through the nervous system. Perceptions are related to the parasympathetic nerve, or our sense of being, and our nervous system responds to our perceptions based upon emotional attachments. Perceptions out of balance with the truth will throw the nervous system out of balance.

Perceptions are like wearing coloured glasses, affecting our view of the world. The story of what happens to us is linked to our perceptions; it is seeing with understanding. I've found that the only way to shift our reality is to change these stories and the feelings associated with them. For example, one of the most difficult perceptions to discern is the difference between perceived injustice and true injustice. Accurate perception empowers us to take the right action, or react in proportion to what happened. This is what we really have control over. Abdu'l-Bahá is reported to have said, 'Thinking about troubles is more difficult than the actual experience.'[28]

Figure 8.1   Links in the chain

Parasympathetic nerve
Perception (being)

Sympathetic nerve
Participation (doing)

Many people have difficulties with money. We talk about their relationship with money and I ask them to tell me their story. Sometimes the story is 'I'm not good enough'. At other times the story is 'I never have any money'. Or, 'I can never find a spouse'. We often don't realize that we can change our stories, or how creative our conscious mind can be. I've seen amazing results through rewriting the stories that are stored in our subconscious mind. The rewriting process puts us in touch with our own creative powers, and the awareness that under every circumstance we can find our old stories and rewrite them. Our free will plays a huge role in this; often we fall prey to the ego out of ignorance in old habitual thinking patterns without realizing it.

Another aspect of this is the examination of our participation in our perceptions. This is related to our sympathetic nerve, or the 'doing' aspect of ourselves (see Figure 8.1). If we have clarity and accurate perceptions, then the question remains, what is a proportional response? For example, if we perceive someone who doesn't like us and slights us, our response can make mountains out of this internally or externally. A healthy response to a slight is slight action, ignoring it internally and externally. We can check to see if our action or reaction is in proportion to the situation. If there is a fire in the house, no internal conflict exists. The clear message within is GET OUT. Humans tend to unite when there is a crisis, because there is no conflict. We even find that the suicide rate drops significantly during wartime. The human mind often creates more drama than necessary over a small conflict compared to a disastrous situation. Keeping our reactions in proportion to the situation safeguards our nerves and mental well-being. This includes taking action where we can. Changing how we participate or don't participate changes the dynamics of our situation. When we don't take action when warranted, or take action that is incorrect, it throws our nervous system out of order because of the internal conflict created.

Mental illness and healing through spiritual powers

The science of the mind has made advances in the past few decades. Mental illness affects both the body and the mind. When assessing mental health, we need to consider the *quality* of its functioning. A true state of health includes the following qualities: clear thinking, a logical sequence of thoughts, rationality, the ability to express oneself clearly, and desire for the good of oneself and others. When these states of mind are out of balance, this leads progressively to greater problems. Cultivating selflessness, humility, and interconnectedness with community safeguards one from grief or fears that cause an overexcitement of the nerves resulting in profound emotions and suffering.

While the soul remains unaffected by mental illness and is always near to its Lord, mental illness can impede our efforts in spiritual progress. 'Abdu'l-Bahá is reported to have said that physical illness (in which he included mental illness) is one of the hardest tests to endure. He also suggests prayer as a remedy:

> Sometimes if the nervous system is paralyzed through fear, a spiritual remedy is necessary. Madness, incurable otherwise, can be cured through prayer. It often happens that sorrow makes one ill, this can be cured by spiritual means.[29]

From my perspective in working with patients, conditions of the mind are the most important to approach in a healing plan. I assess the conditions of thoughts and emotions on a continuum. Some examples of the most out-of-balance conditions in thought include confusion, dullness, lack of concentration, forgetfulness, or difficulties with memory. These conditions are at the deepest level of our being and communicate that a diseased state needs to be addressed. Among the emotional conditions that can result from habitual ways of thinking are anxiety, phobias, grief, apathy and irritability. These symptoms should be assessed by their severity, as they are a dynamic state.

Emotional states vary in their range and expression. The basic emotions I work with are fear, love and grief. Most other emotions stem from these basic ones. Daily living provides a roller-coaster ride on the 'polarity express' going up and down, from love to hate, anger to trust, peacefulness to anxiety. The quality of our emotional experience leads either to happiness or to suffering. The more one is occupied with negative emotions, the more severe the emotional disturbance. Emotional intelligence allows individuals to experience highly evolved emotions such as mysticism, compassion, ecstasy and joy. Positive spiritual emotions enable one to experience unity, to be at one with the vastness of the universe, while the lower animalistic emotions lead to states of separation. This separation creates disharmony within the human temple, disturbing homeostasis.

But emotional intelligence is not often taught, leaving society vulnerable to emotional disturbances from a lack of understanding of healthy ways to experience emotions, build an internal foundation and express oneself with tact. The top three complaints I see frequently in my profession are anxiety, depression and insomnia.

The trick is to be fully detached. Most western individuals confuse detachment with disassociation. Disassociation is the distancing of self, denying connection to someone or something. This leads to unclear thinking. Real detachment is the ability to feel the full range of human emotions without being *imprisoned* by them, or allowing them to determine your response to a situation.

As in all types of illness, Bahá'ís are encouraged to seek the advice of competent physicians, within the balance of the Writings of Bahá'u'lláh. One should use both material and spiritual means to heal a mental illness. Psychology can offer an understanding of how the mind works. A good psychologist with knowledge of the Bahá'í teachings can be an invaluable help in our struggles. The mind can receive great illumination from the Writings of Bahá'u'lláh, and invoke the power contained within His Revelation. The Universal House of Justice explains that

> mental illness is not spiritual, although its effects may indeed hinder and be a burden in one's striving toward spiritual progress . . . Such hindrances (i.e. illness and outer difficulties), no matter how severe and insuperable they may at first seem, can and should be effectively overcome through the combined and sustained power of prayer and of determined and continued effort.[30]

In a letter to a physician, 'Abdu'l-Bahá points out the great effect of spiritual feelings on nervous conditions:

Praise be to God that thou hast two powers: one to undertake physical healing and the other spiritual healing. Matters related to man's spirit have a great effect on his bodily condition. For instance, thou shouldst impart gladness to thy patient, give him comfort and joy, and bring him to ecstasy and exultation. How often hath it occurred that this hath caused early recovery. Therefore, treat thou the sick with both powers. Spiritual feelings have a surprising effect on healing nervous ailments.[31]

The mind reflected in biology

In the science of healing as practised in my profession, a true cure flows from the centre of a person outward, just as the inner life can be reflected in disease. When the mind is disturbed, the body will become disturbed, because changes in the mind scramble the body's intelligence, and tissue changes result, starting in the cell. External disturbances such as improper diet cause more upsets in the body, affecting communication with the mind. There are also conditions where external forces such as grief, depressing tribulation, stress and the like, can affect the body and mind temporarily. If there is an existing internal condition, these effects will develop into disease. If there is no underlying condition, this conditional suffering will yield as soon as the external cause (grief) is removed.

The seat of the mind is the brain. How well it works determines almost every aspect of our daily life. Mind has the ability to determine and create reality, and researchers have proven that our actions and ways of thinking can change the brain's physiology – called neuroplasticity. The brain continuously reshapes and sculpts itself, whether we are aware of it or not, depending upon our ways of thinking and activities.

Since researchers have found that our thoughts can shape our brain, let's examine a recent study about gossip and the brain. Backbiting has repeatedly been condemned by Bahá'u'lláh. The online journal *Science* published a study[32] that reported that negative gossip alters the way the visual system responds to individuals. It doesn't just influence our perception of others, but it actually directs the way we see them visually. The study revealed that the human brain is wired to respond to gossip. This evidence came forth by putting different images in front of each eye at a time. This causes 'binocular rivalry', because the brain can only process one image at a time, so our attention pauses on one or the other, usually the one we deem more important.

The images in front of one eye were neutral faces that were paired with three kinds of gossip: positive, negative and neutral. The other eye had a neutral image, for instance a house. The findings of the experiment were that the brain viewed the people associated with negative gossip for a longer time than people associated with neutral or positive gossip. Lisa Feldman Barrett, the professor of psychology who oversaw the study, interprets this information as protective: gossip helps us predict who is friend and who is foe. Our brains have evolved to rely on gossip.

If gossip is a 'natural tendency of the brain', part of our evolution, then what is the implication of Bahá'u'lláh's teaching on avoiding backbiting? The pull of our natural lower impulses are great. Avoiding gossip when the brain is physically wired to respond to gossip challenges our very brain to change. If thoughts shape the brain, is evolution merely a reflection of habitual gossiping? Refraining from gossip will change the neural wiring of the brain. Obeying Bahá'u'lláh's teachings can feel unnatural at first, because obedience challenges physical restructuring and evolution.

Figure 8.2   *Regions of the brain*

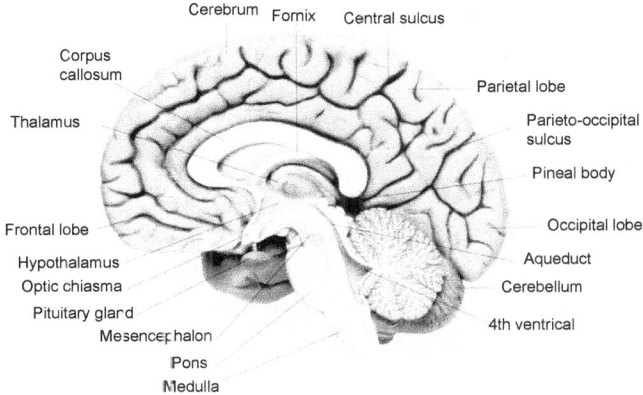

Each region in the brain connects to physiological functions, but also contains spiritual centres. The Bahá'í teachings point out the mind's pivotal role in connecting the soul to the body, creating a unified relationship. Neurologists have labelled the frontal lobe as the 'sweet spot' for spiritual experiences. The frontal lobe is also associated with emotion and memory. It's where we use focus, concentration. During prayer and meditation there is increased activity in the frontal lobe, but decreased activity in the parietal lobe. Why is this so significant? The right parietal lobe defines the self, the 'me'. It generates the self-criticism that is so prevalent in the West. Brick Johnstone of Missouri University says, 'it guides us through physical and social terrains by constantly updating our self-knowledge: my hand, my cocktail, my witty conversation skills, my new love interest . . .'[33] Researchers have found that people with less active parietal lobes are more likely to lead more spiritual lives and have decreased self-focus.

Prayer and meditation stimulate the hypothalamus, suppressing activity in the back of the brain, helping to bury 'background noise'. Andrew Newburg, who for decades has studied the effect of meditation on brains, found that after eight weeks of meditation, twelve minutes per day, participants thought more clearly and were better able to remember things. The new scans and memory tests have confirmed these findings. He says, 'They had improvements of about 10 or 15 percent.'[34] Scans showed a physical change in the frontal lobes, helping to reshape the brain.

During mystical experiences, why does one feel so at one with the universe, intoxicated? Solomon H. Snyder, who founded the Department of Neuroscience at Johns Hopkins University School of Medicine, says that scientists suspect the neurotransmitter serotonin, playing out in parts of the brain dealing with emotions and perceptions.[35]

The brain is where the neurotransmitters, or communicators, are created and sent out all over the body, communicating to every system and every cell. Brain injuries to each or any area usually hinder, and seldom help, the mind's potential; they lessen spiritual experiences and inhibit daily physical living. Brain injuries also greatly affect the families of the injured as well. And, as 'Abdu'l-Bahá told us a hundred years ago, while the mind is associated with the brain, it is not actually in it.[36] As we have seen earlier in this chapter, researchers are finding mind flowing throughout the body.

'Abdu'l-Bahá revealed the weak force of the conscious mind and reminds us that true power lies within the Word of God and the kingdom. He wrote, 'Hypnotism hath a weak influence over bodies, but hath no result, but the power of the kingdom of God is great. If thou canst, endeavour to obtain a share of that power.'[37]

9

PREPARING THE MIND FOR THE FAST

The science of mind, of normality and of the disabilities from which it may suffer, is in relative infancy, but much may be possible to aid you to minimize your suffering and make possible an active life. The last ten years in the therapy of mental disorders has seen important advances from which you may well benefit. Your discovery of the Faith, of its healing Writings and its great purposes for the individual and for all mankind, have indeed brought to you a powerful force toward a healthy life which will sustain you on a higher level, whatever your ailment may be. The best results for the healing process are to combine the spiritual with the physical, for it should be possible for you to overcome your illness through the combined and sustained power of prayer and of determined effort.

The Universal House of Justice[1]

There are no set ways to tame the ego. In the Bahá'í teachings we find that Bahá'u'lláh says, 'Fasting is the supreme remedy and the most great healing for the disease of self and passion.'[2] We consistently struggle between our higher and lower self, whether we are conscious of it or not. Before the Fast, try to become an observer in your daily life. Pretend you are a second pair of eyes and just observe. You may find some snares in your thinking and feelings.

Nutrition: What information do I allow into my mind? Whom do I associate with? What forms of entertainment am I drawn to?
Movement: What negative habits do I need to change? Do I express myself with moderation? When did I last learn a new skill? How often do I smile?
Waste management: Do I forgive myself and others? How do I manage stress?

Rebuilding: How often do I give my mind space to think and reflect? How often do I play? How often am I prone to thinking in absolutes (never, always) rather than responding with unity?

Since it is the mind that chooses our orientation, we can make it a goal to identify habitual patterns of thinking and beliefs that encourage negative behaviour, and specific means of reorienting the mind towards God.

Components of a healthy mind

Healthy neurological development comes from several sources including genetic, cultural, educational and social influences, trauma, physical health, and personality. Like the body systems, our mind has many processes. It seeks nourishment, it needs to digest, then integrate nutrients and eliminate the toxins. Let's take a closer look at these processes, from Table 4.1 in Chapter 4.

Table 9.1 Processes for the mind

Processes	Mind
Nutrition/Respiration	Impressions from the five senses, experiences, imagination
Digestion	*Intelligence required* Comprehension through contemplation, writing a journal, or talking to a 'witness'.
Transformative processes	Assimilating events into memory; identifying negative thought patterns from the ego
Catalysts	Will/submission/acceptance
Elimination	Removal of negative thoughts through forgiveness
Movement	Expressing oneself, social interaction, learning a new skill
Cleanliness	Purifying the mind and intentions/motives
Protection	Obedience to His Laws, avoiding influences of ego, seeking the Middle Way
Resistance	Stubbornness/disobedience/contention

In preparing for the Fast we can promote well-being in the mind, training and strengthening this faculty as well as cleansing and purifying it. Developing our emotional state to bring it into coherence with these aims requires tools, practice, and striving. An unhealthy mind can sometimes stem from physical or spiritual nutrition, digestion or poor elimination. These symptoms can manifest themselves through paranoia, depression, anxiety, impulsive or compulsive behaviours, obsessions, or excessive worry, to name a few. Just as Chapter 6 discussed the various aspects of optimal physical health, this chapter focuses on optimal mental health. If we don't understand what constitutes mental health, how can we know what is important during the Fast?

As previously in this book, this chapter describes my professional experience which has produced results; it also quotes some scientific research as well as some Bahá'í teachings. After studying these components, we can then put them into a systematic approach to the Fast.

Nutrition

Physical food affects the mind

While Chapter 6 discussed the types of food that constitute healthy choices for our bodies, this section looks at healthy foods for the mind. Physical foods can affect the mind. A nutritious diet, keeping in mind when our blood sugar dips, creates well-being for the brain, regulating its processes.

There is another component to eating food, more specific to the mind. Be cautious of consuming foods that have been produced in frustration and anger. The famous quotation attributed to Samuel Hoffenstein, the American poet and screenwriter who wrote *The Wizard of Oz* and *The Phantom of the Opera*, eloquently expresses it: 'My Soul is dark with stormy riot, directly traceable to diet.' Today's farms in the industrialized countries, dependent on agribusiness and supermarket sales, house too many animals confined together, finding ways to grow the animals faster by injecting hormones, and protecting them from disease with antibiotics. These practices create much frustration in the animals so that, for instance, hens housed so closely together have their beaks chopped off in order to stop pecking each other to death.[3] I often wonder if, when we consume eggs from these battery hens, the energy of frustration can enter our system. Not only do we have to physically digest this food, but our minds must digest the emotions associated with the food from that animal. Developing an awareness of what we consume will protect both mind and body.

Non-physical foods

The mind consumes non-physical 'food' through the senses: vision, smell, touch, sense, and hearing. As we have seen, the brain is known to process billions of bits of data per minute. As we go through our day, our brain is bombarded through our senses and must process all this data. What we expose ourselves to determines the strength of the processing required. Living in the age of consumerism, we are exposed to things we choose to be around and also to things we don't choose. For example, magazines, news, television programmes, the Internet or billboard advertisements can prey on emotions of self and desire that will affect the balance of the mind. Even overhearing negative gossip or backbiting is poison for the mind and requires proper processing. Exposing ourselves to harmful people and influences can create mental 'toxins'. Making optimal choices in what we expose ourselves to helps us to avoid mental 'junk food'. In His Writings, Bahá'u'lláh warns, 'guard your eyes against that which is not seemly'.[4]

The mind nourishes itself through building knowledge. We learn about things by studying them or experiencing them. In both methods, our five outer senses take in information and process it through the brain. The section on catalysts below addresses the specifics of how the mind determines the difference between nutrition and waste.

The second type of non-physical food consumed by the mind is emotion. Our brain is hardwired to be empathetic, to identify with others' feelings and moods – especially those whom we identify with and love. Walt Whitman's famous poem 'There Was A Child Went Forth' beautifully expresses nutrition for the mind:

> There was a child went forth every day,
> And the first object he look'd upon, that object he became,
> And that object became part of him for the day or a certain part
>   of the day,
> Or for many years or stretching cycles of years.[5]

We cannot help but build knowledge daily because of our exposure to the outer world. The more rich experiences we expose ourselves to, the more textured, varied and strong will be our intelligence. This is the danger of living a mundane routine life – the mind, like muscles, starts to atrophy, leading to memory loss and fogginess. The environment the mind immerses itself in affects it greatly, because the mind cannot segregate itself totally from its environment. A letter written on behalf of Shoghi Effendi states that one's 'inner life moulds the environment and is itself also deeply affected by it. The one acts upon the other and every abiding change in the life of man is the result of these mutual reactions.'[6]

There are several sources of healthy foods for the mind. Food for thought gives us the sustenance and energy to function. I've come to the conclusion that just as digested physical food energizes our cellular structures, healthy choices in mental food are 'digested' into our memory, making life vibrant. Digesting and absorbing unhealthy mental food causes mental fatigue and indigestion, while too much information will also give us indigestion. Such 'overeating' is one of the most harmful activities for the mind. The phrase, 'I've had a full day' is often used to express the sentiment that the *mind* has enough and it's time to rest.

Some of the healthiest foods that I recommend for the mind include:

- Foods raised on farms close to nature
- Natural scenery
- Textured, fragrant smells
- Enriching experiences
- Changes in environment or routines
- Space to do nothing, nap
- Positive thoughts and visualizations
- Cherishing moments with loved ones
- Exposure to beauty and music
- Analysis
- Puzzles and riddles
- Recognizing and expressing emotion in a healthy way
- Deep breathing
- Humour and laughter
- Fruitful information such as facts, principles and knowledge

Meaningful education is one of the most important aspects in life, and the richest nutrition for the mind. Expose yourself to anything that helps you think, compare, concentrate, calculate, classify, create, memorize, synthesize, visualize, plan or communicate. 'Abdu'l-Bahá spoke about inherited tendencies, personality and character, yet pointed to education as having the greatest influence:

> Through education the ignorant become learned; the cowardly become valiant . . . Through education savage nations become civilized, and even the animals become domesticated. Education must be considered as most important, for as diseases in the world of bodies are extremely contagious, so, in the same way, qualities of spirit and heart are extremely contagious. Education has a universal influence, and the differences caused by it are very great.[7]

What do I feed my mind? Whom do I spend the most time with? When an impulse arises, do I analyse it before I feed it? Am I overexposing my senses in any way?

Digestion

The mind has to 'digest' or *process* the nourishment it ingests through layers of emotion and reason. Rich or difficult experiences are often digested with difficulty, whereas a light and joyful afternoon with friends will be digested quite easily. I've observed that just as digested food in the body is integrated into our tissues, so digested events are integrated into the fabric of our lives. Digestion allows the nutrition to which we expose our minds to be transformed into knowledge and power. Perhaps we can travel across the world to another country, tour museums, listen to lectures and experience the culture, and can take home what we learned about that country and report it. Telling others what we have learned *about* the country denotes nutritional value; however, digestion comes from contemplation on what we learned *from* the experience. What were the lessons involved? How has this impacted my life? What did I think and feel during that experience? I'm now a more textured person from that experience and knowledge.

Weak minds, like weak stomachs, cannot digest rich foods. Just as a weak physical digestion does not fully digest foods so that the body cannot assimilate the nutrients, so the mind cannot assimilate the lessons from events we have not fully processed. Perhaps we still have an old relationship with lingering emotions. Maybe our childhood needs processing. Proper digestion takes place through intelligence and discernment – having a true understanding or perception of events with acceptance. Wisdom allows us to integrate the knowledge we've acquired into proper action – the perfect expression of our true selves.

From the Bahá'í perspective, Bahá'u'lláh tells us that 'Knowledge is as wings to man's life and a ladder for his ascent. Its acquisition is incumbent upon everyone.'[8] And 'Abdu'l-Bahá states: 'Make every effort to acquire the advanced knowledge of the day, and strain every nerve to carry forward the divine civilization . . .'[9] Both spiritual and secular branches of knowledge are to be explored and applied to our professions, arts, crafts and sciences in order to benefit humanity.

Building strong intelligence

These teachings may inspire us to build a strong intelligence or 'digestive tract' for the mind and emotions. It's helpful, therefore, to differentiate between two types of knowledge. One is the mind's knowledge, which is our current focus. It is a pure academic understanding which results in strong intelligence through reasoning, logic and rational discourse. The other is the heart's knowledge. It is an understanding that leads to action. This will be addressed in Part IV on the soul.

Good nutritional choices for the mind build the strong intelligence required for processing. Enriching experiences and education, once digested in the mind, are integrated into the memory. There they become knowledge, or rational intelligence. This knowledge is deposited into a memory bank that can be accessed. Strengthening our intelligence produces the ability to digest a multitude and variety of experiences.

When we have a strong intelligence, our thoughts often interfere and cloud the quality of our emotions, inhibiting their 'digestion'. A common experience for most of us is trying to get the rational mind to help unify our internal processes by consulting our emotions. We try to rationalize the emotion, explain it, blame it, shame it, and often don't understand what we are experiencing because of the interference of our thoughts and struggling to resist. Emotions are not rational and often don't make any sense. We feel things that we 'shouldn't' or are ashamed to admit, or are contrary to logic. An important skill for the rational mind to learn is to stop the stream of thoughts that are racing, riding the strong winds of emotion, and move towards the *energy stream underneath* those thoughts.

- How does it feel? (Emotions need validation because they are real, no matter how ridiculous.)
- If this energy had a voice, what would it say? (It wants to speak and express itself.)
- What does this energy want me to do? (It wants me to take action.)

These simple questions give us pause, allowing us to contemplate the situation, clarify why the thoughts are racing, and help give an intelligent response. Building a strong mind can sometimes divide itself from the emotional flow. However, allowing this strong rational mind and the emotions to consult in a supportive manner builds self-trust, and eternal friendliness towards the self and to others.

Building strong emotional intelligence

Suppressing raw emotions and expressing them with intelligence is by far the largest challenge for most clients I work with and the cause of a lot of imbalance. Therefore, I'd like to share some of the most effective tools I use in my practice, as well as taking a comprehensive look at the emotional field. The most common emotional symptoms I see include anxiety, depression, irritability, anger, dissatisfaction and anguish.

Instead of viewing emotions in the light of good/bad, positive/negative, we can think about them in the following way. In the Bahá'í Writings, certain emotions are related to the world of phenomena, and others to the world of the spirit. 'Abdu'l-Bahá is reported to have said:

> Man possesses two kinds of susceptibilities: the natural emotions, which are like dust upon the mirror, and spiritual susceptibilities, which are merciful and heavenly characteristics . . . The natural emotions are blameworthy and are like rust which deprives the heart of the bounties of God. But sincerity, justice, humility, severance,

and love for the believers of God will purify the mirror and make it radiant with reflected rays from the Sun of Truth.[10]

Spiritual feelings draw a person towards a state of happiness, whereas the 'natural' feelings (described as 'dust' by 'Abdu'l-Bahá) degrade a person and lead to dissatisfaction, leaving them vulnerable to the ego. The more a person feels natural feelings in a waking state, the more out of balance the mind. I've observed that the healthiest individuals can experience a wide range of profound emotional states and yet are not enslaved by them. In these people emotions flow dynamically; they experience a deep serenity and contentment combined with love for self alongside a greater love for humanity and the world.

When difficult situations arise we generally have several emotional responses within. Emotional intelligence allows us to clearly identify our own emotions without mixing them up with another's. It enables us to manage and utilize them in a healthy way, and to not let them dominate us or determine our decisions. Strong emotional intelligence allows us to process and transform the strong winds of negative emotions that accompany the hurts or shocks that life into positive solutions. For example, instead of feeling, 'You are so ridiculous,' one could instead identify the feeling as, 'I feel really intolerant right now.' Then one could have the clarity to process that feeling of intolerance and choose the antidote of patience instead. This clarity provides more confidence and willingness to cooperate with the outer world.

Emotional illness results when we feel trapped by negative feelings so that we express these and become impassioned by them. When we experience strong emotions our first instinct is to shut down, close off and suppress them. First of all, this doesn't work. Once an emotion is in motion, it stays in motion. We have to work extra hard to shut it off and ignore it, and we become even more agitated and tense. Physiologically, this blockage causes insufficient levels of peptide signals to maintain optimal functioning at the cellular level.

Emotions are fast, even faster than our brain cortex can register the reaction. Trying to suppress an emotion is as dangerous to the mind as trying to suppress a fever is dangerous to the body. Research on the immune system has found that unexpressed emotion significantly reduces immune function and raises susceptibility to infections. Expressing emotions improves immunity functionality. Though scientists cannot see the thought 'I'm angry', the results in the body can be measured physiologically by instruments.

Clients have a variety of techniques for avoiding their feelings: throwing themselves into work, a relationship, eating, and even their spiritual practices. Some use meditation to try to avoid a situation. Some become amazing 'spiritual teachers' and can be effective teachers of others. However, the original problem they ran away from remains in the background, causing an imbalance in the system. The more the emotions from the original problem try to arise in various ways, the more often the person tries to avoid the confrontation. The fact is, there is no escape from our feelings, no matter how unpleasant they are: they will find a way to express themselves. The only path is to attain a level of emotional intelligence.

A person with strong rational and emotional intelligence can regulate him- or herself. When the rational and emotional work together this is a state of true health. Daniel Goleman, the American psychologist whose book *Emotional Intelligence* became a bestseller worldwide, developed a framework of five elements that define emotional intelligence. I've listed them below, together with a couple more of my own:

1. *Self-awareness.* Look honestly deep into yourself. Distinguish between a thought and feeling. Label thoughts and feelings, rather than people or situations. Reflect on who you are and what your motives are in your thoughts and feelings. Take responsibility.
2. *Energy.* Feel the energy of the emotion and allow it to be the impetus of empowerment and productive action. Relearn what your emotions are capable of creating.
3. *Empathy.* Make it a practice to simply listen to others without judging. Avoid advising, commanding, controlling, criticizing or lecturing. A high level of empathy towards self and others creates trust and healing.
4. *Validation.* Validate your own feelings and the feelings of others. Discern who you can express your emotions to and receive validation from.
5. *Self-regulate.* Practise controlling emotional impulses. Think before you act. Use thoughtfulness, flexibility and integrity to guide you. Know when to say 'No', or 'I need some time to think'. Identify your thinking habits and the emotions connected to them, and how they determine your responses.

6. *Perspective.* Keep your lifetime goal in mind so that short-term failures don't deter you from this dynamic process of building skills. There is a cycle of crisis and victory to work through.

7. *Social skills.* Learn how to be a team player. Help others develop. Know how to manage disputes as they arise, with tact and grace. Obtain communication techniques and maintain relationships.

When strong emotions do arise, they can initially be difficult to manage. There are some helpful tools to assist in processing strong emotions, or rational thoughts to help develop analytical thinking:

Utilize a trusted person to act as a 'witness', someone who can simply observe, without being involved in the situation. Discuss situations, experiences or thoughts with a witness.

For the *person doing the processing*: First purify your motives so that you simply want to process, not gossip or backbite. Talk about any and all aspects without naming names (even if both you and the witness understand who are the players involved). Talk until your cup is empty. A word of caution: If you need to tell your story more than three times you may gain power and benefit from victimhood. Be careful not to wear pain like a badge, as it strengthens the ego.

For the *witness:* Remain absolutely neutral. Don't give any indication for or against what the person is saying. Simply nod your head and look into the person deeply. Feel compassion. Your job is to try to understand what they are telling you and how they feel. After the speaker has emptied the cup, a simple response of 'that's hard', or 'that's interesting' will suffice. Refrain from commenting, advising or judging. Just 'witness' their reality. The intent here is to allow the speaker to fully hear themselves talk, and process the situation themselves. If you do not interfere, the answer then often becomes clear to the speaker, or they already know what to do.

Write it out. Various studies have found that writing about trauma may be as effective as talking about it. This technique helps those who wish for a more private outlet and don't want to hold back details. Sit down and write a factual account of your story. Write about the feelings and thoughts associated with it. Repeat the exercise for as many days as it seems necessary until you feel a mastery over the situation. Try writing to your higher self, or to God, and if you wish, answer back. Some situations are reoccurring events. One of my clients used to write to her future self, sharing insights, perspectives and advice on how to act when she found herself in that situation. Then when the event happened again, she would write to the hurt one about the past reassurance that she had got through it. Studies show that trauma victims who write about their pain can experience positive psychological changes such as increased blood flow and a boost to immunity that can last for up to six months.[11] If the trauma is extreme, writing about it can sometimes re-traumatize, so it's best to do it when you feel ready and not forced. I've had children write a script with characters about what happened to them. In the script they include the feelings and thoughts of the characters. Then I ask them to rewrite the story, detailing what they'd like to happen in the future, especially focusing on their own character.

Write a letter without intending to send it. When we are angry at an individual or group of individuals, writing a letter to them helps a lot. Ensure that all your points of view are stated, together with the emotions that go with them. When finished, destroy the letter – burn it or delete it.

Sit with strong emotions. A wonderful way to help keep the flow of strong emotions is by sitting quietly, opening the heart to compassion. Reviewing the situation and understanding yourself and others involved will build compassion. Sit and abide with the 'crying child' within, bathing it in compassion. Focus on your breath. Breathe those strong emotions in deeply, and breathe out compassion. When the internal dialogue starts up again on the painful memory, drop the words and find what energy is underneath the words. Sit with that energy and repeat this until it starts to dissipate. This prevents the emotion from damming up, festering or escalating. Repeat this if the resistance arises again. Build a trusting relationship with yourself, that you will not criticize harshly or punish yourself. Allow the emotions to flow without labelling them good or bad. Use the mind to reflect deeply on the situation that has stirred up this particular feeling. Our internal and external environment engenders certain feelings. When we label emotions as negative and resist our reality, we can fall into the clutches of the ego.

It's important to distinguish between emotional response, mood and temperament; these are often mixed up or misinterpreted. Emotions are the most transient, while moods can last for hours or days. Temperament is more linked to genetics and family of origin, more lasting. It's important to decipher these and distinguish between them, in order to understand the dynamic flow and assess the true state of the mind.

I see clients spiritually progress and begin to attain an enhanced level of self-awareness through this practice. They experience many responses to a situation; they become aware that the body may remember anxious feelings in a situation, but the mind can choose a different response from its usual one. As we grow spiritually, our emotional reaction becomes more tempered. For example, our first response to a situation will become less angry. Eventually, when anger is experienced, it may be an indication of a true injustice and a call to action, rather than perceived injustice.

Make a daily practice of digesting the things that happen in your day. If there is 'information overload' or some event that causes great duress, take time to reflect and acknowledge the emotional flow in a healthy, private way. Shoghi Effendi wrote, 'We must not only be patient with others, infinitely patient!, but also with our own poor selves, remembering that even the Prophets of God sometimes got tired and cried out in despair!'[12]

What is my first response to strong emotions? How patient am I with myself and others? How can I build a more compassionate response? How can I build my awareness between my thoughts and feelings?

Transformative processes

The processes discussed in this section come from my own experience; they have to do with refining our perception, assimilating events into memory and identifying negative thought patterns from the ego.

Continuing the analogy with the physical, once food particles are digested by our bodies they are broken down into the smallest particles possible in order to move nutritional elements through the circulation and keep toxins flowing out of the body. In the case of the mind, we have free will to choose nutritional thoughts to integrate into memory and identify positive emotions. The mind can also identify toxic thoughts and emotions that need processing and regulating to move them out. We need to be able to distinguish between these two in order to progress spiritually, as Bahá'u'lláh tells us:

> . . . man should know his own self and recognize that which leadeth unto loftiness or lowliness, glory or abasement, wealth or poverty... The straight path is the one which guideth man to the dayspring of perception and to the dawning-place of true understanding and leadeth him to that which will redound to glory, honour and greatness.[13]

Self-regulation leads ultimately to a sense of well-being. We may understand the transformative processes in the mind as empowering us to choose, having the reins over our will-power. These thoughts can help regulate and influence the body. Some scientific studies in this area can show us how to harness the power of the mind in regaining our health.

Focused thinking can redirect cells, creating a positive physiological response. Injuries recover about twice as fast when the injured person visualizes increased blood flow to the injured part for about 20 minutes each day. Why can't we harness this power for every malady? Why can about 6 per cent of the population go into 'spontaneous remission' after they have determined themselves to beat cancer?[14] Only 5 per cent of individuals 'just quit' smoking and succeed.[15] The same rate is reported by the Harvard Medical School Department of Psychiatry: a yearly spontaneous remission rate of 5 per cent in alcoholism and drug addiction.[16] These statistics are considered 'anomalies' in the data, 'not significant', and are therefore largely ignored by the medical field. It gives me pause. What have these individuals in the 5 per cent harnessed that the average population cannot? The most common sentiment of this 5 per cent population boiled down to: *'I was just sick and tired of _____.'*

The influence of the mind also shows up in how we express our problems in our speech. When I listen to a client's health problems, I see whether they are experiencing the disease or have themselves 'become' the disease. This difference is expressed by 'I have a depressing feeling', or 'I'm depressed'. The first tells me they are aware of a disorder, but the latter tells me they identify with it or enslaved by it. Those who identify with their disease have more difficulty regaining balance.

Working on attaining a high level of self-awareness has its challenges. Identifying positive thought patterns and emotions and distinguishing them from negative ones can be accompanied by a lot of fear. We all have protective personalities which create defensive behaviours, closing us off from perceived danger. This truth is reflected in the behaviour of our individual cells. A cell has both a growth response and a protection response. When it's in protection mode, the messages sent are 'retreat', 'separate' or 'cut off' from the outer world. This response temporarily protects the body from harm, but it also inhibits life-sustaining energy. When this is a chronic state of being, there is a real problem.

Negative thoughts can steal into the conscious mind because they are so habitual. We can increase our awareness and avoid common harmful thought patterns such as:

- absolute thinking (always/never)
- predicting (it's going to be bad)
- assuming (he hates me)
- taking things personally
- blaming and labelling
- taking offence (I have the right to be upset)

Catching these habits is initially uncomfortable and surprising. After working with them for several months or years, it can get frustrating. On this point, we find a lot of encouraging words in the Bahá'í teachings, such as this extract from a letter written on behalf of Shoghi Effendi:

> ... a pessimistic and critical approach (although perhaps fully justified by the situation) produces no results. We, having the power of the Faith to draw on, must always be constructive in our efforts, as this will produce results and attract Divine blessings upon them.[17]

Being overly self-critical will impede our efforts. We must accept the fact that we have until death to refine our efforts, and eternity to spiritually progress. Perseverance and gentleness towards self are the keys to remaining open to change.

In the body, the cell also has a growth response. This enables its walls to remain fluid, openly exchanging information between itself and its environment. This openness expends energy, but the cell also receives energy, remaining in balance. Likewise, in our mental life a constructive positive approach will offset the fear surrounding the task of growth. The first step is to question the validity of thoughts and emotions, measuring them against the Word of God. The second step is to maintain a curious mind and open heart, which helps the mind remain neutral. The third step is to strive to find the higher truth.

We have the opportunity to develop keen insight into our perceptions and search out the truth. Bahá'u'lláh writes:

> In this Day whatsoever serveth to reduce blindness and to increase vision is worthy of consideration. This vision acteth as the agent and guide for true knowledge. Indeed in the estimation of men of wisdom keenness of understanding is due to keenness of vision.[18]

In sharpening our vision, Bahá'u'lláh tells us, justice will aid us to see through our own eyes and not through the eyes of others.[19] I find that in our struggle to remain objective, we must realize that our experiences pass through a gradient of beliefs and experiences, creating obstacles to true objectivity. The mind cannot decipher the *truth* of the situation from *our interpretation* of the situation. Compassionate inquisition into our moods and thoughts helps maintain objectivity.

Unfortunately, most of us habitually lie to others and to ourselves. There is no more blameworthy character trait. In fact, chronic complaining enables us to continue validating a self-lie. In order to purify and strengthen the rational mind we must discipline ourselves to speak the truth to ourselves and to others. When we are about to lie we need to be able to immediately identify our true intention. What is it we really want?

Our perceptions become more accurate when we accept that others have different truths from our own. For example, a person who lives in the northern hemisphere experiences the Fast during spring. It is true that the season is spring, but the idea that the Fast takes place during spring is not the only *truth*, because in the southern hemisphere it's autumn. Our need to be right interferes with our perceptions. The *truth* is that people have different realities.

The result of identifying nutrients in our thoughts and emotions will be reflected in our actions. From a Bahá'í perspective, thoughts are of two kinds, as 'Abdu'l-Bahá makes clear; they either belong to the mind and remain a thought, or they express themselves in action.[20] Psychologists believe that positive stimulating thoughts spur us into action. Identifying toxic thoughts, taking responsibility for them and regulating them to our best ability will help us to feel more confident and take empowered actions. When we identify negative thinking patterns and do nothing about it, it leaves us imprisoned and in stagnation, slowing down 'digestion'.

Some questions to challenge our perceptions include: What is the truth here? How do I act because that is true? How do I lie to myself? Am I willing to hear another's truth?

Catalysts

In the body, enzymes are the catalysts, the forces behind digestion ensuring that the transformative processes take place. Sometimes the body needs to take supplements to put enzymes back. Where are the 'enzymes' of the mind, and do we need supplements?

We may conclude that the catalyst in the mind is the will. Will determines action, and herein lies the definitive battle with the ego. Every human is a victim, to some degree, of self-absorption. The ego feeds off this. Its ignorance and distraction pervades all levels of consciousness. If the mind identifies with the ego, it becomes dark and material, like wastes in the body. If it identifies with the spirit, the mind becomes light and full of nutrition. A letter written on behalf of Shoghi Effendi addresses the subject of the ego:

> . . . the complete and entire elimination of the ego would imply perfection – which man can never completely attain – but the ego can and should be ever increasingly subordinated to the enlightened soul of man. This is what spiritual progress implies.[21]

The ego desperately spends its life building one wall after another because it finds this world to be hostile and dangerous, where everything is separate, as in the cell's protective response. As we look out at the world, the potential for threat and trauma seems ever-present, so we tend to surround ourselves with friendly, familiar things and pleasures. If we maintain this duality, can unity ever be established, I wonder? It's important that we lower the walls around us and acknowledge the oneness of reality (as when the cells stay open in a growth response). The recognition of our interconnectedness allows us to attain unity within ourselves and with others in the external world.

Table 9.2 Remedies for the ego's hidden agendas

Ego's hidden agendas	Remedies in Bahá'u'lláh's Revelation
Complaining or giving excuses. This tactic is used to strengthen the lower self. The underlying emotions can be resentment, anger or grievances.	Show love and kindness to all. Avoid strife and contention, apathy and estrangement.
Being right. The ego will provide all the evidence of being right and point out how others are wrong. The underlying emotions are judgement, misperception, and being opinionated.	Observe the good qualities in self and others. Overlook the faults of self and others (a sin-covering eye). Translate beliefs into action.
Taking a situation personally. This tactic is meant to defend. The underlying emotions are defensiveness, pride, hurt and anger.	Instantly forgive one another. Take no offence. Backbiting and gossip are forbidden.
Being separate or superior. The ego's intention is to keep us 'safe'. The underlying emotions can be fear, prejudice, ignorance or jealousy.	Use consultation for solutions in all matters. Balance justice and compassion.
Keeping control. This gives us the illusion that everything's OK, because it will work out the way we want. Some underlying emotions are fear, anger, greed or suspicion.	Prefer other's good to our own. Conceal the misdeeds of others. Faith and trust in God. Sincerity and purity of motive.
Wanting attention. This keeps us focused on ourselves, whether it's through pity and victimhood, or through triumph. The underlying emotions can be insecurity, neediness, passion, fear of not getting needs met, or anger.	Encourage and assure one another. Firmness in the Covenant. Selflessness and servitude. Purify one's intention.
Attachment to outcome or expectations. This sets us up for disappointment and reaffirms a negative belief pattern. The underlying emotions are doubt, hopelessness, grief and loneliness.	Detach oneself from everything except God. Spiritual progress through patience, prayer and striving. Moderation and the Middle Way. Obedience to His laws.

The ego has hidden agendas and many of our behaviours stem from its selfish desires. Bahá'u'lláh's Revelation, however, contains innumerable remedies; the list in Table 9.2 is by no means definitive, but provides a glimpse of the two paths.

As Shoghi Effendi pointed out, our challenge in this life is to use our free will to create inner discipline over our ego's animal instincts, urges and reactions. Whenever the mind is caught in the clutches of the ego, we can choose to shift into a more open and receptive state of consciousness. The mind is more inclined, as in the pull of gravity, to be absorbed in distractions, preoccupations or vain imaginings.

The mind has qualities of stillness and motion. Most individuals go through extremely difficult periods of darkness, experiencing apathy and stillness. It is our duty as Bahá'ís to strive to overcome this apathy. Our training is analogous to 'Abdu'l-Bahá's description of training horses. He said, they take them into the fields and make them run short distances. The distance is gradually increased until they become thinner and wirier. After months of training their endurance and speed are extraordinary. It was 'Abdu'l-Bahá's desire that all of us be trained to endure great tests, so as to be able to serve the Cause of God continually and without any other desire or motive.[22]

Building will

Our will, our volition, what we want, are all part of our mind. 'Abdu'l-Bahá said:

> Some things are subject to the free will of man, such as justice, equity, tyranny, and injustice, in other words, good and evil actions; it is evident and clear that these actions are, for the most part, left to the will of man. But there are certain things to which man is forced and compelled, such as sleep, death, sickness, decline of power, injuries and misfortunes; these are not subject to the will of man, and he is not responsible for them, for he is compelled to endure them. But in the choice of good and bad actions he is free, and he commits them according to his own will.[23]

It would seem from this teaching that a most valuable use of the rational faculty is to steel one's resolve to find one's shortcomings, then find the spiritual antidote in the teachings to overcome them. Our will is the strongest force determining our actions, and the most challenging to overcome in healing. If one doesn't want to get better, one won't. If one wants to lose weight, but has a stronger affection for food or pain, it will be impossible to overcome. Bahá'u'lláh writes, 'All that which ye potentially possess can, however, be manifested only as a result of your own volition. Your own acts testify to this truth.'[24] And 'Abdu'l-Bahá is reported to have said, 'We all know and admit that justice is good, but there is need of volition and action to carry out and manifest it.'[25]

I've observed that one of the signs of a well-trained mind is a strong will to take the right action. There are small activities one can carry out to train the will and achieve victory over the reins of the horse. An example is to begin training your will on the physical level by acknowledging the impulse to snack, but refusing it. Each time you refrain, your will strengthens. Move on to more difficult tasks, such as being more patient with someone you usually become irritated with.

When our will is weak, the mind becomes self-centred and everything revolves around its desires. Reality becomes filtered through its lens, as shown in Figure 9.1.

Figure 9.1 Me-centred

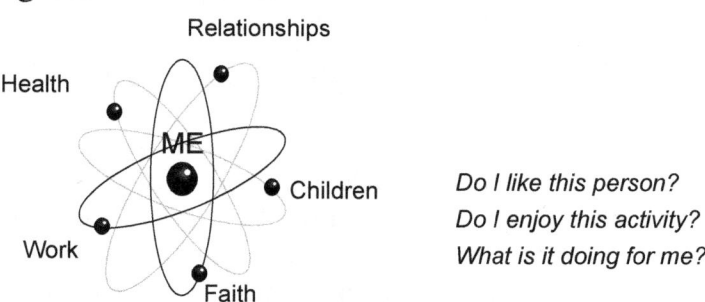

When we become *me*-centred life becomes compartmentalized instead of unified. The mind segregates others and activities according to its passions and dictates. It judges whether the relationship is enjoyable: what is it doing for me? It weighs our job or profession according to what we are and are not getting. We can see even our own bodies as an enemy if we become sick. Our very faith can come under the delusion of pleasure or non-pleasure, as in 'I don't like that activity', or '*those people will be there*'.

When we are God-centred, life revolves around one source and becomes more easily unified. Work is considered worship. Serving our family and children is likened to serving God; this takes judgement out of the activity. We see God in others, rather than their shortcomings. These thoughts take the self out of it all, and our happiest moments are when we are forgetful of self.

Figure 9.2 God-centred

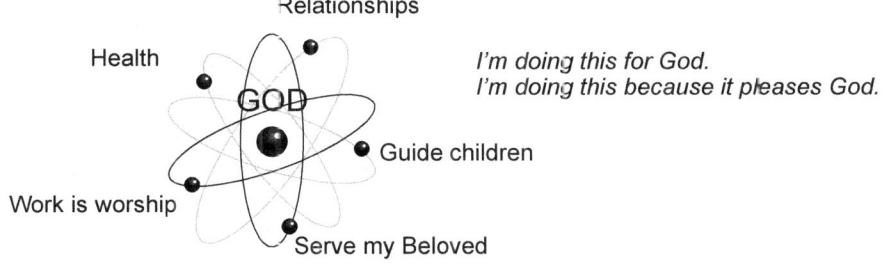

Self-surrender

Bahá'u'lláh gives us the remedy to achieve victory in this battle of opposing forces – surrendering our will to God:

> By self-surrender and perpetual union with God is meant that men should merge their will wholly in the Will of God, and regard their desires as utter nothingness beside His Purpose. Whatsoever the Creator commandeth His creatures to observe, the same must they diligently, and with the utmost joy and eagerness, arise and fulfil. They should in no wise allow their fancy to obscure their judgment, neither should they regard their own imaginings as the voice of the Eternal. In the Prayer of Fasting We have revealed: 'Should Thy Will decree that out of Thy mouth these words proceed and be addressed unto them, "Observe, for My Beauty's sake, the fast, O people, and set no limit to its duration," I swear by the majesty of Thy glory, that every one of them will faithfully observe it, will abstain from whatsoever will violate Thy law, and will continue to do so until

they yield up their souls unto Thee.' In this consisteth the complete surrender of one's will to the Will of God.[26]

'It is a great power to have a strong will, but a greater power to give that will to God. The *will* is what we do; the *understanding* is what we know,' said 'Abdu'l-Bahá to a pilgrim [emphasis added].[27] Surrendering the will always meets internal resistance. Recognizing these resistant forces of the ego is essential to attaining self-regulation. Unless resistance is properly dealt with, it will persist. The resistance stems from our lower nature, or the Evil One, 'he that hindereth the rise and obstructeth the spiritual progress of the children of men',[28] as described by Bahá'u'lláh, and again: 'The Evil One is lying in wait, ready to entrap you. Gird yourselves against his wicked devices . . . Centre your thoughts in the Well-Beloved, rather than in your own selves.'[29]

A tree with deep roots can withstand any wind. Conversely, as we grow spiritually, strong winds are needed in order for the roots to go deep. If resistance is not acknowledged, our consciousness is bound to limitations of the prison of self – our ideas and beliefs. Total surrender requires radiant acquiescence, as 'Abdu'l-Bahá says:

> The afflictions which come to humanity sometimes tend to centre the consciousness upon the limitations, and this is a veritable prison. Release comes by making of the will a Door through which the confirmations of the Spirit come . . . They come to that man or woman who accepts his life with radiant acquiescence.[30]

Reflecting upon these quotations and then looking to science to consider the organs in the body, we see that each cell within that system must acquiesce in the informed decision of the whole. If one cell should stand up and profess its independence or disobedience, disease begins. One of the largest obstacles we face, I think, is how to submit our will to God's teachings when they feel so contrary to us in the moment. When we experience resistance to a person who is continually mean, we may have an impulse to cut them off and protect ourselves, or to lash out intending to push them away. The Bahá'í teachings tell us to treat our enemies with kindness and to forgive them instantly. In the moment, we can acknowledge our resistance on an emotional level, but submit our will and take action as the teachings tell us, to the best of our ability in the moment. Later we can privately process our strong emotional resistance, so that our individual need can be satisfied until a spiritual skill of instant forgiveness can be attained. This prevents us from stuffing feelings away, repressing them. It allows us expression, but in a private appropriate way. When we align our will to God's will and take the correct action in the moment, this immediately attracts the confirmations of Bahá'u'lláh, according to His teachings. 'Abdu'l-Bahá promised that these confirmations could turn 'a gnat into an eagle'. We may then conclude that when we submit our will and take the right action, the experience of those confirmations can be truly amazing.

Radiant acquiescence allows us to accept our situation and obey the Will of God. It opens the door to compassion, allowing us to embrace our situation. It implies dropping resistance and complying with things we cannot change. We don't have to like the situation or agree with it. We must simply change what we can, and accept what we cannot.

There are times when we may find it difficult to surrender to a Bahá'í teaching. If we can't find the will to follow through, then we must use the rational faculty to explore the benefits. I ask my clients to analyse how they benefit from a negative habit or belief, revealing the inner conflict. For example, patients with chronic pain want very badly to resolve their pain, yet often they cannot; in such cases the benefits of physical touch and attention outweigh losing the pain. They are finally getting the attention they need. Some want to lose weight, but keep eating foods that don't benefit them. They will even admit, 'I can see myself go to the cupboard, overeat, and then feel bad later.' The will here has more attraction to the pain and suffering than it does to caring for the self, and sometimes their weight is actually a barrier that keeps the sufferer safe from being intimate with others.

It's hard to believe our negative behaviours have benefits. When you find yourself stuck in the same pattern, try the following exercise:

Example 1. Because I *lose my temper with my spouse*, I get to *have my way*.
Example 2. Because I *have my anxiety every evening*, I get to *avoid chores around the house*.

'Because I _____, I get to _____.'

*Some questions to help tame the ego: **What am I attached to? What do I really need here? How can I best ask for that? What is the Will of God in this situation?***

Elimination

Forgiveness: An essential response

Proper physical elimination ensures a healthy body. Healthy and daily elimination is essential to the mind's well-being, too. Mastering forgiveness allows us to eliminate the burden of our mistakes and prevents us from carrying that pain into the future. One of the ego's favourite ways of separating 'us' from 'them' is by not forgiving. Forgiveness frees us from the needless pain of reliving a hurt over and over. Forgiveness doesn't validate or make a wrong choice right, but it can heal even the most grievous offence. It frees us from the thought that, for example, we never received a proper apology or proper justice, or we are obliged to punish people. While forgiveness is a natural impulse of the soul, it's really the *will* that accepts forgiveness for oneself and decides to forgive others.

The Bahá'ís are to look upon each other with the eyes of compassion and understanding, not with revenge in mind. Bahá'u'lláh asks us to show mercy to our enemies and to see beyond their behaviours, to see truth. If we do otherwise we will be held accountable for our own mistakes. Also, we are only accountable for our own actions, not responsible for the actions of others. Shoghi Effendi reassures us on this point: 'We cannot bear the burden of suffering of others, and we should not try to. All men are in God's hands . . .'[31]

In order to live cooperatively and in unity, we can study the natural world to address humanity's challenge of its lower impulses. Humans have a strong natural inclination to categorize friend or enemy, and this is echoed in the plant kingdom. The following study on plants was carried out by McMaster University in Hamilton, Ontario: the Great Lakes sea rocket plant was studied to see how it reacted with other plants of the same species when sharing a pot. When potted with other plants of the same species, but strangers, they competed with each other for soil nutrients. If researchers potted them with plants that shared their family tree, or 'friends', they instead opted for moderate growth, sharing the nutrients in the pot.[32] I was interested to read this study because I frequently observe how much innate resistance we have to overcome prejudice and separation from others.

How do the plants differentiate? We find similar electronic signalling in the plant kingdom as we do in human cells. This form of communication can even be shared by bacteria. Depending upon the signals they receive, they respond with a growth or protection response. These responses are likened to 'feeling' or energy flow. While plants, animals and bacteria aren't conscious of these 'feelings', they do interpret them. Signals in one living being cause a response in another.

One of the main teachings of Bahá'u'lláh is the oneness of all things. Science is confirming this in all kinds of different ways. For instance, there is the study on flocking by the biophysicist Fritz-Albert Popp, Director of the International Institute of Biophysics, an international network of 19 research groups from 13 countries involved in biophoton research and coherence systems in biology. According to Popp, photon exchange between living beings explains how schools of fish or flocks of birds create perfect and instantaneous coordination. Many experiments on the homing ability of animals demonstrate that it has nothing to do with following habitual trails, scents or even the electro-magnetic fields of the earth, but rather some form of silent communication that acts like an invisible rubber band, even when the animals are separated by miles of distance.

We can even see the influence of thoughts and emotion on water in the well-known – and at the time of writing, highly contested – water studies by Dr Masuru Emoto, which show how the molecular structure of water is affected in response to thoughts, creating varying geometrical patterns.

But apart from scientific discourse and discussion, we know that 'Abdu'l-Bahá said it was not allowable to show kindness when one wished evil, because the thought and feeling associated towards that person was evil, even though kind in outward appearance. He said:

> You must not see evil as evil and then compromise with your opinion, for to treat in a smooth, kindly way one whom you consider evil or an enemy is hypocrisy, and this is not worthy or allowable. You must consider your enemies as your friends, look upon your evil-wishers as your well-wishers and treat them accordingly.[33]

What effect can my thoughts have on others and what does that have to do with forgiveness? The studies briefly described above may show the interconnectedness of all things, and the subtle and constant communication that happens at an atomic level. Any energy we create within us is shared with the collective. We may then see that any thought or action I take will have an equal reaction. What I do and think affects everyone. If I hurt others, I hurt myself; if I help others, I help myself. The essence of the Golden Rule resides in oneness.

Carrying anger and resentment around instead of forgiveness causes disharmony individually and collectively. Our thoughts and emotions affect others on a subconscious level when we are near them. Forgiveness gives us a fresh start every day and the ability to be around others without negatively affecting them.

When past events and the emotions tied to them remain in our consciousness, we have not let them go or eliminated them. Imagine having chronic constipation and how sick your body would be! Suppressed emotions and thoughts find a way of expressing themselves and it will usually be in the mind or the body, creating an imbalance. Emotions unexpressed are like a festering wound with walls of pus around it for protection.

In a letter to the Iranian Bahá'ís in 2009, the Universal House of Justice wrote that

> the proper response to oppression is neither to succumb in resignation nor to take on the characteristics of the oppressor. The victim of oppression can transcend it through an inner strength that shields the soul from bitterness and hatred and which sustains consistent, principled action.[34]

In the same vein, 'Abdu'l-Bahá teaches us to

> look upon our enemies with a *sin-covering eye and act with justice* when confronted with any injustice whatsoever, forgive all, consider the whole of humanity as our own family, the whole earth as our own country, *be sympathetic with all suffering* . . . Our only role is to spread the teachings. If it be accepted, all is well; if not, *leave the people to God.*[35] [emphasis added]

The passages quoted above reflect the power we have in a situation of injustice through opening the mind into forgiveness. We can become sympathetic to all the suffering involved, forgive, take principled action and leave the others to God.

One of the keys to letting go is to acknowledge the emotion in our response to a situation – shame, bitterness, hurt, revenge. Then we can forgive ourselves for being human and having these emotional impulses. We vow to make a fresh start and let it go. We abide with the pain until it's processed. When we find our minds remembering or nursing a past wound, we can immediately focus on our breath, acknowledge the emotion, and bring our mind back to the present moment and use our *will* to forgive and let go.

Forgiveness is only through God

The Bahá'í texts teach us that God is the only one who forgives sins:

> The inmost essence of all things voiceth in all things the testimony: 'All forgiveness floweth, in this Day, from God, Him to Whom none can compare, with Whom no partners can be joined, the Sovereign Protector of all men, and the Concealer of their sins!'[36]

We are encouraged to pray for another's forgiveness. When a client is really stuck in emotion and can't move beyond processing, I advise them to pray for the forgiveness of the person they are struggling with. The intention is to ask God to help both parties see the truth and find their way. Some have childhood dilemmas and traumas they can't move beyond. I've seen amazing spiritual movement and results when one beseeches God for forgiveness for one's enemy. With patience and time, transformation emerges after repeatedly saying these prayers. We can also pray for the souls of our departed parents, to enable their souls to progress in the next world.

This inspiring prayer revealed by 'Abdu'l-Bahá for His enemies provides us with food for thought, in contemplating how to apply it in our own lives:

> I call upon Thee, O Lord my God! with my tongue and with all my heart, not to requite them for their cruelty and their wrong-doings,

their craft and their mischief, for they are foolish and ignoble and know not what they do. They discern not good from evil, neither do they distinguish right from wrong; nor justice from injustice. They follow their own desires and walk in the footsteps of the most imperfect and foolish amongst them. O my Lord! Have mercy upon them, shield them from all afflictions in these troubled times and grant that all trials and hardships may be the lot of this Thy servant that hath fallen into this darksome pit. Single me out for every woe and make me a sacrifice for all Thy loved ones. O Lord, Most High! May my soul, my life, my being, my spirit, my all be offered up for them. O God, My God! Lowly, suppliant and fallen upon my face, I beseech Thee with all the ardour of my invocation to pardon whosoever hath hurt me, forgive him that hath conspired against me and offended me, and wash away the misdeeds of them that have wrought injustice upon me. Vouchsafe unto them Thy goodly gifts, give them joy, relieve them from sorrow, grant them peace and prosperity, give them Thy bliss and pour upon them Thy bounty.

Thou art the Powerful, the Gracious the Help in Peril, the Self-Subsisting![37]

Forgiveness in daily practice

So what does to forgive really mean? Its dictionary definition is 'to cease feeling resentful', and the Bahá'í teachings ask us to do it instantly. For some of us that can take great effort and courage. I find it important to recognize that there can also be anger towards the self, because resentment can also stem from not taking action when it was required, or taking the wrong action in a situation and carrying guilt. The ego traps us into thinking we cannot accept God's forgiveness for something terrible we've done. In healing, forgiveness is a way of living. In one study, researchers found that when people talked about being betrayed, their blood pressure increased and their breathing became shallower. Those who had a forgiving nature saw their bodies come back into balance much faster than those who refused to forgive the person involved.

Take no offence in the first place

The ultimate quest is to not be offended in the first place. 'Abdu'l-Bahá asks of us,

> Act in such a way that your heart may be free from hatred. Let not your heart be offended with anyone. If some one commits an error and wrong toward you, you must instantly forgive him.[38]

The Greatest Holy Leaf, the daughter of Bahá'u'lláh, describes more in depth how not taking offence may be manifested in our lives. She faced great sorrows throughout her life and consoled all those who suffered, even those who showed her great cruelty. One of the early American Bahá'ís who had several opportunities to observe the Greatest Holy Leaf in action wrote after her passing:

> You were sure that if one tried to hurt her she would wish to console him for his own cruelty. For her love was unconditioned, could penetrate disguise and see hunger behind the mask of fury, and she knew that the most brutal self is secretly hoping to find gentleness in another . . .
>
> Something greater than forgiveness she had shown in meeting the cruelties and strictures in her own life. To be hurt and to forgive is saintly but far beyond this is the power to comprehend and not be hurt . . . She was never known to complain or lament. It was not that she made the best of things, but that she found in everything, even in calamity itself, the germs of enduring wisdom. She did not resist the shocks and upheavals of life and she did not run counter to obstacles. She was never impatient. She was as incapable of impatience as she was of revolt. But this was not so much long-sufferance as it was quiet awareness of the forces that operate in the hours of waiting and inactivity.[39]

A large source of hurt in my clients stems from other people's opinions, observations and thoughts on their actions. However well-intended, these can often be unhelpful when they hit a wound, and some comments can be downright thoughtless, judging, rude and sometimes cruel. If we tape-recorded our own unguarded comments to others we would want to take a lot of them back! Bahá'u'lláh admonishes us that speech requires moderation:

> For the tongue is a smouldering fire, and excess of speech a deadly poison. Material fire consumeth the body, whereas the fire of the tongue devoureth both heart and soul.[40]

> The Great Being saith: Human utterance is an essence which aspireth to exert its influence and needeth moderation.[41]

If we take another's words or actions personally, a part of us agrees with them, or we have a sensitivity to that issue. It's all about 'me' and when we take the me out of it, the truth is that other people's actions and words are always about *themselves*. A well-known teaching in the Buddhist tradition is that everyone lives in their own world and illusions, and this world is revealed whenever we speak or take action. Even if someone directly insults or injures us, it's really about the other person's own struggle, stress or poison they need to get out of their own system. On the other hand, if someone tells you how wonderful you are, it still isn't about you. If someone complains about a friend for their hour of consultation, I take their case as though they are talking about themselves, because they are simply revealing to me their sensitivities and what they don't like in themselves. We reveal so much about ourselves in our complaints and criticisms of others.

There's a significant level of freedom you attain when you stop personalizing everything around you. It allows you space to instantly forgive. Therefore, if someone feels compelled to comment about your life, you can simply observe how *they* revealed where their soul is on the continuum of eternal progress. We are all on this path somewhere, and our words reveal where. 'Abdu'l-Bahá confirmed this:

> Man's speech is the revealer of his heart. In whatever world the heart travels, man's conversation will revolve around that center. From his words you can understand in what world he is travelling, whether he is looking upward toward the realm of light or downward to the nether world, whether he is mindful or unaware, whether he is awake or asleep, whether he is alive or dead.[42]

Is there any emotional 'background noise' in my head? What lingering thoughts or feelings have I not dealt with? Have I fully embraced what happened to me and the part I played in that event? What thoughts keep recurring and what are the feelings associated with those thoughts? Does an event or person in my past still anger me?

Cleanliness

Purifying our intentions and motives, and humility

Hygiene has been one of the main contributors to the health and increasing longevity of populations in the last two centuries. Cleanliness pushes toxins out of the body. It enables things to renew and prevents disease and its spread. The mind, too, requires cleanliness for its health. Purifying our intentions is one aspect of cleanliness for the mind, leading us to the core of self-regulation. Humility also contributes to cleanliness of the mind. According to the Bahá'í teachings, servitude is the highest station we can attain today and humility clears the path to servitude.

Bahá'u'lláh encouraged us to search out our own imperfections and not the imperfections of others. Nothing is more fruitful for our spiritual growth than the knowledge of our shortcomings. Spiritual progress depends on this knowledge; it keeps us humble and prevents us from blaming others for our own mistakes. It helps us to build on what we are doing right while balancing this with an acknowledgement of our challenges.

In the natural world, water cannot flow if the ground is level with or higher than itself; it can only flow to an area which is lower. The Revelation of Bahá'u'lláh is like a great mountain. Making ourselves lowly and humble, emptying the cup of ego, creates space that is lower for the Holy Spirit to flow into. The ego builds itself up to become higher, preventing the waters of the spirit from flowing into our vessel.

Bahá'u'lláh admonishes the 'wayfarer' not to exalt himself above others:

> Rather must he regard himself as standing at all times in the presence of his Lord. He must not wish for anyone that which he doth not wish for himself, nor speak that which he would not bear to hear

spoken by another, nor yet desire for any soul that which he would not have desired for himself.[43]

He also inform us that the seeker

> must never seek to exalt himself above any one, must wash away from the tablet of his heart every trace of pride and vainglory, must cling unto patience and resignation, observe silence, and refrain from idle talk.[44]

Pride is a dangerous type of self that prevents us from having the open-mindedness that helps us grow. George Vithoulkas in his book *The Science of Homeopathy* assesses disease in the mind, echoing the beautiful quotation from the Writings of Bahá'u'lláh above: 'Selfishness and acquisitiveness are the primary factors that derange the mind. Freedom from selfishness and acquisitiveness will naturally lead to a healthy state of mind.'[45] Selfishness is the natural tendency of the mind. Our will must continually paddle against this strong current.

Science now offers explanations for why the brain feeds self-centredness. Normal thinking relies on a defence mechanism in the brain which protects our core beliefs. It kicks in when facts are presented to us that do not fit our belief models, by automatically rejecting the new information. It prevents us from open rational thought. When new facts are presented to us, or if someone is trying to be helpful to point out a negative behaviour, this creates *cognitive dissonance*, a type of discomfort. This mechanism helps us to achieve equilibrium from the dissonance by dismissing the information contrary to our beliefs. Our brain even goes so far as to perceive the person delivering the facts as an enemy. These studies help us to better understand that humility is a practised skill, to override the defence mechanism in the brain. The resistance to hearing new information, especially information contrary to one's current beliefs, can be painful. Humility prevents our defence mechanisms from interfering with self-regulation and balance in the mind.

A recent study in the *Boston Globe* concluded that facts do not determine our beliefs, but that it's our beliefs that determine which facts we'll accept. George Lakoff demonstrated in his studies that we are not born with an ideology, but socialized into it as children, usually by parental figures.[46] Bahá'u'lláh's teaching of the independent and unfettered search after truth – that is, not following blindly in our parents' footsteps, challenges the very wiring of the brain. 'Abdu'l-Bahá sets forth this key teaching:

> Another new principle revealed by His Holiness Bahá'u'lláh is the injunction to investigate truth – that is to say, no man should blindly follow his ancestors and forefathers. Nay, each must see with his own eyes, hear with his own ears and investigate the truth himself in order that he may follow the truth instead of blind acquiescence and imitation of ancestral beliefs.[47]

In my professional work I teach self-regulation as a fundamental practice. A self-regulated person checks in throughout the day and cleanses the mind of all 'blind followings'. Minds can fundamentally change through continued open investigation, awareness, effort, prayer, and striving to refine our understanding of what is true. This practice cleanses the self of delusions and habits. It is when we are in selfless action and service that we receive the breaths of the Holy Spirit and are free from the prison of self.

One of the most important factors behind our actions is motivation. I often ask clients to examine what they really needed when they were behaving in a particular way. For example, when we feel hurt but really want validation, we can lose our temper. Our intention was to express our hurt, but we failed to do it with tact because we gave in to our impulse to protect ourselves through anger.

Cleansing our intentions is vital to our connection to God and our spiritual growth. Bahá'u'lláh states, 'Every act ye meditate is as clear to Him as is that act when already accomplished.'[48] Checking our intentions keeps us aware of what we are doing and why with more purity. Reviewing our past actions and thoughts is helpful in weighing them in the balance of intention. What did I really want when I acted that way? What was I really trying to say?

Some questions to help realign the mind with humility: Do I value the thoughts of others? What is my intention by doing/saying . . . ? Can I admit my mistakes? Am I willing to share and receive?

Movement

One of the tools I use is 'movement for the mind'. The science of healing confirms the necessity to exercise the brain if it is to remain healthy. There are many activities to strengthen its endurance, which can be compared to aerobic exercise for the body. Both body and mind also need strength training. This manifests itself in the mind through learning new skills that challenge our ways of thinking. The body needs stretching, and the mind attains that through stretching its limits and boundaries. Let's take a look at a few examples to help exercise the mind.

Play and creativity. Many people severely lack this stimulation in their lives. They go to work, take care of their family and obligations, then sleep. This becomes a passive, reactive and robotic way to live and a source of dissatisfaction. But creativity is one of the critical aspects of health for the mind. Magic unfolds when the mind enters the realm of eternity while playing or creating; these activities allow the mind to connect to the spiritual realms. The mind can manifest what is seen in the unseen, creating beauty, inspiration and invention.

Our health depends upon us engaging in some activity that allows us to lose all track of time, space and sense of who we are. In such activity our energies are fully immersed in the present moment; all our attachments – thoughts, worries and concerns – are left behind This place in the mind is a vital part of being in balance, and needs visiting daily, even if it's only for a short amount of time.

Learning a new skill. Intelligence is one of the greatest gifts given to humanity and distinguishes us from animals. Similar to bones and muscles, knowledge provides structure and movement, creating a core belief system.

Strength training in the body requires resistance through weights. Think of your state of mind when you receive a new phone or learn a new job. The mind first encounters resistance, in a wide range of responses from exhilaration to frustration. Some long for the old phone or the past job – old routines. This resistance is indicative that a new network of neural connections is being created in the brain. The more neural connections the brain creates, the more we gain protection from memory loss. (For further research, look up 'neural redundancy'.) Learning a different language or computer program is a perfect example of this process.

Any activity that allows you to experience some resistance will give your neural pathways a workout. Just like weights and barbells, you can determine how much resistance you would like for your workout. Incorporate various routines, mess up your routines, your comfort zones. Use memory games, puzzles, a new hobby, avoid the calculator for a day. Create opportunities to challenge the mind and ways of thinking. A simple example would be to try wearing your watch upside down or on the other wrist for a few days.

Social connectivity. A healthy mind maintains connectivity to community. Ideally, the community should be diverse in culture, generations, religious backgrounds and so on. Create a support system of at least five individuals who understand, listen to you and sincerely desire your well-being. Socialization keeps our neurons firing and our brain connectivity active.

The need for society is also reflected in the Bahá'í texts. 'Abdu'l-Bahá teaches us:

> . . . man cannot live singly and alone. He is in need of continuous cooperation and mutual help. For example, a man living alone in the wilderness will eventually starve. He can never, singly and alone, provide himself with all the necessities of existence. Therefore, he is in need of cooperation and reciprocity.[49]

Like any other aspect of health, our choices between healthy or toxic influences pertain also to our social connections. The Bahá'í Writings offer some insights into our choice of company. Bahá'u'lláh admonishes us to examine our associations and their ramifications for our spiritual progress: 'The company of the ungodly increaseth sorrow, whilst fellowship with the righteous cleanseth the rust from off the heart.'[50] Shoghi Effendi has clarified that

> In the passage 'eschew all fellowship with the ungodly', Bahá'u'lláh means that we should shun the company of those who disbelieve in God and are wayward. The word 'ungodly' is a reference to such

perverse people. The words 'Be thou as a flame of fire to My enemies and a river of life eternal to My loved ones' should not be taken in their literal sense. Bahá'u'lláh's advice is that again we should flee from the enemies of God, and instead seek the fellowship of His lovers. [51]

In commenting on these words of Bahá'u'lláh, Adib Taherzadeh writes:

> The word 'ungodly' should not be misunderstood. An ungodly person may profess belief in God, while many who regard themselves as agnostics or atheists may not be ungodly in reality. An ungodly person is one who through his friendship, knowingly or unknowingly, prevents a believer from following the dictates of his faith and becomes a barrier between him and his God.[52]

There is an easy way to check our associations. After leaving someone's presence do you feel depleted or radiant? Of course, people will always have bad days and need a dear one to listen, but in general, if you feel drained after repeatedly being with someone, make a point of setting a clear boundary and choosing to associate with those who generally uplift your spirit. This disciplines the mind to associate with heavenly attributes, and not the material world.

'Abdu'l-Bahá was always very practical. His advice to Juliet Thompson was:

> You must try to associate with those who will do you good and who will be the cause of your being more awakened, and not with those who will make you negligent of God. For example, if one goes into a garden and associates with flowers, one will surely inhale the beautiful fragrance, but if one goes to a place where there are bad-scented plants, it is sure he will inhale an unpleasant odor. In short, I mean that you will try to be with those who are purified and sanctified souls. Man must always associate with those from whom he can get light, or be with those to whom he can give light. He must either receive or give instructions. Otherwise, being with people without these two intentions, he is spending his time for nothing, and, by so doing, he is neither gaining nor causing others to gain.[53]

Smiling and yawning. One of the things Bahá'u'lláh loved was a 'face wreathed in smiles'. Bahá'u'lláh would always smile at the mention of Mary Magdalene, as 'Abdu'l-Bahá described: 'There was one name . . . that always brought joy to the face of Bahá'u'lláh. His expression would change at the mention of it. That name was Mary of Magdala.'[54]

According to Newberg and Waldman's book *How God Changes Your Brain*, smiling promotes the health of the brain and provides exercise for it. Yawning also helps the brain to process information, so I welcome my clients to yawn; it helps a sleepy brain to process and retain what's being discussed. It can sometimes, though, be an indication of resistance to the materials presenting themselves, or of too much material. Yawning can be a polite way of the brain shutting down or needing to process information.

Reflect on organizations, groups, clubs, places of work and books you read, and ask: Does it uplift me? Do I feel whole and connected by doing this? Does this serve a greater purpose?

Protection

Everything in nature has a protective response. The body needs protection, and the mind needs protecting too. Bahá'u'lláh revealed prayers of protection for many reasons. Some protect us from external enemies, and others protect us from the internal influences of the ego. These influences swing us like a pendulum, from happy to sad, between good and bad, between judging and victim.

In one of the prayers revealed by Bahá'u'lláh, He asks for protection from external influences: 'Shield us, then, O my God, from the mischief of Thine enemies, and assist us to help Thy Faith, and to protect Thy Cause, and to celebrate Thy glory.'[55] He has also revealed prayers for protection from our own selves:

> Keep us safe, then, through Thine unfailing protection . . . from them whom Thou hast made to be the manifestations of the Evil Whisperer, who whisper in men's breasts.[56]

And in another prayer,

I implore Thee, O my God, by Thy mercy that hath surpassed all created things, and to which all that are immersed beneath the oceans of Thy names bear witness, not to abandon me unto my self, for my heart is prone to evil. Guard me, then, within the stronghold of Thy protection and the shelter of Thy care.[57]

Seeking the middle way

External and internal influences can create a roller-coaster effect of emotions. The path of protection between the extremes is a middle path, known in most religions and philosophies as the 'middle way'. The Buddha describes the middle way as a path of moderation between the extremes of sensual indulgence and self-mortification. Self-indulgence pursues desires and gives in to earthly temptations. At the other end of the spectrum, self-mortification is based on living without feelings and without enjoyment of any kind. The middle way is based on the principle of moderation. In the Bahá'í teachings, Bahá'u'lláh confirms this: 'In all matters moderation is desirable. If a thing is carried to excess, it will prove a source of evil.'[58]

A protected mind possesses moderation, a middle way in perceiving the world and expressing itself. Bahá'u'lláh teaches us how to reach this:

> Lament not in your hours of trial, neither rejoice therein; seek ye the Middle Way which is the *remembrance of Me in your afflictions and reflection over that which may befall you in future.* Thus informeth you He Who is the Omniscient, He Who is aware.'[59] [emphasis added]

Another directive is given by Bahá'u'lláh in the passage from the Kitáb-i-Íqán popularly known as the Tablet of the True Seeker, in which He encourages us to remove both extremes of love and hate before seeking the truth. For love may blind us, while hate may repel us from the truth.[60]

Shoghi Effendi's vision of the Bahá'í Faith as reflecting the middle way has been described by his wife, Amatu'l-Bahá Rúḥíyyih Khánum:

> So often he would say: this is a religion of the golden mean, the middle of the way, neither this extreme nor that. What he meant by this was not compromise but the very essence of the thought conveyed in these words of Bahá'u'lláh Himself: 'overstep not the

bounds of moderation; whoso cleaveth to justice can, under no circumstances, transgress the limits of moderation.' We live in perhaps the most immoderate society the world has ever seen . . .[61]

In our quest to seek the middle way, understanding the unity of the relationship of extremes is essential. We can examine the concept of yin and yang, for example, where yin represents feminine energy, and yang represents masculine energy. This concept is over three and a half centuries old. Traditional Chinese medicine developed this system to treat the body as a whole, seeking the unification of body and mind through balancing these two opposing forces. Nothing in the universe is wholly yin or wholly yang. In their book *Between Heaven and Earth*, Harriet Beinfield and Efrem Korngold explain that the interaction between yin and yang

> reflects the interaction of matter and energy. Their dependence on each other renders them inseparable. Yin and Yang are interdependent and cannot exist in isolation. Each balances the other and contributes to the harmony of the body as a whole.[62]

I've observed that the energies in the Fast are conducive to finding harmony as a whole, offering us sustained protection from polarization.

Familiar paths

The infinity symbol shown in Figure 9.3 is a helpful tool I use to explain the 'path' of polarities, the prison of self. This is usually a well-worn path, a thinking pattern we churn over and over again in our minds, back and forth in a vicious cycle. It's a looping pattern, where the ego will treat our consciousness like a ping-pong game: Should I or shouldn't I? I want to do this, but I'm afraid. I want to resolve this matter, but it never works! The consciousness goes back and forth, never resting in the centre. This prison of self often results in disempowerment, lack of momentum and confusion. Clients of mine often say, 'I'm stuck, I don't know what to do.' As we saw in Chapter 8 (Figure 8.1) one end of the infinity symbol can represent the parasympathetic nerve and the other the sympathetic nerve. Like yin and yang, consciousness moves between the two, creating balance.

In the Bahá'í Writings we find this explanation by 'Abdu'l-Bahá:

> The powers of the sympathetic nerve are neither entirely physical nor spiritual, but are between the two (systems). The nerve is connected with both. Its phenomena shall be perfect when its spiritual and physical relations are normal.[63]

Figure 9.3   An infinity of polarites

1. Friend (*they are good to me*)
2. Good (*that brings me joy*)
3. Yin (*I feel...*)
4. Gluttony (*I deserve...*)
5. Past (*I should have...*)
6. Only justice (*judging thoughts*)

1. Enemy (*I'm not treated well*)
2. Bad (*that brings me pain*)
3. Yang (*I think...*)
4. Deprivation (*I'm not worthy*)
5. Future (*what if...*)
6. Only compassion (*only 'loving'*)

In Figure 9.3, I included the vortex to represent my understanding of how the soul associates with the body. It can be found only in the middle way, between the two polarities. When we find the stillness in the middle, we are essentially standing in the eye of the storm, calm, peaceful, connected to our inner wisdom. Bounty and confirmations as well as information from the next world can come through this vortex to us in meditation, as discussed more thoroughly in the next chapters on the soul. The trick is to not swing out too far on either side, because our humanness will pull us into polarity throughout the day.

These polarities can be seen in virtues. For example, compassion in one polarity could be non-existent, while in the other it could be too much compassion. Too little leads to unfeeling and too much indicates that we avoid conflict at all costs and don't set boundaries when needed. Somewhere in the middle lies true compassion.

Shoghi Effendi gave an excellent example of the well-worn path many of us walk between the past and the future. The present moment is the middle way. He commented, 'Think about what you have to do today, and not speculate about the past and future. Forget the past, don't brood over it, it paralyzes us.'[64]

In polarities, one end is sometimes worse than the other, as 'Abdu'l-Bahá revealed:

If haste is harmful, inertness and indolence are a thousand times worse. A middle course is best, as it is written: 'It is incumbent upon you to do good between the two evils,' this referring to the mean between the two extremes. 'And let not thy hand be tied up to thy neck; nor yet open it with all openness . . . but between these follow a middle way.[65]

If we further examine polarities, we may see the infinity sign as a whole – the ends are not separate from each other. Even though the ego may pull us out of the middle to one extreme or the other, it's still a whole. So even though we see attraction/aversion, or good/bad, as opposites, in the oneness of reality our spirit is able to see goodness in the bad or bad in the good. Because there is extreme wealth, there is extreme poverty. In the poor, we see the effects and consequences of extreme wealth, while conversely, in extreme wealth we are able to see that because of extreme poverty the resources are pooled in one place. One aspect of Bahá'u'lláh's teaching is intended to reduce the distance between the wealthy and the poor.

Another example of wholeness in polarities may be found in nature: beautiful fruits served on a platter are fragrant, but if they are left out for a day or two will spoil and become smelly compost. Yet in the foul-smelling compost bin lies the potential for the fruit tree to be nourished. Looking at polarities as a whole integrates the mind and preserves us from compartmentalizing our world.

The middle way in relationships

An untrained mind caught in polarity results in absolute thinking, as discussed above. It judges our experiences as good or bad, avoiding things labelled bad or painful, wanting what is good or brings pleasure. Herein lies the vicious cycle of continual suffering. As we can easily observe, this is particularly the case in relationships. Our lack of moderation leads to hurtful situations with one another, especially in the exchange of words. As we have seen above, Bahá'u'lláh gave us a remedy:

> Human utterance is an essence which aspireth to exert its influence and needeth *moderation*. As to its influence, this is conditional upon refinement which in turn is dependent upon hearts which

are detached and pure. As to its moderation, this hath to be *combined with tact and wisdom* as prescribed in the Holy Scriptures and Tablets.

Every word is endowed with a spirit, therefore the speaker or expounder should carefully deliver his words at the appropriate time and place, for the impression which each word maketh is clearly evident and perceptible. The Great Being saith: One word may be likened unto fire, another into light, and the influence which both exert is manifest in the world. Therefore an enlightened man of wisdom should primarily speak with words as mild as milk . . . [66] [emphasis added]

A black and white view of the world causes division. If we examine the following Hidden Word in light of our personal relationships, we could save ourselves a lot of emotional ups and downs:

O Son of Man! Sorrow not save that thou art far from Us. Rejoice not save that thou art drawing near and returning unto Us.[67]

We often are so offended if a friend or spouse has temporarily withdrawn, and are so happy when they want to be with us because we feel wanted and important. These attachments cause emotional swings and can cause a ping-pong affect within the relationship itself.

Sorrow, thou art far
(HATE)

Rejoice, thou art near
(LOVE)

Another path to the middle is balancing justice with compassion, as Shoghi Effendi has pointed out:

A God that is only loving or only just is not a perfect God. The Divinity has to possess both of these aspects as every father ought to express both in his attitude towards his children. If we ponder a while, we will see that our welfare can be insured only when both of these divine attributes are equally emphasized and practised.[68]

I've observed that personal relationships based only on justice or only on compassion stem from a mind swinging from one extreme to another, creating disharmony and unpredictability for the other person. Too much compassion may result in passivity, smiling and being 'nice' when you don't feel like it. Too much justice results in swinging on the pendulum of reward and punishment, being critical one day and complimentary the next, or even nagging. This creates mistrust and apprehension with each other. Balancing justice and compassion creates harmony within the mind, and within the relationship.

Training to prevent our minds from thinking or feeling negative about others is the best protection for our relationships. This is a simple directive, but not easy to carry out. The mind is prone to dwell on what it is not getting and on the faults of the other person, rather than on solutions, which is the middle way. If we regularly use consultation, and balance justice and compassion in our relationships, we can remain in the middle. If each party prefers the other's good, then the relationship is elevated to the divine. This is a vast topic and I have only touched upon it, with the aim of stimulating more dialogue and research.

Work and service in balance

Staying in the middle provides clarity of vision, understanding, and perception. The outcome is wisdom and discernment in thought and action. An example of this perfect balance involves our professional lives and our service to the Faith, which protects us, maintaining sustainability. In a letter written on behalf of Shoghi Effendi, he recommends, 'As you rightly suggest, the middle path, that is to say practising one's profession and also teaching the Cause is the best way for you to follow.'[69]

Obedience as a sunscreen

Just as a good sunscreen protects the skin from harmful rays, so firmness in the Covenant and obedience to Bahá'u'lláh's laws we might define as the best protection one can find for the human mind. This requires, however, the submission and training of the mind. The Western mind has been moving towards humanism for a long time: obedience is not a natural impulse or even admired. It's popular to say that 'religion is for dummies, for those weak-minded people who need to be led'. This view can be easily refuted, but it is nevertheless understandable in today's world, as Adib Taherzadeh comments:

> As the moral and spiritual values in life decline today, a great many people all over the world look upon the word 'obedience' with suspicion and fear. They regard this word to be synonymous with dictatorship, blind acceptance, religious fanaticism and all sorts of fettered beliefs. The majority of those who hold this view are among the honest, open-minded and enlightened peoples of the world . . . A great many people now rebel against the idea of obedience and they are quite justified in doing so. However, when we study the way of life in human society, we note that man wholeheartedly obeys any person or institution that speaks with the voice of truth and has authority to do so. The same person who shuns the word 'obedience' blindly obeys instructions issued from certain authorities in his daily life. For example, a man not knowing the way to a city follows blindly the road signs and never questions their authenticity. The reason for this blind obedience is that he accepts the authority of the body which has placed the signposts. The same is true of a patient who unquestionably obeys his doctor's prescription even to the extent of letting him amputate a limb. Again, this is because he has faith in the physician and accepts his advice without any hesitation.
>
> Obedience is a natural step for man to take provided he finds the truth.[70]

There is an illuminating letter on the subject of obedience from the Universal House of Justice:

> In considering the effect of obedience to the laws on individual lives, one must remember that the purpose of this life is to prepare the soul for the next. Here one must learn to control and direct one's animal impulses, not to be a slave to them. Life in this world is a succession of tests and achievements, of falling short and of making new spiritual advances. Sometimes the course may seem very hard, but one can witness, again and again, that the soul who steadfastly obeys the law of Bahá'u'lláh, however hard it may seem, grows spiritually, while the one who compromises with the law for

the sake of his own apparent happiness is seen to have been following a chimera: he does not attain the happiness he sought, he retards his spiritual advance and often brings new problems upon himself.[71]

Bahá'u'lláh warns us:

> The Lamp of God is burning; take heed, lest the fierce winds of your disobedience extinguish its light. Now is the time to arise and magnify the Lord, your God. Strive not after bodily comforts, and keep your heart pure and stainless.[72]

Like a good sunscreen, obedience protects the mind from the harmful rays of its own vain imaginings and elevating itself. It blocks stubbornness, disobedience and contention, and preserves us from getting burned.

I believe that the Fast offers us a chance to connect with the multiple facets and latent powers of the mind, a chance to discipline it and aid our spiritual progress.

10

RECOMMENDATIONS FOR THE FAST

Since there are no specific recommendations in the Bahá'í teachings for the mind during the Fast, this chapter includes general ideas I use as a healing practitioner that can be applied during this time and which draw on the energies of the Fast. Quotations from the Bahá'í Writings also illuminate some of the key points of healthy living. The actions recommended here can help cleanse the mind of old habits, create integration and wisdom, and continue our efforts to maintain balance throughout the year. They are offered simply as examples, a starting place for your own plan, creativity and ingenuity. The recommendations are framed in different ways to accommodate various learning styles, so there are some overlaps among them. You may wish to take just one or two during each Fast, and build on them every year. New habits take time and patience to integrate into one's lifestyle.

Cleansing and calming our conscious mind

As a health practitioner, I find that the energies of the Fast are conducive to cleansing our mind of old resentments, hurts, traumas or hidden agendas. These tend to be attachments associated with the emotions of hurt, anger or desire, expressing themselves in habits and tendencies. During the Fast we can identify such habits which create suffering and try to eliminate them.

Fasting from negative impressions

The mind is inundated by email, the Internet, television, radio, telephones and mail. This is a good time to question what junk food we allow into our minds. Limiting the amount of time we spend with these influences provides some additional space needed during the Fast to focus on our spiritual growth.

Shoghi Effendi eloquently testified that

> Bahá'ís should seek to be many-sided, normal and well-balanced, mentally and spiritually. We must not give the impression of being fanatics but at the same time we must live up to our principles.[1]

Here are a few ideas for fasting from the many negative influences that bombard us daily.

Select optimal 'nutritional' choices in:
- television, computer, video games, phone calls, books
- exposure to advertisements, even billboards
- radio or talk show programmes, Internet – where do you seek information about the world?'

'Fast' from:
- complaining, giving excuses, gossiping, backbiting
- taking things personally
- assuming you know what others are thinking
- blaming others for your problems
- being separate or superior, wanting control, wanting it your way, wanting attention, and being right
- feelings of anger, passion, ignorance, prejudice, greed, envy, jealousy, resentment, suspicion, insecurity, and defensiveness
- lying
- thinking in absolutes (always, never, every time, everyone)
- expecting the worst
- self-abasement and beating yourself up (should, have to, you must)
- judging / labelling yourself and others

Healing crisis

The practice of refraining, or training the ego, usually leads to resistance, so be prepared. Watch how you react to initial attempts to fast from your usual intake of Internet surfing, television, etc. Ask yourself, 'How do I contribute to this situation?' The resistance will manifest itself in various forms. Just before the mind surrenders, you may find a healing crisis or a climax of discomfort in these forms:

- emotional turmoil
- irritability to influences that don't normally bother you
- mood changes
- anxiety
- depressive feelings
- insomnia
- sleepiness
- nervousness
- sensitivity
- uneasiness, or underlying feeling that something isn't right

During the day, some of these symptoms can be relieved by the use of essential oils. If you are participating in the Fast, you can't eat or drink anything while the sun is up, so here are some alternatives. Lavender oil can be used directly on most skin types. Other essential oils should be used in a carrier oil such as jojoba, coconut, olive or almond. Use one tablespoon of carrier oil to one drop of essential oil. Rub it into the wrists, elbows, soles of the feet. Place one drop of lavender on the temples for a calming effect. Ylang ylang or jasmine can bring about a joyful feeling. Insecurity can be relieved by an essential oil called neroli. Anger and irritation can be soothed by citrus scents such as bergamot, orange or lemon. As a last resort, you can place a dropper full of Bach Rescue Remedy on your tongue to help calm nerves or high anxiety.

As you may remember, some of these symptoms have also appeared in the recommendations for the body in Chapter 7. Some of them arise from the body resisting its cravings, detoxifying itself and resisting its carnal impulses. These symptoms can be exacerbated if you are not getting enough sleep, too. Ensure that you discipline yourself to go to bed early enough to attain enough restful sleep for the next day. Many feel out of sorts during the whole Fast simply because they are not sleeping enough. If symptoms last more than three days, you can identify it as a new symptom. If you have any questions, check with your doctor or psychologist.

Rebuilding the mind

Building intelligence and realigning

A strong mental 'digestion' can withstand many tests. With right thinking and knowledge, we can readily digest our experiences.

- Listen to your inner voices. Listen to others when they talk to you.
- Does your internal dialogue assist you in attaining your divine bounty? Does it reflect divine principles and truths?
- Practise maintaining a state of gentleness and curiosity.
- Build on your strengths and acknowledge them.
- Get organized at home and at work.
- Include stimulation, meaning, and sparks of creativity in your weekly schedule.
- Engage in meaningful, uplifting conversations.
- Challenge your feelings and reactions. Find a way to heal and replace these thought patterns with new healthier responses to your environment.
- Surround yourself with people who build you up.
- Give and receive physical affection.
- Practise focusing the mind in the present. The easiest way is to tune into your five senses: smell, sight, touch, taste, sense.
- Focus on activities listed in Chapter 9 in the sections on nutrition and digestion.
- Get plenty of laughter.

Systematizing conflict and stress management

Choosing the best course of action during conflict helps to eliminate the great stress that conflict produces. In the Writings of Bahá'u'lláh we find the following advice:

> One should not ignore the truth of any matter, rather should one give expression to that which is right and true. The people of Bahá should not deny any soul the reward due to him . . . [2]

In reflecting on this, I conclude that the truth of any matter applies both internally and externally. A clear mind expresses what is right and true, but it is only through prayer and contemplation, consulting the soul, that one can determine what is right and true. Assessing the truth in the situation is the first step. Acknowledge your own responses to the conflict and determine to stick to the truth. Then determine the best response. There is a wide range of possible responses to conflict – from doing nothing to aggressively controlling the situation. Take into consideration your own capacity at the time, how much effort you are willing to put into the stress/conflict, and assess if it's really worth the energy. Consider the limits in others' capacities in the moment as well, and this is harder to assess.

Bahá'u'lláh reassures us, 'Whoso cleaveth to justice, can, under no circumstances, transgress the limits of moderation.'[3] As long as we hold fast to the cord of justice, our actions will be within the bounds of moderation. But we must not become attached to what our mind believes 'justice' looks like, or we will put limits on what the spirit can express in a particular situation. That would leave us inflexible. As always, the Master is our exemplar; he was able to express a wide range of emotions and actions pertaining to justice in various situations.

When we are trying to be kind or compassionate it is often helpful to simply become listeners. Countless people who have finally voiced their concerns and grief to another have experienced relief that they were able to change their situation eventually for the better. Understand that your feelings of discomfort in the moment can indicate a need for change, so don't be too influenced by them.

If there is a particular repeated sticky situation, create some phrases ahead of time, such as 'Can you give me some time to think about that?' This gives you time to process your initial emotional response and gather your thoughts. Don't allow another's emotions or opinions to knock you out of empowerment and clarity. Above all, maintain self-control; communicate with civility and cordiality.

Minimize a wildfire from spreading. Try to let out your strong emotions privately or with the persons involved in the conflict, to minimize the energy surrounding you. Involving others outside the circle only adds fuel to the fire.

Integrating the ego

Self-discipline will integrate our ego, which seeks to separate divide, and constantly create internal emptiness. As 'Abdu'l-Bahá described, 'some souls are ignorant, they must be educated; some are sick, they must be healed; some are still of tender age, they must be helped to attain maturity, and the utmost kindness must be shown to them.'[4]

Keep a state of curiosity and compassionate inquisition into your life. Acknowledge that your thoughts are real, and that they have a physiological effect. When the mind dwells on a thought, it's an indication that our internal processes are divided and need integration. Imagine this internal process as different 'fragments' of the self longing for unity.

Ego can be expressed in exalting ourselves over others, in ambition, in envy. It is also reflected in self-abasing thoughts and unworthiness, or indulging in shame. In particular, the Western mind is prone to this self-bashing, overly critical internal dialogue that paralyses our spiritual growth. Creating an internal dialogue that reflects the God-given nobility of human beings and is conducive to spiritual growth is an essential tool. Bahá'u'lláh confirms this in the Hidden Words: 'I created thee rich, why dost thou bring thyself down to poverty? Noble I made thee, wherewith dost thou abase thyself?'[5] Again He admonishes us to 'Hear no evil, and see no evil, abase not thyself, neither sigh and weep.'[6]

We must overlook our weaknesses and submit the reins to God. 'Abdu'l-Bahá tells us: 'One must never consider one's own feebleness, it is the strength of the Holy Spirit of Love, which gives the power . . . the thought of our own weakness could only bring despair,'[7] while Shoghi Effendi 'strongly urges you not to dwell on yourself. Each one of us, if we look into our failures, is sure to feel unworthy and despondent, and this feeling only frustrates our constructive efforts and wastes time.'[8]

While our spiritual growth is dependent upon knowing our own selves – our weaknesses, strengths, and our true station – the trick is not to indulge them; I have found that this is the middle path. Bahá'u'lláh admonishes us, 'Be not careless of the virtues with which ye have been endowed, neither be neglectful of your high destiny.'[9] The station of the true believer in this day is great indeed, He writes:

> Such is the station ordained for the true believer that if to an extent smaller than a needle's eye the glory of that station were to be unveiled

> to mankind, every beholder would be consumed away in his longing to attain it. For this reason it hath been decreed that in this earthly life the full measure of the glory of his own station should remain concealed from the eyes of such a believer . . . If the veil be lifted, and the full glory of the station of those who have turned wholly towards God, and in their love for Him renounced the world, be made manifest, the entire creation would be dumbfounded.[10]

With such reassurance, we must try to overcome our faults but not dwell on them, and keep our minds turned towards the kingdom, drawing down the power of the Holy Spirit.

The essential quality of integrating the ego is to become aware of what you do and think, and then learn to stay present through it. When your mind focuses on the 'story' and spins out negatively, embrace the fact that that's where you are and interrupt the thought by recognizing it as the mind generating 'noise'. Drop down into the body and connect to the energy associated with these thoughts. Sit with this energy and feel compassion for where you are. Repeated negative thoughts are simply well-established fear-based habits or anger habits created in the brain as neural pathways. When you are attached to something or are sensitive about someone's comments and you struggle, it's important to look at the root of the attachment and your suffering, to stay present without pushing it away or closing off. If you can learn to stay with your own suffering gently, you will eventually integrate the ego. It will be more difficult to buy into the ego's lies as well. If you don't deal with it, it will become a monster.

Spiritual progress is dependent upon discipline, effort and striving, while love is dependent upon attraction and is magnetic. The mind has the power to work in both realms. This is where the rider can lovingly take care of the horse without letting the horse be in control or whipping it relentlessly for a few mistakes. Some self-reflecting questions to help us rise to our station might include: What would I do/say/think if I were in the presence of Bahá'u'lláh? Does this response draw me nearer to God? If I follow this thought, or this action, what will be the result? In a couple of years? When the mind is stuck, we can use the techniques listed in Table 10.1, balancing the yin (feminine) and yang (masculine) energies. (Bear in mind that these are simply my personal recommendations; the concepts of yin and yang are not part of the Bahá'í teachings.)

Table 10.1 What to do when the mind is stuck

Energy	Technique	Detail
Yin	Give it a voice	Sit in a quiet and undisturbed place. Turn towards the part of you experiencing pain or discomfort and acknowledge, validate it. Feelings are real, no matter how 'silly' they may seem. Sit with compassion and allow the feeling to express itself until it empties its cup. There will be a physical response to this – a sigh, a shifting of posture. Acknowledge how painful or difficult the circumstances are. Recognize the self's current capacity in the present moment.
Yin	Nurture and reassure	After the cup is empty, embrace this painful part of self and feel love and compassion. These thoughts represent fragments of hurts, impressions or emotional shocks, often in our past. Healing comes when the rational mind practises gentleness and mercy to the self. If a child gets hurt, you would stop and care for it, holding it as long as it needed to be held – do the same for yourself.
Yang	Education	After nurturing, empower the self with education. Take responsibility for the change required. Internal processes require a barometer to hold our actions up to some measurement. The barometer for the ego is the will of God, found in the sacred writings. When the brain produces irrational thoughts, the rational faculty can reeducate it with these teachings and redirect our actions. Reflect on your past actions, make a new plan and try to implement it.
Yang	Discipline	Once a fragmented thought has been expressed, acknowledged, nurtured and reeducated, discipline is required to prevent any injustices from reoccurring. If they choose to return (like complaining), *gentle but firm* discipline is required. These negative thought patterns can paralyse us into destructive habits. When thoughts are allowed to fester, they can act like badly behaved children. A strong will is required to overcome the impulses of reliving the past.
Yin/Yang	Prayer and striving	Shoghi Effendi said that to try is to persevere. Call on the Kingdom for continual help. A continual process of victory, crisis, prayer and striving, patience and endurance steadies growth and draws the confirmations of the Kingdom.

Rewriting core beliefs

Challenging our core beliefs is part of creating a healthier way of thinking, in alignment with the divine will. Our actions tend to be grounded in auto-pilot programmes or core beliefs that were developed by our inherited tendencies through genetics and by our early environments. The behaviours we witnessed then have influenced how we act today. Unless there was a traumatic event or specific life experience that persuaded us NOT to act in a certain way, humans have a tendency to have patent responses to their environments. This is not living consciously or intentionally. Figure 10.1 is a diagram of typical daily programming.

Figure 10.1 Actions on auto-pilot

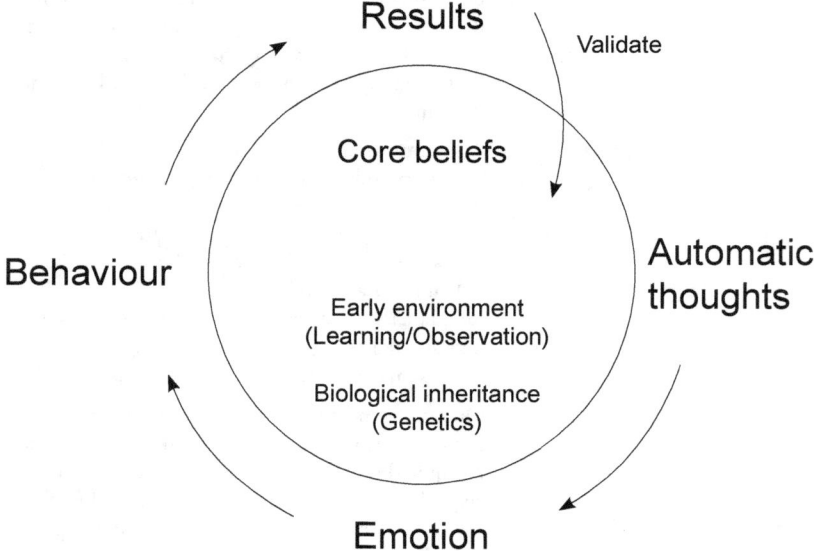

When we encounter an event in the external world, we have an automatic thought that responds. This thought is associated with an emotion, which ultimately affects our actions. The result is to keep us safe by self-validating our core beliefs (this person always makes me mad, that political party is wrong, etc.).

Living more intentionally is dependent upon open-mindedness in reviewing the truth and facts about an event. It also involves challenging our automatic responses. When your mind is in the present moment, you will have an awareness of how you are responding to a situation, by your emotional quality. However, if your mind is somewhere else, you will be aware of the emotions faster than the thoughts. The emotional power will prompt you for a patent behaviour because it's a physiological response at the cellular level.

Figure 10.2   Searching for truth

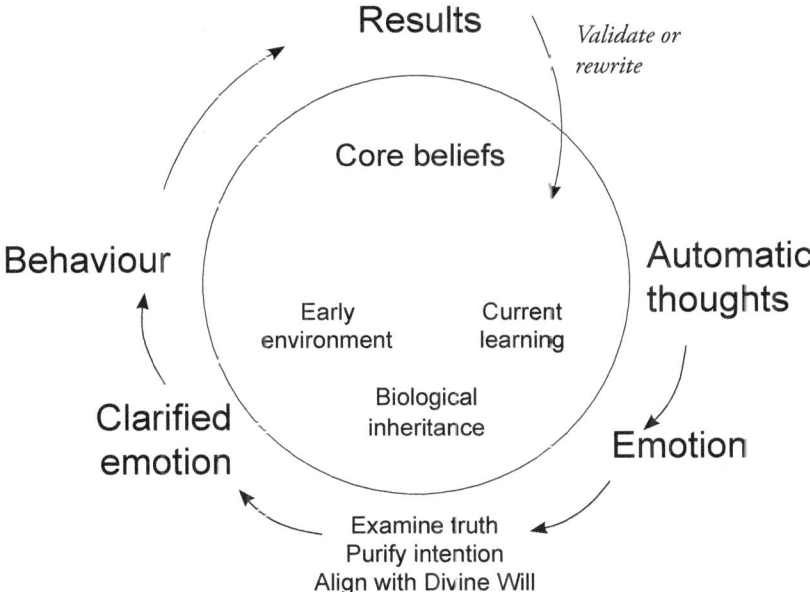

Developing a habit of searching for the truth of the situation (assessing the accuracy of your perceptions) is helpful. Do the best you can in the moment. Under heated emotions, it's good to take as much time as possible, and revisit when you've cooled down. Find out what your intentions are in the situation, ensuring that you are coming from a place of pure intent. Research the Writings, and a *clarified emotional* quality will be associated with these thoughts. Clarified emotions often bring relief to the initial emotional response, not necessarily replacing it. Remember, anger is sometimes warranted in unjust situations and is a call to action. Moving beyond the anger is the trick.

Actions based upon this model will lead to spiritual growth and healthier patterns of thinking. When developed as a habit, you will find your core belief systems re-analysed over time and your 'automated thoughts' will be updated eventually through a series of crises and victories. Biological and God-given personality traits never totally disintegrate, but can be transformed into more healthy patterns of action and ways of perceiving the world.

Specific conditions

In my practice I see many people who sense something is wrong with them, who have pain that moves from one spot to another or changeable symptoms that can't be identified by medical standards. I interpret this as an imbalance of the system and early warning signs of a deeper condition of the organism that will eventually express itself as a disease. Friends, family or healthcare practitioners can sometimes tend to dismiss these symptoms, particularly in the early stages. Contemplating how the behaviour of the organism can change at a cellular level enables us to see how thoughts and emotions affect our body in various ways, including our heart rate and immunity levels. We see an increasing number of studies, for instance on the relationship of forgiveness and blood pressure.[11]

When treating the whole person, two concepts on how thoughts relate to disease are particularly important. First, wrong thinking in itself cannot bring on a horrible disease. Negative thinking can be related to an imbalance in the system or a shock experienced earlier in life – therefore, an expression of the present diseased state. Thinking positive thoughts to combat this will produce few effective and lasting results. It's a great start, but doing only positive thinking merely palliates the situation; additional work is required. Second, the imagination can affect the body to a great extent. Some clients come in imagining themselves to be sick, and this can bring on a mild illness. These illnesses can often be cured through correcting the wrong thinking, bringing in another perspective, or through reassurance and prayer. A skilled practitioner will need to discern between the two conditions, because they present themselves similarly.

No soul is exempt from illness; it is one of the tests and bounties offered from the Kingdom. Even the most holy souls become ill; this is not a reflection of their mind, but is an imbalance in the physical world. The most unproductive question in illness is 'why?' Instead, we can focus on the opportunity or gift the disease presents, and how to use the power of the mind and emotions to transform ourselves. When the body becomes imbalanced, we can contemplate the symbolic nature of that condition. What part of the body is affected and what is its purpose? In this way, the body reveals what lies hidden in the mind.

Some examples of specific conditions

One of the assignments I often give clients is to answer the question, 'Who is talking?' For example, if you say, 'I'm hungry,' who is talking? The physical body itself could have multiple parts expressing hunger – the brain on low blood sugar, or the stomach that feels empty. 'I'm hungry' could also be the mind expressing boredom and wanting entertainment. It could also be expressing a deeper emotion of emptiness that needs nurturing and feeding. One simple phrase can mean different things.

If you think of your body as your best friend trying to convey a message to you to pay attention, one of the ways of hearing that friend is by analysing what the body part does, its symbolic nature, and then equate it to the internal imbalance of the mind that accompanies physical ailments. They are both an expression of the diseased state of the entire organism. For example, I see people who have a lot of wonderful ideas yet never put them into action. Years later, this same situation may be found in their bowels: they have many urges yet nothing comes out! Both mind and body are expressing the essence of the disease in different ways.

The following examples are some of the most common ailments affecting mind and body. If you suffer from them, ask yourself some of the related questions:

Allergies: The symbolic nature of allergies is to resist something in the environment. What am I so irritated about? How can I accept myself more fully? Is there someone/something I'm 'allergic' to?

Anxiety: Anxiety bleeds our energy into the future. It's a lack of trust; it is fear-based thinking, causing stagnation and imprisonment. Why don't I trust life's process? What is stuck in my past? Am I really being threatened? Am I afraid of new ideas?

Back pain: The back carries a lot of weight, supports the body and is energetically connected to relationships, money and love. We often hear the phrase, 'Get off my back!' What weight am I carrying? How can I become more secure about my finances? How can I bring more love and support into my life?

Cancer: Cancer cells no longer acquiesce to the greater mind. The cells multiply and masquerade so that the immune system overlooks them. What grief can I process? What hidden grievances can I forgive? Am I acting authentically, or putting on a mask? Am I caretaking, overdoing things? Have I lost hope? Can I let go of controlling life?

Chronic pain: Chronic conditions haunt society, representing resistance to a high-paced lifestyle and constant changes. The condition in the body and the thoughts that go with it are stuck. What unresolved needs do I need to fulfil? How do I punish myself? How can I be more flexible and accept change?

Chronic fatigue: Feeling tired all the time and unable to interact normally represents resistance to something. Symbolically we could be avoiding something. How am I resisting my future? How can I relieve boredom? (I don't want to do/face _____)

Colds and flu: These are temporary setbacks, or signs that we are overdoing it. How can I use moderation? When can I provide the rest and relaxation I need?

Depression: Symbolically we are spiritually bleeding into the past, lamenting, or regretting. Depression often hides anger. Does my depression allow me to avoid facing something? What is my hopelessness? How can I give myself permission to feel? How can I expand my perceptions? Am I angry with myself because I have not dealt with a situation or person?

Heart disease: The heart loves, nourishes, nurtures, expresses spiritual emotions and processes the lower emotions. Our language speaks to illness: I have a 'broken heart' or 'my heart is heavy'. How can I bring joy into my life? How can I keep my heart open? In what ways can I soften my heart and not be so rigid? How can I process my emotions past and present?

Indigestion/gas: Symbolically, something is not sitting right; there is resistance to accepting something. Our language conveys the mind's connection to the gut: 'I can't digest that.' 'That feels like a punch in the gut.' 'My stomach is in knots.' How can I help my mind better digest ideas and events? In what ways can I move my heart into trust rather than fear?

Inflammation/swelling: 'I'm all heated up' – unprocessed emotions that are stuck, anger that is fear-based. How can I be more peaceful in my thinking? In what healthy ways can I express my anger? How can I move any stuck or congested idea(s)?

Insomnia: Sleep is how we nurture, restore and rejuvenate ourselves. It is at night that we process the day. Deprivation of sleep interrupts life at a deep level. What/who don't I trust? What do I need to control? Have I put too much on my plate? Can I learn to say 'no'?

Rashes: Redness symbolizes irritation, resentment, repressed anger, frustration. How can I better manage my feelings of irritation? What am I attached to? What emotions have I repressed? Am I mad I'm not getting my way?

Weight gain: Putting on weight allows us to add another layer to who we are, hiding the vulnerable part or filling up emptiness. What do I need to cover? How can I take responsibility for my boredom? What anger can I release? How can I embrace who I am, including my soul?

PART IV

THE SOUL

11

FASTING FOR SPIRITUAL PURPOSES

> The highest station destined for man is to be illumined by the 'spirit of faith', which comes through recognition of the Manifestation of God for the age and through obedience to His commandments. To attain this station is the very purpose for which God created man.
> *Adib Taherzadeh*[1]

The following chapters reflect my current understanding of the workings of the soul from my study of the Bahá'í Writings. However, we are trying to understand something we cannot fully understand and so I shall be drawing on several different kinds of metaphor. We are striving to manifest the invisible in this material realm. How can words explain the invisible? Think of how truly challenging it is to explain even a spiritual experience.

Parts II and III have discussed qualities associated with the mind and body. The soul cannot be wholly separated from the discussion, for body, mind and soul are as three expressions of one reality: a human being. The soul is the animating force of the body and can observe its manifestations. However, these mere reflections and shadows can never fully reveal the true nature of the soul, because Bahá'u'lláh says the soul is a 'mystery, a sign of the revelation of God'.

From the Bahá'í Writings we understand that, unlike the mind and body, the soul is exempt from decline. Bahá'u'lláh tells us:

> Verily I say, the human soul is exalted above all egress and regress. It is still, and yet it soareth; it moveth, and yet it is still. It is, in itself, a testimony that beareth witness to the existence of a world that is contingent, as well as to the reality of a world that hath neither beginning nor end.[2]

The soul is also exempt from maladies and sickness. Bahá'u'lláh says a sick person shows signs of weakness because of the 'hindrances that interpose themselves between his soul and his body, for the soul itself remaineth unaffected by any bodily ailments'.[3] The soul is always intact, regardless of the condition of the body and the mind. It is the animating force of the body, and can enlighten the mind.

From this, we may conclude that the problem arises when there is some kind of impediment between the soul and the body. Spiritual illness results in many conditions: apathy, estrangement, contention, pride, Covenant-breaking, and many others. It's a condition of a 'mistunement' between the soul and the body. These conditions have also been pointed out in the Writings of Bahá'u'lláh as barriers to unity. There are many gems of mysteries and laws revealed in the Revelation of Bahá'u'lláh that *finely tune* the soul to the body and cause our spiritual progress while we are here on earth. For example, 'Abdu'l-Bahá said that prayer is one of the means used to heal spiritual illness. These laws and gems are the things to focus on for spiritual health.

Bahá'u'lláh's laws also enable our soul to recognize, draw nearer and worship God by 'carrying forward an ever-advancing civilization' in this life. And we also need to acquire the forces necessary for the next life – these constitute 'health' for the soul as well. The soul is 'the first among all created things to declare the excellence of its Creator, the first to recognize His glory, to cleave to His truth, and to bow down in adoration before Him'.[4]

'Abdu'l-Bahá said that the soul is not of this world or any substance of it, but made up from an indivisible single substance. It 'has neither entered this body nor existed through it'.[5] It is like the wind. We cannot see the wind, yet we know it's there because we see evidences of it and the results of it.

'Abdu'l-Bahá offers a beautiful analogy of the human condition:

> like that of a ship which is moved by the power of the wind or steam; if this power ceases, the ship cannot move at all. Nevertheless, the rudder of the ship turns it to either side, and the power of the steam moves it in the desired direction . . . in all the action or inaction of man, he receives power from the help of God; but the choice of good or evil belongs to the man himself.[6]

Reading this, I am encouraged to try continue the analogy:
- The ship is like the body.
- The wind is the Holy Spirit and God's assistance.
- The captain is the mind, deciding the best course of action.
- The instrument panel is like the Covenant guiding us where to steer the ship.
- The weight of the cargo is our ego, attachments, our insistent self.
- The engine of the ship is faith and love, desire to serve.

Relationship of the soul and body: Rider and horse work together

In Parts II and III we have referred several times to 'Abdu'l-Bahá's metaphor of the rider and its relation to the horse:

> The spirit, or human soul, is the rider; and the body is only the steed.[7]

Anyone experienced with horses knows that *balance and unity* give the best ride. The intention to unify the horse and rider, body and soul, is imperative when it comes to spiritually progressing. The Fast provides the opportunity to do this.

The spirit is predisposed to virtue, while the material is predisposed to ignorance and desire. When the rational mind turns towards God, it struggles to control the soul. When it succeeds in directing the rider, the soul becomes attuned to the divine, but if it is the ego that makes the decisions the soul becomes corrupt and inclined to the material world. It is through this relationship that free will is exercised, that choices are made in response to external impressions and experiences. When the mind chooses forgiveness over resentment, the soul has an opportunity to progress.

As we saw in Part III, the mind brings the unknown into the known, the hidden into the light of day. The mind acquires knowledge through the perception of the senses. The soul, on the other hand, acquires knowledge through prayer, meditation, dreams, intuition, inspiration and imagination. While the mind is restricted by information coming from the material world, the soul has unlimited potential and is free from any earthly hindrance in acquiring information. The mind, however, can assist the soul and work with the heart to reflect spiritual qualities into this life. 'Abdu'l-Bahá explains:

> The outward powers are five: the power of sight, of hearing, of taste, of smell and of feeling.
> The inner powers are also five: the common faculty, and the powers of imagination, thought, comprehension and memory.[8]

The soul also contains the outer powers. For example, while we are asleep the auditory nerve may be motionless, but we still hear. Our eyes may be closed, but we still see and have vision. This reflects the beautiful similarity of the rider and the horse because they both have the outer senses. They both have eyes, but use them to process information differently. The horse needs to learn to submit to the rider's discretion and judgement.

Happiness is attained when the rider and horse achieve unity and balance. Happiness is a spiritual state; 'Abdu'l-Bahá is reported to have said that it is 'dependent upon the susceptibilities of the heart and the attitude of the mind'.[9] Therefore, when the soul receives the purity of the mind it is free from ego, and in turn, the soul will share with the mind divine mysteries and realities from the spiritual world.

The soul's beginning

We learn from the Writings that the soul emanates from the worlds of God and comes into existence at the time of conception. The fertilized egg becomes a magnet, attracting the soul like the light in a mirror, reflecting it into creation. The infant gradually acquires the capacity of manifesting its spirit; its body becomes the instrument by which the soul's qualities may be expressed. The soul receives virtues and bounties from the Holy Spirit and gives them to the body, similar to the process where our senses take information and give it to the inner faculties to be deposited into memory, to be utilized later. The soul can act without the body, like vision without eyes, hearing without ears, but it also functions through the various organs of the body. The seat of the soul is in the heart – the container of the Revelation, just as the seat of the mind is in the brain, but not found in the brain. 'Abdu'l-Bahá confirms this:

... the mind has no place, but it is connected with the brain. The Kingdom is also like this. In the same way love has no place, but it is connected with the heart; so the Kingdom has no place, but is connected with man.[10]

Pre-ordained capacity of the soul

Bahá'u'lláh tells us, 'Unto each one hath been prescribed a pre-ordained measure, as decreed in God's mighty and guarded Tablets.'[11] Each soul has a pre-ordained capacity and its own individual uniqueness – just as in nature there are also no repetitions. In physics, we see that the universe doesn't usually manifest perfect symmetry. Slightly imperfect symmetries make the world organized and more pleasing to the eye.

The soul contains latent potential for virtues. Children show various capacities and personalities, even in the womb. These differences are not attributed to good or evil, but simply to differences in degree. Even though each one of us has varying gifts, each soul is equally capable of manifesting all the attributes of God. 'Abdu'l-Bahá describes differences in personality:

> Personality is of two kinds. One is the natural or God-given personality which the western thinkers call individuality, the inner aspect of man which *is not subject to change*; and the other personality *is the result of acquired arts, sciences and virtues* with which man is decorated. When the God-given virtues are thus adorned, we have character . . . It is evident that we have two modes for the expression of life, – individuality and personality, – the former becomes as the son of God and the latter the son of man. As we have shown, the personality of some is illumined, that of others is dark . . . the personality of man is developed through education, while his individuality which is divine and heavenly should be his guide.[12] [emphasis added]

This inborn unique individuality and inherently good qualities largely depend upon how we express that individuality. Tendencies and character can change, depending upon our education, training and experiences.

Purpose of the soul's existence in this world

In discussing the various gifts given to humanity, Bahá'u'lláh tells us that the greatest of these is perception and understanding, so that each soul has the capacity to know and recognize God:

> Know thou that, according to what thy Lord, the Lord of all men, hath decreed in His Book, the favours vouchsafed by Him unto mankind have been, and will ever remain, limitless in their range. First and foremost among these favours, which the Almighty hath conferred upon man, is the *gift of understanding*. His purpose in conferring such a gift is none other except to enable His creature to know and recognize the one true God – exalted be His glory. This gift giveth man the power to discern the truth in all things, leadeth him to that which is right, and helpeth him to discover the secrets of creation. Next in rank, is the power of vision, the chief instrument whereby his understanding can function. The senses of hearing, of the heart, and the like, are simlilarly to be reckoned among the gifts with which the human body is endowed.[13] [emphasis added]

Our priorities in this life are to know and worship God and prepare for the next life. Bahá'u'lláh informs us that

> The Prophets and Messengers of God have been sent down for the sole purpose of guiding mankind to the straight Path of Truth. The purpose underlying their revelation hath been to educate all men, that they may, at the hour of death, ascend, in the utmost purity and sanctity and with absolute detachment, to the throne of the Most High.[14]

Our preparation for the next life is compared to the child in the womb. The embryo develops organs and senses to use when it is born, i.e. ears, lungs, eyes. These faculties are specifically developed for life outside the womb without the child realizing their true purpose. This infant also has a 'veil': it is unable to see the world in which it is to be born, yet it has sensations from all the life going on outside its mother's womb.

When 'Abdu'l-Bahá was asked what the purpose of our lives is, he answered, 'To acquire virtues.'[15] After the child is born it must develop the virtues and perfections that are required for the heavenly Kingdom.

Those faculties, like faith, will only be realized, fully utilized, once we are born into the next life. 'Abdu'l-Bahá discusses this next life, the 'real world':

> Know thou that the Kingdom is the real world, and this nether place is only its shadow stretching out. A shadow hath no life of its own; its existence is only a fantasy, and nothing more; it is but images reflected in water, and seeming as pictures to the eye.[16]

This life is like a school for our training:

> Out of the wastes of nothingness, with the clay of My command I made thee to appear, and have ordained for thy training every atom in existence and the essence of all created things.[17]

Capacity and readiness are a requisite for spiritual growth. Each soul has a natural *inborn capacity* and an *acquired capacity*. The acquired capacity changes through training and education, through sciences and arts, through conscious effort, through striving and sincerity: 'All that which ye potentially possess can, however, be manifested only as a result of your own volition. Your own acts testify to this truth,' writes Bahá'u'lláh,[18] and again makes it clear that 'Success or failure, gain or loss, must, therefore, depend upon man's own exertions . . . The greater the effort exerted . . . the more faithfully will it [the soul] be made to reflect the glory of the names and attributes of God.'[19] 'Abdu'l-Bahá is reported to have said:

> Without capacity and readiness, the divine bestowal will not become manifest and evident . . . Therefore, we must develop capacity in order that the signs of the mercy of the Lord may be revealed in us. We must endeavour to free the soil of the hearts from useless weeds and sanctify it from the thorns of worthless thoughts in order that the cloud of mercy may bestow its power upon us.[20]

'Abdu'l-Bahá clarifies that we are not responsible for our *inborn* capacity, but our acquired capacity is where we'll be held accountable. For example, a flower is not blameworthy because its inborn capacity is not an animal and cannot display the qualities of an animal. But it is a pity if it does not reach its acquired capacity as a flower – growing, blooming, and providing nectar.

> But the material beings are not despised, judged and held responsible for their own degree and station. For example, mineral, vegetable and animal in their various degrees are acceptable; but if in their own degree they remain imperfect, they are blamable, the degree itself being purely perfect.
> The differences among mankind are of two sorts: one is a difference of station, and this difference is not blameworthy. The other is a difference of faith and assurance; the loss of these is blameworthy, for then the soul is overwhelmed by his desires and passions, which deprive him of these blessings and prevent him from feeling the power of attraction of the love of God. Though that man is praiseworthy and acceptable in his station, yet as he is deprived of the perfections of that degree, he will become a source of imperfections, for which he is held responsible.[21]

While we are acquiring capacity in this life we experience tests, just as a school tests a student's readiness. This is paralleled in physics. When something begins motion it meets immediate resistance, for instance air resistance. Tests and difficulties for the human being arise when the soul recognizes its Creator and begins its spiritual growth. When we make efforts to love God and serve Him, we will be tested. Growth stems out of our suffering, but Bahá'u'lláh reassures us that 'God hath never burdened any soul beyond its power'.[22]

'The mind and spirit of man advance when he is tried by suffering. The more the ground is ploughed the better the seed will grow, the better the harvest will be,' said 'Abdu'l-Bahá.[23] Difficulties lead us to search for spiritual meaning and encourage us to engage in constructive behaviour. Shoghi Effendi explains:

> Failures, tests and trials, if we use them correctly, can become the means of purifying our spirit, strengthening our characters, and enable us to rise to greater heights of service.[24]

The soul is tested through various means; among the most common are health, relationships, children, finances and faith. Of these five,

'Abdu'l-Bahá mentioned ill-health as being the most difficult to endure. Some tests are a result of man's choices, his free will; God's foreknowledge of events does not cause them: 'The trials of man are of two kinds. (a) the consequences of his own actions . . . (b) other sufferings there are, which come upon the Faithful of God.'[25]

Shoghi Effendi said that there are tests for punishment and tests for educational purposes; there are accidents, and there is cause and effect.

> Suffering is both a reminder and a guide . . . In every suffering one can find a meaning and a wisdom. But it is not always easy to find the secret of that wisdom. It is sometimes only when all our suffering has passed that we become aware of its usefulness.[26]

'Abdu'l-Bahá summarizes these ideas:

> The more one is severed from the world, from desires, from human affairs, and conditions, the more impervious does one become to the tests of God. Tests are a means by which a soul is measured as to its fitness, and proven out by its own acts. God knows its fitness beforehand, and also its unpreparedness, but man, with an ego, would not believe himself unfit unless proof were given him. Consequently his susceptibility to evil is proven to him when he falls into the tests, and the tests are continued until the soul realizes its own unfitness, then remorse and regret tend to root out the weakness.
>
> The same test comes again in greater degree, until it is shown that a former weakness has become a strength, and the power to overcome evil has been established.[27]

The cycle of spiritual growth

The horse and rider must endure these tests in life in order to progress. From my own work with clients, I find that most tests appear to result from one's own actions. We are immersed in a tumultuous world where cultural influences, temptations, distractions, confusion and little resolution to practical problems compound the test. I often see a test as a result of the state of the world, and the client's ego adds a mountain of emotion to the test because he or she becomes trapped in the illusion of resolution or in other traps. Our own worst enemy is within ourselves.

Spiritual growth can be cyclical, as reflected in the quotation from 'Abdu'l-Bahá's reported words in the quotation above. It's also reflected in creation. Just as a flower opens with the light of morning and closes with the fading light of evening, spiritual growth ebbs and flows as well. Even the changing seasons prove that cycles are inherent to material life. We encounter tests and difficulties and learn many lessons rapidly. With reflection, we can harvest the skills learned while we were enduring the test. We then enter a period of time where things seem to 'even out'. This is an indication of the opportunity to apply the skills we've learned to creating a new habit and integrating it into our memory. At the end of this cycle, our minds begin to look for the 'next thing', which is an indication of intuitive knowledge of the next 'training period' beginning soon.

Spiritual development is an organic cyclical process obtained through victory and crisis. Intimate relationships between humans flow like this as well, because they centre around the heart. The heart centre, like a lotus flower, opens and closes depending upon the situation one is in. When we are with people we consider friends, our hearts open. When we are in the company of strangers or those we'd consider enemies, our hearts close. It's no wonder 'Abdu'l-Bahá exhorted us to see none as strangers. When we experience joy or pain in our closest relationships, it is the soul that is affected:

> If we are caused joy or pain by a friend, if a love prove true or false, it is the soul that is affected. If our dear ones are far from us – it is the soul that grieves, and the grief or trouble of the soul may react on the body.
>
> Thus, when the spirit is fed with holy virtues, then is the body joyous; if the soul falls into sin, the body is in torment!
>
> When we find truth, constancy, fidelity, and love, we are happy; but if we meet with lying, faithlessness, and deceit, we are miserable.[28]

There is further discussion of this later in this chapter, in the section 'A metaphor for the soul reflected in biology'.

After death: Separation of the soul from the mind and body

The cycle of spiritual growth continues after death. Since the soul acts in the physical world through the help of the body, when the body dies the relationship between the soul and body disintegrates. The soul itself, on the other hand, cannot suffer disintegration or destruction. Bahá'u'lláh assures us that 'it will endure as long as the Kingdom of God, His sovereignty, His dominion and power will endure',[29] and that

> If the soul of man hath walked in the ways of God, it will, assuredly, return and be gathered to the glory of the Beloved . . . It shall attain a station such as no pen can depict, or tongue describe. The soul that hath remained faithful to the Cause of God, and stood unwaveringly firm in His Path shall, after his ascension, be possessed of such power that all the worlds which the Almighty hath created can benefit through him. Such a soul provideth, at the bidding of the Ideal King and Divine Educator, the pure leaven that leaveneth the world of being, and furnisheth the power through which the arts and wonders of the world are made manifest.[30]

Bahá'u'lláh tells us that a soul 'sanctified from the vain imaginings of the peoples of the world . . . liveth and moveth in accordance with the Will of its Creator.'[31] And 'Abdu'l-Bahá is reported to have said:

> Those who have passed on through death, have a sphere of their own. *It is not removed from ours*; their work, the work of the Kingdom, is ours; but it is sanctified from what we call 'time and place'. Time with us is measured by the sun. When there is no more sunrise, and no more sunset, that kind of time does not exist for man. Those who have ascended have different attributes from those who are still on earth, yet there is no real separation.[32] [emphasis added]

The most frequent question I receive from clients about the loss of a loved one is if they will see them again, and how long it may take after death to see them. 'Abdu'l-Bahá answered that 'this would depend upon the respective stations of the two. If both had the same degree of development, they would be re-united immediately after death.'[33] He further reassures us:

The difference and distinction between men will naturally become realized after their departure from this mortal world. But this distinction is not in respect to place, but in respect to the soul and conscience. For the Kingdom of God is sanctified (or free) from time and place; it is another world and another universe . . . And know thou for a certainty that in the divine worlds the spiritual beloved ones will recognize one another, and will seek union with each other, but a spiritual union. Likewise a love that one may have entertained for anyone will not be forgotten in the world of the Kingdom, nor wilt thou forget there the life that thou hadst in the material world.[34]

The soul's infinite journey

Bahá'u'lláh assures us:

When the soul attaineth the Presence of God, it will assume the form that best befitteth its immortality and is worthy of its celestial habitation. Such an existence is a contingent and not an absolute existence, inasmuch as the former is preceded by a cause, whilst the latter is independent thereof. Absolute existence is strictly confined to God, exalted be His glory.[35]

Some of the comments made by 'Abdu'l-Bahá create a sense of wonder:

The outer expression used for the Kingdom is heaven; but this is a comparison and similitude, not a reality or fact, for the Kingdom is not a material place; it is sanctified from time and place. It is a spiritual world, a divine world, and the centre of the Sovereignty of God.[36]

But the paradise and hell of existence are found in all the worlds of God, whether in this world or in the spiritual heavenly worlds.[37]

Even in the physical world, modern science acknowledges unseen dimensions and parallel universes within them. Einstein's theory of relativity acknowledges a fourth dimension and explains that energy and matter curve space and time. This theory indicates that matter and energy are manifestations of the same force, just as light can act as a wave or a particle. Lisa Randall, in her book *Warped Passages*, acknowledges that science speculates that other dimensions include folds and warps, so that they escape detection. Some studies suggest that we may be closer than we thought to infinite versions of our own world in parallel worlds – even down to millimetres apart; that these other worlds contain space, time and other forms of matter, and that we just happen to live in one of these dimensions. Science is beginning to examine the existence of these worlds through mathematical equations and theorizing.

We find in Bahá'u'lláh's Writings references to 'worlds besides this world', although we cannot know whether Bahá'u'lláh was referring to the idea of 'parallel universes' briefly outlined above:

> Know thou of a truth that the worlds of God are countless in their number, and infinite in their range . . . Verily I say, the creation of God embraceth worlds besides this world, and creatures apart from these creatures. In each of these worlds He hath ordained things which none can search except Himself, the All-Searching, the All-Wise.[38]

However, science cannot explain the mystery of the soul, nor has it yet explained the 'essential reality' of these physical phenomena, as 'Abdu'l-Bahá eloquently testifies:

> When we consider the world of existence, we find that the essential reality underlying any given phenomenon is unknown. Phenomenal, or created, things are known to us only by their attributes.[39]

The most important evidence emerging in the field of physics is the 'unified principle.' Many physicists are coming to the conclusion that the natural world, its diverse and distinct phenomena, is actually governed by a single set of physical laws. This clearly parallels the truth in the Writings of divine unity of all things.

Divine unity and its mysteries can be known by human beings only metaphorically, through the symbolism in the world of creation. Some interesting analogies can be found in the sciences. In mathematics, the nonlinear, ironically, is the 'straight path': nonlinear equations are fundamental because nature produces curves. The Einstein equation was nonlinear; it described the curvature of the universe. Climate also isn't linear, for when the wind blows stronger in one region, another is immediately affected. In economics, tables are usually presented and described in linear ways, but the market fluctuates just as the weather does. These truths revealed in nature and in human affairs might teach us that the straight path in our spiritual life will have many 'curve balls'. We may therefore conclude that the unity of all things is reflected in the truth that when one is affected, all are affected.

Though time appears to pass in a linear fashion, upon closer examination we can see that it really moves in spheres. In working with people over the last couple of decades, I've observed that we seem to evolve in layers: although the core of us, our inborn capacity and individuality (our essence) are constant, the changeable variable is our acquired capacity developed through our choices. It's as though we orbit around a pivotal point. In Part III we used the concept of polarities to describe how we attain the middle path; the diagram of the infinity symbol could also apply to our spiritual cycles or relationships, as described earlier. As on a pendulum, sometimes we are in and then out, close and then far. I find clients sometimes in the 'in-between' spaces, or feeling lost. This means they are on the outermost edge, the furthest point, and it brings feelings of apathy and estrangement. Anything associated with the heart can have a movement similar to the one shown in Figure 11.1.

Figure 11.1 The movement of spiritual proress

Our life path orbits around a pivotal point, the soul. Our individuality is at the core, and our actions, or acquired capacity, will revolve around it. As for time passage, this diagram shows our childhood as the centre. As we age, we revolve around core issues.

A metaphor for the soul reflected in biology

In examining the Bahá'í texts written by the Báb and Bahá'u'lláh we can see the high station accorded to the heart. In his book *Gate of the Heart*, Nader Saiedi comments:

The concept of 'heart' (*fu'ád*) is one of the most important principles in the writings of the Báb. The station of the heart is the highest stage of created being's existential reality. It is the reflection of divine revelation itself within the inmost reality of things.[40]

Here are a few of Bahá'u'lláh's statements on this theme:

> The spirit that animateth the human heart is the knowledge of God . . .[41]

> Thy heart is My home; sanctify it for My descent.[42]

> That the heart is the throne, in which the Revelation of God the All-Merciful is centered, is attested by the holy utterances which We have formerly revealed. Among them is this saying: 'Earth and heaven cannot contain Me; what can alone contain Me is the heart of him that believeth in Me, and is faithful to My Cause.'[43]

> All that is in heaven and earth I have ordained for thee, except the human heart, which I have made the habitation of My beauty and glory . . .[44]

> Were the eye of the heart to open, it would surely perceive that the words revealed from the heaven of the will of God are at one with, and the same as, the deeds that have emanated from the Kingdom of divine power.[45]

It's interesting that Baha'u'llah describes the heart as 'the throne in which the Revelation of God is centered' and the 'habitation of My beauty and glory'. When we turn to science and examine the latest research that is emerging, we also find this reflected, although of course in a focus on the heart's interaction with the body. The internationally recognized nonprofit research organization, Institute of HeartMath, concludes that the heart

> functions as a sophisticated information encoding and processing center, and possesses a far more developed communication system with the brain than do most of the body's major organs. With every

beat, the heart not only pumps blood, but also transmits complex patterns of neurological, hormonal, pressure and electromagnetic information to the brain and throughout the body. As a critical nodal point in many of the body's interacting systems, the heart is uniquely positioned as a powerful entry point into the communication network that connects body, mind, emotions and spirit.[46]

In studying human biology, we learn that approximately 60 per cent of heart cells are neural cells. Scientists have discovered that the heart's signals have a significant effect on the brain's cognitive and emotional functions, continuously influencing how people perceive and respond to the world as well as how they feel.[47]

From a simple hierarchal perspective, the most important organs to the organism are the heart and the brain – insignificant damage to these organs can significantly destroy life. The heart can produce an electromagnetic field that is 5,000 times stronger than the brain's and can be detected by instruments up to 10 feet away. Just as the brain processes what we perceive through the senses, so the heart processes unique EM bandwidths through complex signals experienced as emotions. Waves of information continually flow out from matter around us, and the heart is able to perceive the information embedded in the electron waves. This information is then passed to the brain for analysis and translation.[48]

What exactly makes the human heart pump remains a mystery. Information can be found about pacemaker cells, and 'electrical impulses' discharging at a given rate, but emotional reactions and hormonal factors can also affect heart rate. The heart affects and works with the entire body in instantaneous communication. It ensures that enough blood passes through the complex series of arteries, veins and capillaries bringing nourishment to all organs of the body as well as offering a highway for nutrients and toxins to travel. Optimal health depends upon the quantity and quality of blood. There is an analogy to this in the spiritual teachings: reading the revealed Word of God brings nourishment to all parts of our being; it is our 'lifeblood'.

In trying to understand how the human heart can reveal spiritual truths, I thought about the heart and its four chambers, two on the right and two on the left. Both sides are separate pumps, while working as one. The right side receives oxygen-poor blood and sends it to the lungs, releasing carbon dioxide and obtaining oxygen. The left side pumps blood into the organs and tissues of the body. Symbolically the right side of our body relates to the traditional 'masculine' quality of activity – the active exchange of blood with the lungs. The left side of the body relates to traditional 'feminine' energy or nurturing, providing the body with fresh blood.

Figure 11.2 The heart: Right and left, upper and lower

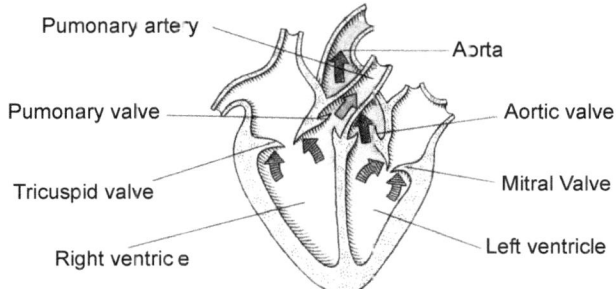

The heart also has upper and lower chambers. The upper chambers receive oxygen-poor blood and pump it to the lower chambers. The walls of the ventricles (lower chambers) are thicker and contain more cardiac muscle than the walls of the atria (upper chambers), enabling the ventricles to pump oxygen-rich blood out to the lungs and the rest of the body. Oxygen-poor blood, or blood that has already circulated throughout the body, returns to the heart to receive oxygen from the lungs.

Symbolically, we receive 'oxygen' from the breaths of the Holy Spirit by breathing in the fragrances, or sacred Writings, of Bahá'u'lláh. When we read His Writings in the morning and in the evening, we fill our spiritual 'blood' with oxygen, which nurtures our whole being. When we stop reading the Writings our spiritual 'blood' becomes oxygen-poor, making us feel spiritually lethargic and apathetic.

According to the ancient art of the chakra system, there is a 'high heart' and a 'low heart', like the upper and lower chambers of the physical heart. The high heart contains the *seat of the soul*. It has the qualities of compassion, unity, love and joy. The low heart, however, is the point of access of the lower self and appetites of lust, power, passion, envy, attachment, etc. We could further examine the significance of the lower chambers of the heart being thicker in walls, like veils of the ego. Could it also be a reflection of the denseness of matter and physical reality? The need for strength to overcome the ego? The upper chambers of the heart have thin walls, perhaps a reflection of the thin veil that exists between this world and the next . . . and the upper and lower hearts are so close in proximity that it's often hard to distinguish their voices.

Turning to the Baháʼí Writings, we see that ʻAbduʼl-Bahá clarifies how the heart has two influences:

> What is inspiration? It is the influx of the human heart. But what are satanic promptings which afflict mankind? They are the influx of the heart also. How shall we differentiate between them? The question arises: How shall we know whether we are following inspiration from God or satanic promptings of the human soul? Briefly, the point is that in the human material world of phenomena these four are the only existing criterions or avenues of knowledge, and all of them are faulty and unreliable. What then remains? How shall we attain the reality of knowledge? By the breaths and promptings of the Holy Spirit which is light and knowledge itself. Through it the human mind is quickened and fortified into true conclusions and perfect knowledge.[49]

Reflecting further on this, I find that the valves of the heart, too, are worth investigating for a spiritual analogy. The heart has valves that keep blood flowing in **one direction** through your heart. They open to let blood flow through and then close to prevent blood from flowing back. The four heart valves can be grouped by their job:

- *Atrioventricular valves* control blood flow between the heart's upper and lower chambers.

- *Semilunar valves* control blood flow out of the heart. Blood flows to the lungs through the pulmonary valve, and to the rest of the body through the aortic valve.

In thinking about the flow of blood, I wondered if the spiritual truth hidden in this reality reflects the two energies that cannot abide in the heart together. Atrioventricular valves may show us how love and fear cannot reside in the same heart, just as selfish desires and heavenly virtues cannot. So what are we to make of our sometimes conflicting feelings, as the Elizabethan poet and composer Thomas Weelkes picturesquely put it?

> These things seem wondrous, yet more wondrous I,
> Whose heart with fear doth freeze, with love doth fry.

While we can act from a place of love, feeling love and faith and connected to the spirit, this only means that the soul has the reins over the horse and is expressing itself clearly through the nervous system of the body. The rider will still be aware of the fear of the lower heart and feel the fear simultaneously. There is a barrier, or valve, that is preventing the fear (or ego) from acting through the nervous system. This is how a warrior feels in battle when carrying out a courageous and valiant deed. In the moment, he may be possessed by fear (frozen), and yet act from a place of great strength and faith.

If the heart has trust, then the 'valve' closes off fear. In the Writings of Bahá'u'lláh we read:

> Hast thou ever heard that friend and foe should abide in one heart? Cast out then the stranger, that the Friend may enter His home.[50]

Oxygenated blood (like a heart filled with prayer) cannot reside in the heart along with blood that has already been in circulation and is oxygen-poor (like a heart filled with desires). If the (spiritual) heart has even a trace of envy, the 'valve' closes to the spiritual world, as Bahá'u'lláh explains:

> Know, verily, the heart wherein the least remnant of envy yet lingers, shall never attain My everlasting dominion, nor inhale the sweet savours of holiness breathing from My kingdom of sanctity.[51]

He also tells us that self and God cannot abide in the same heart:

> Wouldst thou have Me, seek none other than Me; and wouldst thou gaze upon My beauty, close thine eyes to the world and all that is therein; for My will and the will of another than Me, even as fire and water, cannot dwell together in one heart.[52]

Meditating further on this analogy, I wondered if the semilunar valves reveal a wonderful truth. Like blood flowing out of the heart, sacrificing our lower nature to build character and reflect heavenly virtues is necessary. Selflessness, or 'giving your blood', is the key to attaining the Kingdom and true happiness. The aortic valve feeds blood to the rest of the body and is like the fear of God which is an 'indomitable army'. Bahá'u'lláh advises us to fear only God; the only fear the heart should possess is the fear of God. In our analogy, the fear of God will allow the heart to remain in the high heart, it is like the backflow valve that shuts off other fears. 'And if he feareth not God, God will make him to fear all things; whereas all things fear him who feareth God.'[53]

The open heart

The human experience offers us the opportunity to remember who we are, our true selves. With clients I often refer to this as the 'authentic self' or 'true self'. I feel that this may correspond to is the higher self 'Abdu'l-Baha encourages us to consult with during meditation, to listen to and pose questions to. Maintaining an open heart can be challenging, given the myriad influences in our lives. Our first response generally is to close the door, to protect ourselves. The lower self helps to shut others out, maintaining the 'us and them' mentality.

When we stifle or suppress our emotions, our body responds with fright or flight. It creates anxiety and panic or depression. When we feel these emotions, we can understand that we may need to address strong emotions we have not dealt with. Suppression closes the heart and bottles up stress. 'True happiness depends on spiritual good and having the heart ever open to receive the Divine Bounty,' 'Abdu'l.Bahá tells us.[54] I see so many clients of great spirituality who are ashamed of their humanity, the dark places within themselves, and who restrict or suppress it. Embracing our humanity is the key to an open heart, especially embracing our weakness, fully accepting the entirety of our humanness. We all struggle and battle within ourselves, it's what makes us equal and allows us to honour one another on a profound level.

When we live mindfully, in the present moment with awareness, we can tune into our body and mind's energies and join the spiritual energies available to us. We know when we are closing down, because our chest may feel constriction, our muscles may tense and tighten, or we may feel emotionally defensive. These are all signs that the door of our heart is closing. When the spiritual heart is closed, there is no way our true self can act in this world, nor access the spiritual energies offered to us. 'Abdu'l Bahá writes:

> Never lose thy trust in God. Be thou ever hopeful, for the bounties of God never cease to flow upon man. If viewed from one perspective they seem to decrease, but from another they are full and complete. Man is under all conditions immersed in a sea of God's blessings. Therefore be thou not hopeless under any circumstances, but rather be firm in thy hope.[55]

Here is an indication that when our heart is closed, from one perspective all hope is lost. From another perspective, we are immersed in a sea of God's blessings, as if we are under water. Whatever problem my clients present, I ultimately hear them saying, 'Where is the water?' and yet I can see that they are immersed in it! When our heart is open, we can drink from this ocean. When our heart is closed, we feel as though we are going to drown. My recommendation to clients is that it's not our job to find blessings and bounty, but simply to open up and receive the blessings that are always present.

In the Hidden Words, Bahá'u'lláh writes, 'Love me that I may love thee. If thou lovest Me not, My love can in no wise reach thee.'[56] I conclude from this that if our hearts remain open and in tune with the higher self, the seat of the soul, the sea of blessings can freely come in and pass through like a channel. There is movement both ways. The Holy Spirit can act through us, and grace can flow out of us when we teach or serve humanity; and we too can also receive the breaths of the Holy Spirit when the heart door is open.

There are many ways to keep the door of the heart open, including prayer, meditation, reading the Writings, serving and teaching. I have found that there are also some practical ways we can remember our true selves and act from our higher self. Integrating what we have learned by engaging the mind and body keeps the heart open. In my practice I teach some of the ideas listed below; they will be discussed further in the next chapter.

- Breathing deeply brings us to the spirit. It helps our defences drop and relax, so that we are able to love ourselves and others in a true sense of the word.
- Connect to your body. Observe sounds around you, the colours, the bottom of your feet on the floor, your feelings, the taste in your mouth, the smells that surround you. This integrates the energies of the soul, mind and body.
- Know your true self and what it loves, what brings it joy. Be who you authentically are in the moment, with crystallized discernment. Check in with your true self before speaking or acting. Take time to get in touch with your feelings.
- Surround yourself with those who are in touch with their true selves and validate, support and strengthen your own.
- Keep clear boundaries within yourself and between yourself and others. Take time for real rest and relaxation when needed. Call yourself to account when you say yes when you really mean no. Express your needs tactfully, and act in a manner that honours your soul. For example, backbiting slams the door of the heart closed and deprives us of all grace – it's like throwing garbage on our inner holy shrine. Act as though you are tending the holy places and gardens when interacting with yourself and others.
- Face the tests and misfortunes of life with an open attitude, faith and patience. Recognize with wisdom that our soul's lessons lie where we feel victimized, frustrated, pain, resistance, irritation, struggle and loss. Examine these situations closely, hunting for gems in the midst of dust. Ask yourself: what can I learn from this experience?
- Embrace your strong emotions with fortitude and compassion.
- Have the courage to stand up for what is just.

We will always have 'baggage' and ego issues to deal with, as long as we live. But the gifts we brought into this world are found in what we truly love, and not in an ego sense of love and passion. 'Abdu'l-Bahá reminds us:

> Know thou of a certainty that Love is the secret of God's holy Dispensation . . . the Holy Spirit's eternal breath that vivifieth the

human soul . . . the unique power that bindeth together the divers elements of this material world, the supreme magnetic force that directeth the movements of the spheres in the celestial realms. Love revealeth with unfailing and limitless power the mysteries latent in the universe.[57]

12

PREPARING THE SOUL FOR THE FAST

> Baha'u'llah has specified no procedures to be followed in meditation, and individual believers are free to do as they wish in this area, provided that they remain in harmony with the teachings, but such activities are purely personal and should under no circumstances be confused with those actions which Baha'u'llah Himself considered to be of fundamental importance to our spiritual growth. Some believers may find that it is beneficial to them to follow a particular method of meditation, and they may certainly do so . . . while they may appeal to some people, they may repel others.
> *The Universal House of Justice*[1]

This chapter draws on my own experience and the results of my experience with clients. In the spirit of the quotation above, we need to keep in mind that our spiritual path is personal and that we are free to choose what methods we incorporate in our lives to draw nearer to God, so long as these methods are in harmony with the teachings.

The energies of the Fast are potent. About two weeks before it begins, we can start paying particular attention to what spiritual 'foods' we are attracted to, or if there is a lack of attraction or direction. We can observe and reflect on our attachments. To what or to whom are we attached? We can assess where our time is being spent. Are there certain spiritual concepts we would like to deepen during the Fast? This is a great time to prepare our spirit for renewal and awakening for the new year.

Nutrition: Am I reading the Word of God in the morning and evening? What else am I doing to feed my spirit?
Movement: Do I serve humanity? Do I apply the teachings to my life? Do I maintain an 'open heart policy'?
Waste management: Do I regularly assess my attachments to things,

people, ideas, expectations and attributes? Can I translate the Revelation into action?

Rebuilding: How often do I pray every day? Do I consider myself to be in the presence of my Lord at all times? What virtues and divine qualities can I build upon?

'Abdu'l-Bahá wrote:

> this material fast is an outer token of the spiritual fast; it is a symbol of self-restraint, the withholding of oneself from all appetites of the self, taking on the characteristics of the spirit.[2]

While we are physically preparing our kitchens and bathrooms for the Fast by eliminating harmful items and replacing them with healing ones (as outlined in Chapters 6 and 7), we can notice how (and if) our environment builds and supports the acquisition of divine attributes. Observe at work, home and play the temptations and distractions, those things that may symbolize 'selfish desires'. Look around you and ask: What would constitute 'selfish desires' in my life, internally and in my external environment, and how can I reset them to lead to a higher direction? Maybe you would like to prepare a small booklet of Writings on certain attributes, so as to have them readily available for study during the Fast. Be sure to 'stock your pantry' with books and readings that will assist you.

Components of spiritual health

A healthy spirit continually cleanses itself of the self and ever advances towards God. Focus on building a strong relationship to your soul. 'Abdu'l-Bahá wrote to an inquirer: 'You have written about the weakness of your body. I ask from the Bounties of Bahá'u'lláh that your spirit may become strong, that through the strength of your spirit your body also may be healed.'[3]

When the heart expresses selfish desires and blots out the splendours of the soul, the result is spiritual illness. I've often observed that this pattern is similar to that in the body when the tongue's sense of taste is attached to junk foods and does not have a taste for healthy foods. Table 12.1 shows the chart from Chapter 4 as it pertains to the soul.

Table 12.1 Processes of the soul

Processes	Soul
Nutrition/respiration	Daily writings, prayer, music
Digestion	*Yearning required* Reflection and meditation
Transformative processes	Assimilating spiritual knowledge into understanding; recognizing attachments.
Catalysts	Desire/sacrifice/faith
Elimination	Releasing of attachments to material world, Kingdom of Names
Movement	Servitude, teaching, actions aligned with God's will
Cleanliness	Purifying and cleansing the heart/desires
Protection	Avoiding the 'ungodly' and things that spark passion and desires of the self; contentment
Resistance	Apathy/estrangement/heedlessness

As already mentioned, a spirit out of balance can portray apathy, estrangement or dissension. The following discourse attempts to provide some glimpses out of the vast Revelation of Bahá'u'lláh that offer revitalizing and regenerative powers for the Fast, focusing on optimal spiritual health.

Nutrition

Spiritual food

In our physical lives we usually eat because our stomach feels empty, but sometimes for entertainment or comfort or self-abuse because we feel empty emotionally. Many of my clients eat out of compulsion or loneliness, for various reasons. Sometimes they keep weight on to build walls between them and another person, or between them and their own empowerment. Through consultation, we discover what part of them is in pain; and whatever lonely, scared or angry part of them we find, I ask them when they are reaching for food to open their hearts and reach instead for the part of them that is in pain. I walk them through the process of asking this part what it needs, giving it some compassion and discipline. I ask them to embrace this part of themselves that wants their attention; to converse with it, love it and build their will to aid it to submit to the greater good of the body. When we love ourselves and have our hearts open we are connected to our higher, more authentic self. I ask my clients to connect with their authentic self to help them choose foods that are going to properly nourish the body and in the correct proportions. When we begin the journey of loving ourselves in the true sense, these types of habits can be addressed.

During the Fast we can to choose appropriate foods for the soul, just as we do for the body. The body receives nutrition through ingesting food, through respiration and absorption through the skin. During the Fast we should ensure that we open our hearts to optimal nutritional food for the soul, and the best nutrition comes from the Writings of the Manifestation of God for this day. 'Abdu'l-Bahá defined spiritual food as follows:

> The Spirit breathing through the Holy Scriptures is food for all who hunger. God Who has given the revelation to His Prophets will surely give of His abundance daily bread to all those who ask Him faithfully.[4]

> In reality thou art spiritually hungry and athirst for the Water of Life. Therefore I send thee spiritual food and bestow upon thee the Water of Life Eternal. That food is the divine advices and exhortations revealed in the Tablets and the spiritual outpourings of the breath of the Holy Spirit. I hope ere long it will reach thee and thou wilt behold what an exhilaration and beatitude it produceth and what cheerfulness and serenity and what heavenly emotions it createth.[5]

The Bahá'í Writings also use the metaphor from respiration, 'breath' and 'inhale'. Bahá'u'lláh characterized His laws and ordinances as 'the breath of life unto all created things'. In His Most Holy Book, He reveals:

They who recite the verses of the All-Merciful in the most melodious of tones will perceive in them that with which the sovereignty of earth and heaven can never be compared. From them they will inhale the divine fragrance of My worlds – worlds which today none can discern save those who have been endowed with vision through this sublime, this beauteous Revelation.[6]

We also find the concept of 'absorption' in the Bahá'í Writings. Absorption in the spiritual realms helps fill the soul and leaves no room for self and desire, as 'Abdu'l-Bahá writes: 'Be thou so wholly absorbed in the emanations of the spirit that nothing in the world of man will distract thee.'[7] He uses the same analogy in a prayer that 'this material realm may absorb the rays of the world of spirit'.[8]

The inspiring story of Dhabíh, a faithful follower of Bahá'u'lláh, conveys the nature and potency of spiritual food.

> As was customary at that time of day, their host had provided several trays of various fruits and sweetmeats. Dhabíh was invited by Bahá'u'lláh to partake of the food but he begged most humbly and earnestly to receive instead, through Bahá'u'lláh's bounty, a portion of spiritual food from the unseen treasury of His divine knowledge. Favourable to his plea, Bahá'u'lláh summoned Dhabíh to sit before Him and hearken to His words – words of incomparable power and awe which were filled with spiritual significance and which, according to Bahá'u'lláh's testimony, no one is capable of describing.
>
> By hearing the utterances of Bahá'u'lláh on that day, Dhabíh was transformed and worlds of spirit were opened before his eyes. After this meeting he remained in a state of spiritual intoxication, wholly devoted to Bahá'u'lláh, his love for Him intensifying with the passing of each day.[9]

This story conveys the power of the Word of God, even to the extent that the soul '. . . hath been called forth by the Word of God'.[10]

As we sit to read the sacred verses, we recognize the vastness of Bahá'u'lláh's Revelation and the implications of it on all the worlds of God. He writes:

> . . . is not the object of every Revelation to effect a transformation

in the whole character of mankind, a transformation that shall manifest itself both outwardly and inwardly, that shall affect both its inner life and external conditions?[11]

So potent and universal is this revelation, that it hath encompassed all things visible and invisible.[12]

Through the movement of Our Pen of glory We have, at the bidding of the omnipotent Ordainer, breathed a new life into every human frame, and instilled into every word a fresh potency. All created things proclaim the evidences of this world-wide regeneration.[13]

My holy, My divinely ordained Revelation may be likened unto an ocean in whose depths are concealed innumerable pearls of great price, of surpassing lustre. It is the duty of every seeker to bestir himself and strive to attain the shores of this ocean, so that he may, in proportion to the eagerness of his search and the efforts he hath exerted, partake of such benefits as have been pre-ordained in God's irrevocable and hidden Tablets.[14]

As we pick up our book to read, let us remember, reverently and humbly, the true transformative power of these words.

Recitation of the sacred texts morning and evening

As the body awakens to another day we can also welcome our spirit, acknowledge its presence and give thanks. Our bodies and physical eyes face the sunrise, and our spiritual eyes open the heart to send out love and gratitude, connecting to the abundance and grace that surround us. We care for our human temple as a holy and sacred site, cleaning it and nourishing it. If we awaken suddenly and jump into our day without any intention or thought or connection to the Beloved, our spirit becomes neglected. When this happens every day, I and perhaps many others have found that our body may give us feedback by becoming fatigued or manifesting some pain.

In the Kitáb-i-Aqdas Bahá'u'lláh asks us to partake of spiritual food daily by reciting the verses of God every morning and evening. Recitation literally means to read, or repeat, something prepared or committed to memory. Memorization comes in handy if you are in a situation without access to books. Reciting the sacred texts has a specific intention – to listen to what the Creator is asking us to do. God reaches out to us in the Writings, like the sun reaching earth with its rays, providing heat and light. Bahá'u'lláh commands us:

> Recite ye the verses of God every morn and eventide. Whoso faileth to recite them hath not been faithful to the Covenant of God and His Testament, and whoso turneth away from these holy verses in this Day is of those who throughout eternity have turned away from God. Fear ye God, O My servants, one and all. Pride not yourselves on much reading of the verses or on a multitude of pious acts by night and day; for were a man to read a single verse with joy and radiance it would be better for him than to read with lassitude all the Holy Books of God, the Help in Peril, the Self-Subsisting. Read ye the sacred verses in such measure that ye be not overcome by languor and despondency.
>
> Lay not upon your souls that which will weary them and weigh them down, but rather what will lighten and uplift them, so that they may soar on the wings of the Divine verses towards the Dawning-place of His manifest signs; this will draw you nearer to God, did ye but comprehend.[15]

In reflecting on what Bahá'u'lláh is asking us to do, we may understand it in the context of the physical body. Once the physical body has woken up, it needs nourishment to enter the day. Likewise, the soul needs a spiritual breakfast to enter the material world. It's like turning on the GPS in your car; we need to ensure that we are properly connected to the source of all being, and will receive a roadmap for the day. Taking time to enter our day with intention is essential to well-being, especially during the Fast. It's helpful to form the habit of turning our soul to its Creator in the early hours of the morning. In the evening we will feel hungry again. Through this one command, Bahá'u'lláh ensures that the hearts of the peoples will be given adequate nourishment.

The passage quoted above not only tells us when to read the Writings, but *how*. As Bahá'u'lláh so lovingly points out, we should not lay not upon our souls that which will weary them and weigh them down, but rather 'what will lighten and uplift them, so that they may soar on the wings of the Divine verses towards the Dawning-place of His manifest signs; this will draw you nearer to God, did ye but comprehend'.[16] It's interesting that in the Tablet to a Physician, He writes that overeating is harmful to the body. It seems to be the same with the spirit: if we 'overeat' or over-read the verses, it will be more harmful than profitable. He also warns against the 'excessive piety' of reading too much. Gauging how much spiritual food we need is like sitting quietly while eating and paying attention to your stomach. There are certain sensations or indicators that tell us when to stop eating, and we need to learn them.

When we read, we search for the truth and use the Word of God to transform ourselves individually and collectively. Bahá'u'lláh exhorts us to

> Meditate upon that which hath streamed forth from the heaven of the Will of thy Lord, He Who is the Source of all grace, that thou mayest grasp the intended meaning which is enshrined in the sacred depths of the Holy Writings.[17]

And again:

> O peoples of the world! Cast away, in My name that transcendeth all other names, the things ye possess, and immerse yourselves in this Ocean in whose depths lay hidden the pearls of wisdom and of utterance, an ocean that surgeth in My name, the All-Merciful.[18]

I've observed that when we open our hearts to the Word of God, we receive our daily bread and strengthen our muscles to keep the door open. Maintaining balance in the quest for truth and transformation is important. A flight into spiritual realms shouldn't propel us away from the cares of the world, but should inspire us to be of service to others. It should help us to ground our energy and be ready to serve. Walking around floating and disassociated won't help anyone, even the self. Because the Revelation is seated in the heart, it may be interesting to contemplate after reciting the verses – whether in privacy or attending meetings – How much more do I *love*? Or, how much more do I *know*?

Prayer: *The most potent spiritual food*

Prayer is the essential tool to spiritual progress, and opens the heart to the Kingdom. In prayer, we welcome the Kingdom and the Holy Spirit to interact with our true self. Bahá'u'lláh writes in the Arabic Hidden Words, 'Forget all save Me, and commune with my spirit.'[19] During prayer, energies flow in and energies flow out as He promises, telling us that when a believer prays in a spirit of true devotion, 'the scattering angels of the Almighty shall scatter abroad the fragrance of the words uttered by his mouth, and shall cause the heart of every righteous man to throb'.[20]

Prayer and supplication build the ladder for the soul to ascend. It's the only direct approach to God. The Báb likened prayer to a 'river of milk' that 'floweth through the depths of prayers and supplications'.[21] The more we drink this food, the more the soul advances. As we develop the capacity of focus and concentration during communion, we build our capacity to receive the influx of the Holy Spirit, enabling us to penetrate hidden mysteries.

Prayer and fasting are both devotional acts we perform to draw closer to God. Shoghi Effendi writes of prayer:

> The Bahá'í Faith, like all other Divine religions, is thus fundamentally mystic in character. Its chief goal is the development of the individual and society, through the acquisition of spiritual virtues and powers. It is the soul of man that has first to be fed. And this spiritual nourishment prayer can best provide . . . The believers . . . should fully realize the necessity of praying. For prayer is absolutely indispensable to their inner spiritual development . . .[22]

The intention of prayer is to commune with God. Recitation of the Writings, like reading Tablets, has the intention of hearing what God asks of us. Many read Tablets to begin meetings, when prayers are more appropriate. Prayers are us talking to God, and reading His Writings are listening to Him speaking to us. We often in prayer ask something of God, but the purest form of prayer is one that is free from desire, one that praises and glorifies our Creator.

Bahá'u'lláh has given us a specific Bahá'í rite, or ritual – obligatory prayer. It is one of the laws of His Dispensation. He says that if we have to make a choice between this prayer or reading the Writings, the obligatory prayer takes precedence. He has also revealed many other prayers for various purposes which can be used at any time.

Just as a midday meal provides the most nourishment for the body, enabling us to have enough stamina to get us through the day, I've observed that this is also true for the soul. The obligatory prayer is the heartiest meal because it is a law of Bahá'u'lláh. Bahá'u'lláh revealed three obligatory prayers: a long, a medium-length and a short one. Each believer is free to choose which prayer is said, so long as it's done daily. Bahá'u'lláh sets this out in the Kitáb-i-Aqdas, together with the instruction to turn to the Qiblih, the most holy spot:

> We have enjoined obligatory prayer upon you . . . When ye desire to perform this prayer, turn ye towards the Court of My Most Holy Presence, this Hallowed Spot that God hath made the Centre round which circle the Concourse on High, and which He hath decreed to be the Point of Adoration for the denizens of the Cities of Eternity, and the Source of Command unto all that are in heaven and on earth.[23]

THE SHORT OBLIGATORY PRAYER
TO BE RECITED DAILY BETWEEN NOON and SUNSET

I bear witness, O my God, that Thou hast created me to know Thee and to worship Thee. I testify, at this moment, to my powerlessness and to Thy might, to my poverty and to Thy wealth. There is none other God but Thee, the Help in Peril, the Self-Subsisting.

Bahá'u'lláh

Here are some reflections concerning the quality of prayer:
1. **Reverence**. 'When you wish to pray you must first know that you are standing in the presence of the Almighty.'[24]
2. **Union of prayer and practice**. We cannot pray every day for better health and not change our eating patterns.
3. **Ask for the right things.**. Shoghi Effendi clarifies this:

> The true worshipper, while praying, should endeavour not so much to ask God to fulfil his wishes and desires, but rather to adjust these and make them conform to the Divine Will.

Only through such an attitude can one derive that feeling of inner peace and contentment which the power of prayer alone can confer.[25]

4. ***Pray with feeling***. 'Abdu'l-Bahá is reported to have said, 'If there be no love or spiritual enjoyment in prayer, do not pray. Prayer should spring from love, from the desire of the person to commune with God.'[26] He was asked how to acquire this love when one is not in a receptive mood but immersed in worldly affairs. He answered:

> . . . the power of will draws you into this condition – this state of ecstasy. By a force of will and an effort of mind, man turns his attention to God, to His knowledge, His wonderful creation, His wisdom and His Omnipotence, and then thinking frequently and deeply of Him, attains the state of love, of desire for prayer, of supreme ecstasy.[27]

5. ***Try praying aloud***. 'Abdu'l-Bahá is reported to have said:

> Why should it be necessary for him to repeat prayers aloud and with the tongue? One reason for this is that if the heart alone is speaking, the mind is more easily disturbed. But repeating the words so that the tongue and heart act together enables the mind to become concentrated. Then the whole man is surrounded by the spirit of prayer and the act is more perfect.[28]

> Prayer is both attitude and word; it depends upon the soul-condition. It is like a song, both words and music make the song. Sometimes the melody will move us, sometimes the words.[29]

6. ***Turn towards the point of adoration***. There are certain conditions for prayer. For the obligatory prayers, for example, we turn towards the 'point of adoration' which is the Shrine of Bahá'u'lláh in 'Akká. This reinforces the symbolism of a flower which reaches towards the sun to receive its nutrients.

7. ***Pray in private***. The obligatory prayer is a time when we confess

our insignificance before God and our humility; this is easier to do in private. Some parents find it helpful to pray in front of their children so that they understand its reverence and importance.

8. **Wash away the world.** Perform ablutions (the washing of hands and face) prior to prayer. The ablutions help the mind wash away the things of this world. It's a time when we cross the threshold into the next world to focus our mind on God. Focusing our mind on prayer requires longing and attraction, for our prayers have greatest effect when our mind and heart are pure. If we have no access to water, we can say, 'In the name of God, the Most Pure, the Most Pure' five times.

Prayer is another avenue to opening the heart. It is a natural impulse. When we fall in love with someone, it's impossible to keep from mentioning their name. When you love another, don't you wish to express it? Prayer is simply conversation with your Beloved. 'Abdu'l-Bahá reassures us:

> Spirit has influence; prayer has spiritual effect. Therefore, we pray, 'O God! Heal this sick one!' Perchance God will answer. Does it matter who prays? God will answer the prayer of every servant if that prayer is urgent. His mercy is vast, illimitable. He answers the prayers of all His servants . . . But we ask for things which the divine wisdom does not desire for us, and there is no answer to our prayer . . . God is merciful. In His mercy He answers the prayers of all His servants when according to His supreme wisdom it is necessary.[30]

Music as a spiritual food

In this new age, Bahá'u'lláh 'specifically proclaimed that music, sung or played, is spiritual food for soul and heart', as 'Abdu'l-Bahá reminds us.[31] When we feel joy the nerves are affected by the vibration and this can produce health. Music is a chief instrument in creating a state of joy: in the Kitáb-i-Aqdas Bahá'u'lláh advises us:

> Let your joy be the joy born of My Most Great Name, a name that bringeth rapture to the heart, and filleth with ecstasy the minds of all who have drawn nigh unto God. We, verily, have made music as

a ladder for your souls, a means whereby they may be lifted up unto the realm on high . . .'[32]

When a client is really stressed out, I often suggest they breathe in deeply, and on the exhale, make the sound 'Ahhhh'. If you put your hand to your mouth, you can exhale 'cool' breath, or 'warm' breath. (When you slow down your breathing and exhale from the abdominal muscles, the air feels more moist and warmer than your hand temperature. If you pucker your lips and blow faster, the moisture is blown away, just as the wind blowing on a hot day feels cool. A fast breath blows moisture and heat away from the body.) Try it. When you are tense and your heart is closed off, or you feel strong emotion or defensive, try exhaling, saying 'Ahhh' with warm breath. It helps to quickly open your heart, centre your energies, relax the body and bring clarity to the mind. When your heart opens your defences can't be up, they have to drop. This is the time to call on your true self to think, act or speak.

In all forms of human vocalization, nothing can rival intoning. Using your voice can enhance your mood and memory. In his book *The Mozart Effect* Don Campbell, the founder of the Institute of Music, Health and Education, writes that intoning 'balances brain waves, deepens the breath, reduces the heart rate, and imparts a general sense of well-being'. Campbell has correlated certain sounds with specific effects on the body:

1. ***Ahhh*** immediately evokes a relaxation response.
2. ***Eee or Ay*** is the most stimulating of vowel sounds; helps with concentration, releasing pain and anger
3. ***Oh or om is*** considered the richest of sounds; it can increase skin temperature and relax muscle tension

Daniel Amen in his book *Change your Brain, Change your Life* recommends intoning for 5 minutes a day for two weeks. He notes that children hum when they are happy. As the sound activates your brain, you will feel more alive and your brain will feel more tuned in to the moment.'[33]

How does one intone? When reciting meaningful passages out loud, try to elongate the vowels as you are reading. Then attempt to utter the phrases in a musical tone, changing pitch. Bahá'u'lláh encourages us to intone and elucidates its effects:

Intone, O My servant, the verses of God that have been received by thee, as intoned by them who have drawn nigh unto Him, that the sweetness of thy melody may kindle thine own soul, and attract the hearts of all men. Whoso reciteth, in the privacy of his chamber, the verses revealed by God, the scattering angels of the Almighty shall scatter abroad the fragrance of the words uttered by his mouth, and shall cause the heart of every righteous man to throb. Though he may, at first, remain unaware of its effect, yet the virtue of the grace vouchsafed unto him must needs sooner or later exercise its influence upon his soul. Thus have the mysteries of the Revelation of God been decreed by virtue of the Will of Him Who is the Source of power and wisdom.[34]

Digestion

After we take in physical nutrition our bodies must digest and process the food. In the same way, as we pray and read the Writings, our spirit must process through the heart what we've read. Meditation and reflection allow the heart to process the spiritual nourishment it's just received. They bathe the Word of God in the light of the heart, giving it life, purpose and depth. They process it into what we can glean from it prior to moving it into action.

Divine breezes flow freely when the heart is opened. While intelligence is dependent upon mental capacity, heavenly understanding is dependent upon an open heart and freedom of spirit. 'Abdu'l-Bahá writes:

> It is incumbent upon you to ponder in your hearts and meditate upon His words, and humbly to call upon Him, and to put away self in His heavenly Cause. These are the things that will make of you signs of guidance unto all mankind, and brilliant stars shining down from the all-highest horizon, and towering trees in the Abhá Paradise.[35]

What is true thinking? Bahá'u'lláh in His writings asks us to 'ponder in thy heart'. This has led me to reflect that most of us believe the stream of consciousness we tune into is 'thinking', but I've found that in fact it is all too often simply memory recall, a regurgitation of the past. When this is the case, we generally 'think' about a problem but are inhibited in finding a solution. Only when we seek the heart through meditation or reflection can we receive inspiration from the soul and experience true 'thinking'. Quieting the stream of consciousness helps to best hear these divine breezes. Sometimes the best 'aha' moments come in the shower or driving to work, when we are stationary and zoning out. This is why meditation is so important; if we don't do it, our spirit has to fit in when our schedule allows.

In his book *Through Time into Healing*, Brian Weiss tells the story of how Thomas Edison came to his inventions through meditative techniques:

> While sitting in a certain chair, Edison used relaxation and meditation techniques to reach the state of consciousness that is between sleep and wakefulness. He would hold some ball bearings in his closed hand, palm down, while resting this hand on the arm of his chair. Beneath his hand he kept a metal bowl. If Edison fell asleep, his hand would open. The ball bearings would fall into the metal bowl and the noise would awaken him. Then he would repeat the process over and over again.[36]

'Abdu'l-Bahá tells us:

> Bahá'u'lláh says there is a sign (from God) in every phenomenon: the sign of the intellect is contemplation and the sign of contemplation is silence, because it is impossible for a man to do two things at one time – he cannot both speak and meditate.[37]

In my experience, meditation allows the heart to open. It finds the stillness already present. All conversations have pauses, and the mind focuses on those pauses in our conscious stream. We identify with the observer within, and in the silence we can witness the internal dialogue. It's in the stillness that we receive bursts of inspiration from the heavenly Kingdom; in the stillness we draw closer to the Creator, to our true nature. It bridges the gap between realities. We should not try to suppress the stream of consciousness, for it will not cease, but to try initially to focus the mind away from the noise of the stream.

Meditation allows us the powerful tool of reflection – another way to process things we have ingested through the mind and spirit. 'One hour's reflection is preferable to seventy years of pious worship,' says a Muslim tradition quoted in the Bahá'í Writings.[38] How can we progress if we don't reflect on results? Without reflection, we become reactionary and animalistic instead of intentional. Intelligence requires contemplation; connecting the mind to the heart creates the pathway to understanding. It's not possible to purify the mind simply by thinking about it. Emotions can't be conquered by the mind; but reflection provides a bridge from the mind to the spirit to release these forces. We can use the space to hover outside the well-worn paths we continually walk, reflective in our actions, thoughts and feelings. Our daily routines and relationships create neural pathways which our thoughts run over and reinforce into patterns, our beliefs and then actions. Meditation breaks up these habitual ways of thinking and feeling. We can explore better pastures, in touch with inner resources that can create new roads of thought and belief. This is true transformation – when we take what is unseen, jewels from the Writings, and turn them into new roads ultimately leading to action.

Reflection is an impetus to change. It spawns inventions and discoveries; it brings things from the unseen world to the seen. Bahá'u'lláh confirms this in the following verse:

> O people of Bahá! The source of crafts, sciences and arts is the power of reflection. Make ye every effort that out of this ideal mine there may gleam forth such pearls of wisdom and utterance as will promote the well-being and harmony of all the kindreds of the earth.[39]

After time for reflection, we must consult with ourselves to create a pathway to deeper understanding. When systematic time is dedicated to this, it builds a relationship to our higher self, training our minds to trust the information we receive from the spirit and to differentiate between the higher and lower promptings of the heart. 'Abdu'l-Bahá specifically describes this process of meditation:

> It is an axiomatic fact that while you meditate you are speaking with your own spirit. In that state of mind you put certain questions to your spirit and the spirit answers: the light breaks forth and the reality is revealed.

You cannot apply the name 'man' to any being void of this faculty of meditation; without it he would be a mere animal, lower than the beasts.

Through the faculty of meditation man attains to eternal life; through it he receives the breath of the Holy Spirit – the bestowal of the Spirit is given in reflection and meditation.

The spirit of man is itself informed and strengthened during meditation; through it affairs of which man knew nothing are unfolded before his view. Through it he receives Divine inspiration, through it he receives heavenly food.

Meditation is the key for opening the doors of mysteries. In that state man abstracts himself: in that state man withdraws himself from all outside objects; in that subjective mood he is immersed in the ocean of spiritual life and can unfold the secrets of things-in-themselves. To illustrate this, think of man as endowed with two kinds of sight; when the power of insight is being used the outward power of vision does not see.

This faculty of meditation frees man from the animal nature, discerns the reality of things, puts man in touch with God.

This faculty brings forth from the invisible plane the sciences and arts. Through the meditative faculty inventions are made possible, colossal undertakings are carried out; through it governments can run smoothly. Through this faculty man enters into the very Kingdom of God.

Nevertheless some thoughts are useless to man; they are like waves moving in the sea without result. But if the faculty of meditation is bathed in the inner light and characterized with divine attributes, the results will be confirmed.

The meditative faculty is akin to the mirror; if you put it before earthly objects it will reflect them. Therefore if the spirit of man is contemplating earthly subjects he will be informed of these.

But if you turn the mirror of your spirits heavenwards, the heavenly constellations and the rays of the Sun of Reality will be reflected in your hearts, and the virtues of the Kingdom will be obtained.

Therefore let us keep this faculty rightly directed – turning it to the heavenly Sun and not to earthly objects – so that we may discover the secrets of the Kingdom, and comprehend the allegories of the Bible and the mysteries of the spirit.

May we indeed become mirrors reflecting the heavenly realities, and may we become so pure as to reflect the stars of heaven.[40]

Meditation, as prescribed by Bahá'u'lláh, is thus an important tool during the Fast. I use it as a time to process many 'toxins' that are creating a blockage with the body, causing a mistunement. Are there toxins such as resentments or anger that remain in your system? Are there events that happened that need processing? I think of how Shoghi Effendi said the Fast is

> essentially a period of meditation and prayer, of spiritual recuperation, during which the believer must strive to make the necessary readjustments in his inner life, and to refresh and reinvigorate the spiritual forces latent in his soul.[41]

Benefits of meditation

The benefits of meditation on the mind, body and soul are innumerable. Next to breathing properly, it's the first prescription I make professionally for insomnia, anxiety, anger or depression. It's a true unifier and an indispensable resource during the Fast.

Meditation allows our parasympathetic nervous system (nurturing) to dominate over our sympathetic nervous system (fright/flight). The role of the nervous system in causing disease is mentioned by 'Abdu'l-Bahá, who said that 'the cause of the entrance of disease into the human body – is either a physical one or is the effect of excitement of the nerves'.[42] 'Thus an illness caused by affliction, fear, nervous impressions, will be healed more effectively by spiritual rather than by physical treatment.'[43] And further:

> Sometimes if the nervous system is paralyzed through fear, a spiritual remedy is necessary. Madness, incurable otherwise, can be cured through prayer. It often happens that sorrow makes one ill, this can be cured by spiritual means.[44]

The modern lifestyle tends to over-stimulate the sympathetic nerve, leading to various spiritual illnesses such as insomnia, panic-disorder, chronic fatigue and others. Meditation will help to balance our systems.

Figure 12.1 Balance between the sympathetic and parasympathetic systems

Sympathetic nerve 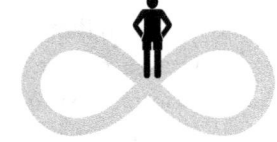 Parasympathetic nerve

I have found that meditation has the following specific benefits:
- ***It reduces stress***. It is the most effective method for reducing stress because it allows us to release emotions that are stuck in modes that subvert the flow of biochemicals in the mind/body. This is done without conscious awareness.
- ***It has healing physiological effects.***
  - It leads to deep relaxation: four to six hours of sleep are needed to attain the same level of relaxation experienced during a period of meditation lasting 12 minutes.
  - It produces alpha brain waves, reverses autoimmune disease, decreases oxygen consumption, lowers metabolic rate, slows breathing and heart rate, dramatically reduces pain, and improves mood in chronic pain.
  - Biology stays younger. R. K. Wallace and his associates spent over a decade studying meditators. He found that on a cellular level, this group was significantly younger biologically than others in their chronological age group. How much younger correlated with how long they meditated, i.e. those who meditated twenty minutes per day for ten years were ten years biologically younger.[45]
- ***It balances the mind.***
  - Meditation keeps us in the present moment and maintains balance so that our energy is not expended on the past (depression) or in worrying about the future (anxiety).
  - It leads to mindfulness. In this quiet place, we become aware of and observe ideas, thoughts, emotions and sensations from the body. We can more clearly see how we play our part in life, and we become empowered by this clarity of information in meditation. Our mind is fully connected to the body and to the spirit.

- It connects mind to divinity. Daily practice helps prevent the ego from building boundaries and offers freedom from the prison of self. Connecting to the soul is merely a doorway where we are no longer confined to self.
- **It allows the soul to bestow heavenly food through inspiration.** Meditation trains the mind to give the reins over to the soul, gaining mastery over the self. It opens and connects the heart to the Holy Spirit.

Meditation styles

Most of my clients have no clue as to what meditation is, how to do it or how to benefit from it. In a workshop it is this area that generates the most questions.

There are no specific or prescribed guided meditations or formulas in the Bahá'í Faith. One is free to meditate in any way. Shoghi Effendi wrote:

> There are no set forms of meditation prescribed in the teachings, no plan, as such, for inner development. The friends are urged – nay enjoined – to pray, and they also should meditate, but the manner of doing the latter is left entirely to the individual.[46]

With this in mind, you may like to try the suggestions in Table 12.2 on the next page. The goal overall is to sit with awareness, turn our hearts towards the Kingdom and allow the heart to open and observe what presents itself. Meditation is not a time for talking, but for listening and observing. The Bhagavad Gita describes deep meditation as being 'like the flame of a candle kept in a windless place'.[47]

Table 12.2 A basic 'recipe' for meditation

1. Posture should be straight, aligned and comfortable. You can lie down, but not if you are sleepy.
2. Do some deep yoga breaths, at least 10. You can breathe into your nose for about 4 counts, and exhale 4 counts out of the mouth. You can incorporate intoning if you'd like to try it. After about 10 deep breaths, gently breathe normally, but focus on your breath reaching below your belly button to your abdomen on the inhale. Most of us breathe into our chest and don't go any deeper. Babies naturally breathe from their bellies, yet most adults need to relearn it.
3. Make the intention to open the heart and access the higher self. Feel its energies, the energies of the Kingdom. This is communing.
4. Early morning can be a productive time for meditation, just before sunrise if possible. Avoid meditation immediately before sleep, as the body will begin to confuse the two intentions.
5. If you feel drowsy during meditation, take a brisk walk before it, or shift your posture. Ensure the room is well ventilated.
6. Stay in the middle. Emotions that arise may be painful or blissful. Don't be a bee caught in its own honey ('I just love this intoxicating feeling'), or stuck in poison ('I'm so uncomfortable with this anger arising'). Keep the mind focused. Extreme emotion can be worked through with a brisk walk. Avoid riding the pendulum swinging back and forth.
7. Keep an open mind. As you practise meditation more and more, the relationship you develop with it will evolve. The mind will require great concentration initially to keep focused.
8. Practise meditation in daily life. Notice when you are rushing, when you are trying to do several things at once. Have mastery of where your attachments form and attention goes:

    > Be watchful lest the concerns and preoccupations of this world prevent you from observing that which hath been enjoined upon you by Him Who is the Mighty, the Faithful.[48]

Be aware of excessively stimulating your senses. All these factors lead to 'spiritual bleeding' and diffusion of our vital energy.

Now that you have a basic recipe, you may wish to try some of the following specific methods of meditation:

Transcendental meditation

Transcendental meditation (TM) is one of the best ways to train the busy mind. It uses the technique of repeating a phrase, sometimes called a mantra. While we remember that 'there are no set forms of meditation prescribed in the teachings', Bahá'ís are enjoined to call upon the power of God through the 'Greatest Name', *Allah'u'Abhá,* meaning 'God the Most Glorious'. In the Kitáb-i-Aqdas, the Most Holy Book of Bahá'u'lláh, we are instructed to call upon the power of the Greatest Name 95 times a day.[49] The Greatest Name has influence on both physical and spiritual matters. It can be used for invocation if in trouble, for comfort, protection, illumination or unity.

When repeating a phrase in transcendental meditation, your mind tends to wander off. If you are using this technique, gently bring your mind back to the mantra. If you wish to train the mind and practise concentration, start at 10 minutes and then increase your time by one-minute increments per week up to 20 minutes or however long you wish to train. Some find it helpful to imagine thoughts like clouds, simply watching them pass through. The mind will have difficulty in concentrating at first, but after time it will deepen. You may notice a small difference in your ability to focus after six weeks of training. Be patient with the process, you are receiving benefits even if the mind wanders all around.

Once you've acquired some level of concentration, focus on attracting the heart to the Kingdom. In this state, you can commune with the Spirit of God, asking for meanings to verses or other questions from your day. This one practice has helped numerous clients of mine to improve their brain power, to focus and discipline their thought processes. I recommend it for everyone.

Simulation training

Simulation training is a meditative technique I readily prescribe that helps an individual train for a certain event or situation. Athletes in training run events in their minds; the Olympic programmes use this technique. Buddhist monks train in this way for greater compassion. The purpose of the technique is to examine the range of responses in a given situation, choose one, and accustom our bodies to habitually respond with that attribute.

Another helpful meditation for changing a situation is to review an event that reoccurs in your life (such as responding with compassion rather than anger). Perhaps you respond angrily when your spouse habitually does something that annoys you, and wish to change your response to a more virtuous one. You can explore the range of possible responses – how it would appear and feel to do something different. When you've decided what virtue to apply to the situation, bring something to mind that inspires you to feel that virtue. (For example, people often choose the image of a hurt child or animal to evoke feelings of deep compassion.) Hold that in your body and mind for several minutes. Now replay the situation you'd like to change in your mind. When it's time for your response, pull up that virtue and hold it for several minutes while visualizing yourself responding in this way – the action. This helps your brain and cells to 'rewire themselves' so that when you are actually faced with the real-life situation you will more easily respond. This can apply to many situations – overeating, losing your temper, holding resentment towards a boss.

The best simulation builds attributes like compassion. When the mind comes to a quiet place, focus on an image that will stimulate your feelings of compassion. Feel the compassion – where it connects in your body, the texture of the feeling, the temperature. Experience it for several minutes. Move on to focusing on a neutral image for which you feel neither hostility nor love. Try to feel the same amount of compassion. Do this for several minutes. When you have mastered that skill, move on to something you consider an enemy. Bring it into your awareness and pay attention to the change in your energy. Try to bring up compassion. Move between the three levels until there is a seamless transition. As long as you are in the mode of compassion, that object or person will not be able to threaten you in any way. You will remain in the higher heart, experiencing that person or thing. Focus on your breath during this meditation in order to stay connected with yourself.

Bring yourself to account

What we do and what we give time to is inherently reflective of our subconscious beliefs and priorities. You will only know your real priorities when you look back on your week and reflect on how you spent your time, and how you reacted to your environment. In the Bahá'í teachings there is another helpful remedy, given to us by Bahá'u'lláh, Who enjoins us in the Hidden Words:

> Bring thyself to account each day ere thou art summoned to a reckoning; for death, unheralded, shall come upon thee and thou shalt be called to give account for thy deeds.[50]

I've found that this single remedy encourages accountability, and has been an amazing tool for spiritual transformation. Our minds are so trained to see what is wrong and blame others for it that it takes time to train the mind to first ask, 'What is my responsibility in this?' This question is appropriate in every situation. Taking the time to reflect upon our actions and words at the end of each day, we can better see where we are aligned with God's Will, and where we are out of line. Build on what is working and what you are doing right first. As you pull up events from the day, give praise and thanks for an action that was praiseworthy. This helps keep an open heart. Find in your day when you truly were caring or compassionate, when you gave more patience than you had. These are strong heart qualities and high emotional intelligence. Ask God to help you to act on that quality for the rest of your life. If you find an action to transform, pray for forgiveness and ask for guidance and strength to do better. In this way, we have only a 'twenty-four hour' guilt policy. Once we take account of our actions with God at the end of the day, we can release the events and strive to do better next day, not carrying the past into it.

This essential tool of bringing ourselves to account helps us to live mindfully and consciously of our words and choices. It's one of the most powerful tools I've used with clients. When we honestly look at our own actions, words and thoughts, ask for help, and acknowledge the things we are doing well, it promotes us to spiritually progress on a more rapid level, and not carry the past into our lives, bundling emotions and becoming ill either mentally or physically. It creates physiological integrity, knowing your true intentions and creating unity in all our systems.

Transformative processes

In looking to the body to understand the invisible, we know that after we have eaten, the body digests and processes the food into the smallest particles possible. The body decides between what is nutrition – assimilating molecules into the cells – and toxins, removing them. We may draw the analogy that we take in our spiritual food in a similar manner, reading the Writings and digesting them through reflection and meditation. This allows us to decipher their 'nutritional content', which is usually the guidance needed in our present moment. Our hearts assimilate that spiritual food into understanding. If we find resistance, for instance through our attachment to the way we have viewed the world, in our response to readings or prayers we can make the intention to remove them.

When my clients finally have that 'aha' moment, I often find that it has resulted from a deeper understanding about themselves or another person. It's amazing to me how helpful it is for people to hear another perspective or the higher truth of a situation. The truth penetrates on such a deep level that an understanding transforms the heart and opens the door to the vast possibilities. This truth must be brought forth with gentleness and tact, or it can be like a sword and cut deeply. Just understanding a wife's or husband's perspective on a situation, or why she or he is acting in a certain way, can bring healing relief to many. When a person understands why they feel a certain way, or what the resistance is behind their behaviour, it often brings instant liberation. Understanding is yet another tool to keeping the heart's door open.

When we research the Bahá'í Writings, we find incredible words about creation. In the Tablet of Wisdom Bahá'u'lláh writes:

> Know thou, moreover, that the Word of God – exalted be His glory – is higher and far superior to that which the senses can perceive, for it is sanctified from any property or substance. It transcendeth the limitations of known elements and is exalted above all the essential and recognized substances . . . It is God's all-pervasive grace, from which all grace doth emanate.[51]

The process of creation emanates from the Word of God. Bahá'u'lláh describes this as follows:

> The world of existence came into being through the heat generated from the interaction between the active force and that which is its recipient. These two are the same, yet they are different . . . Such as communicate the generating influence and such as receive its impact are indeed created through the irresistible Word of God which is the Cause of the entire creation, while all else besides His Word are but the creatures and the effects thereof.[52]

There exists in the body the same process as described in this quotation. The heat produced in the body during transformative processes in digestion allows certain molecular functions to respond faster. I like the analogy that when the mind interacts with the Word of God, the heat generated from the interaction can be a type of cleansing of the heart generated from its 'active force' and transformation of the reader's consciousness. We can recognize this material world as the world of shadow, and through the Word of God, connect to the vibrant creative force that is connected to the heart. In this process, the 'motionless' (material) encounters the heat of the Word and becomes active.

In my experience, spiritual transformation focuses primarily on the process that takes the Word from the pages into a deep and rich understanding that leads to spiritual knowledge, eventually affecting the way we perceive reality in the mind and changing our actions. To understand the Word of God means to uncover its true meaning, and is dependent upon the capacity of each individual reader. In his seminal book *Gate of the Heart* Nader Saiedi points out that a recurrent theme of the Báb's Writings is that 'a single verse, a single word, or a single letter of the divine Word potentially discloses all spiritual mysteries'.[53] Bahá'u'lláh quotes a Muslim tradition: 'We speak one word, and by it we intend one and seventy meanings; each one of these meanings we can explain.'[54]

We may conclude, then, that rational thinking alone is not sufficient for understanding and becoming attracted to the Kingdom of God. We must also open the heart, or 'inner perception'. 'Abdu'l-Bahá wrote about the effects of reading with the inspiration of the Holy Spirit:

> I now assure thee, O servant of God, that if thy mind become pure from every mention and thought and thy heart attracted wholly to the Kingdom of God, forget all else beside God and come in

communion with the Spirit of God, then the Holy Spirit will assist thee with a power which will enable thee to penetrate all things, and a Dazzling Spark which enlightens all sides, a brilliant Flame in the zenith of the heavens, will teach thee that which thou dost not know of the facts of the universe and of the divine doctrine.[55]

The level of understanding is wholly dependent upon the capacity and perception of each individual. Individual transformation is also dependent upon our understanding, and our subjective understanding of the virtues. Someone who treasures servitude will come to a different personal interpretation of the Writings from a person who is strong in justice. This is clearly one of the reasons why in the so-called 'Tablet of the True Seeker' Bahá'u'lláh states, 'He must so cleanse his heart that no remnant of either love or hate may linger therein, lest that love blindly incline him to error, or that hate repel him away from the truth.'[56] Many of us have experienced this through studying prayers together and hearing the varying thoughts about the meaning of these divine words.

Ultimate transformation may come from viewing the texts in the light of unity and through purification of the heart, instead of an academic understanding from the perspective of limitation and conflict. In a letter from the Universal House of Justice concerning seeming conflicts in the Writings, they clearly state:

> In attempting to understand the Writings, therefore, one must first realize that there is and can be no real contradiction in them, and in the light of this we can confidently seek the unity of meaning which they contain.[57]

Any sacred text must be viewed as coming from one and the same source – divine unity. In a Tablet written to Mírzá Sa'íd, the Báb emphasizes:

> Such conclusive truth hath been revealed through the gaze of the heart, and not that of intellect. For intellect conceives not save limited things. Verily, bound by the realm of limitations, men are unable to gaze upon things simultaneously in their manifold aspects . . . [mind, body, soul] No one can recognize the truth of the Middle Way between the two extreme poles except after attaining unto the

gate of the heart and beholding the realities of the worlds, visible and unseen.[58]

Here the Báb draws our attention to the middle way again, warning against going to extremes. He also points out we are unable to fully understand the Writings simultaneously through all the various expressions of a human being – mind, heart, thoughts, love, hate. This is why it is not permissible to be in conflict or contention with one another over diverse interpretations of the Holy Word. Keeping in mind one's limitations (our pre-ordained capacity) in understanding the truth protects us from pride and facilitates the process of transformation, because it places us in servitude and selflessness, both essential qualities for allowing the truth to penetrate our hearts.

In Bahá'u'lláh's Writings two types of knowledge are referred to in the original texts in Arabic. One word is '*el*' and the other '*erfan*'. They are both translated into English as 'knowledge'. However, the first refers to understanding and knowledge of the mind, while the latter, *erfan*, refers to a deep understanding which has penetrated the heart. Knowledge of spiritual truths comes from the heart, not the mind. These differences are reflected in one of Bahá'u'lláh's Tablets: 'The Great Being saith: The man of consummate learning and the sage endowed with penetrating wisdom are the two eyes to the body of mankind.'[59]

The mind is the place of intellect, and the heart is the place of love. Bahá'u'lláh quotes the Muslim tradition: 'Knowledge is a light which God sheddeth into the heart of whomsoever He willeth.'[60] Imagination, thought, comprehension and memory are gifts of the spirit which emanate to the brain. Therefore, the mind is assisted by the soul's direct knowledge or inner perception, its intuition. This information is immediate (sometimes like a lightning flash) and independent of anything physical. If this relationship remains inactive it becomes vulnerable to atrophy, like muscles unused. Bahá'u'lláh writes: 'When the fire of love is ablaze, it burneth to ashes the harvest of reason.'[61]

To illustrate this relationship, I often explain the catalyst in spiritual growth – faith – with the following metaphor. Like faith, knowledge is planted in the soil of the heart like seeds in the farmer's field. Tests and difficulties plough this soil until its deep rows create fertile ground for these seeds to be planted. Once planted, the light of the mind nurtures these seeds and the dawn of understanding sprouts into tender shoots. It is this essential relationship of the mind and heart that brings certitude and firm belief to the soul, and it is why a purely intellectual approach to spiritual development cannot bring fruition to these young plants. Anyone can be well versed in the sacred teachings, but without the heart, absolute certitude is missing. The heart, like the mind, is a focal point influencing our quality of life. It can choose to love the material world, which will lead to attachment to material things, or it can choose to love God and the spiritual. This is done by placing the Revelation of God into the heart and releasing all attachments except to God. The most difficult attachment is to the self and one's own knowledge. Once the heart obtains humility, it can receive the knowledge of God and attain spiritual intoxication from reading the Writings. Releasing these attachments creates certitude, from which spiritual qualities of contentment and acceptance can bud, and thus an inner joy and happiness.

The following list of qualities is one I use to help assimilate our spiritual 'nutrition' and identify toxins (attachments):

Purifying and sanctifying the heart

Here are Bahá'u'lláh's words:

> No man shall attain the shores of the ocean of true understanding except he be detached from all that is in heaven and on earth. Sanctify your souls, O ye peoples of the world, that haply ye may attain that station which God hath destined for you . . .[62]

> He must so cleanse his heart that no remnant of either love or hate may linger therein . . . [63]

In order for the breezes of divine confirmation to flow into our heart we must first clean the lens of our camera, so that we can take a perfect snapshot of the spiritual truths in what we are reading. Oftentimes, we will need to pull the lens back to get both a greater perspective and a close-up analysis.

Submitting our will to the Will of God

Adib Taherzadeh writes:

It is, of course, natural that a believer may not understand the wisdom of a certain teaching, or may have difficulty in adjusting his own views on an issue to the teachings of the Faith. The way to resolve such a conflict is to study the Holy Writings further and to discuss the problem with knowledgeable believers. But if every approach fails, and the person does not succeed in reconciling his views with the teachings of the Faith, the only sure way to bring confirmation to his soul is to carry out Bahá'u'lláh's exhortation . . . According to this, two steps must be taken. First, not to reject those teachings which the individual cannot comprehend. This can be done through having faith in the truth of the Word of God and becoming humble before Him. Indeed, the believer becomes filled with heavenly strength when he can acknowledge in his heart that man is a fallible being, whereas the teachings of God are based on truth. To insist that one is right in his views and opinions is to erect a barrier between himself and God. The mere acknowledgement of one's imperfections and inadequacies is a major stepping-stone to resolving the conflict and finding the truth.

The second step is to pray ardently that God may open to one's heart 'the portals of true understanding'. This is a stage in which the light of knowledge will shine within the heart of the believer and he will be 'apprised' of the things he could not comprehend earlier. The knowledge of God and a true understanding of His teachings can come about when the believer approaches Him in a spirit of utter humility and submissiveness, and opens his heart fully to the outpourings of His Revelation. Then and only then will the vernal showers of His unfailing grace cause the tree of knowledge and wisdom to grow within the heart, and enable him to bring forth, in the fullness of time, the fruit of understanding. When this stage is reached, the individual will be aided to comprehend the truth of the Word and discover the manifold mysteries that are enshrined within God's Revelation. Knowledge of spiritual truth comes through the heart of man. The intellect will then grasp the subject and reason will emerge.[64]

This passage may help us see that in opening the heart by meditating on the teachings we come to deeper understandings of the mystery of their meanings and how to apply them with action to our daily lives.

This understanding of the heart penetrates deep within us. We are like the diver plunging into the great ocean. When a pearl is uncovered, we love it and want to know everything about it; we think about what to do with it outside the ocean. In parallel, when we fully understand a teaching and know how it looks in the material world, we have properly digested that food. We allow the teaching to become integrated into our heart, transforming our life and belief systems. We think about how to turn it into action. This helps us to strive to understand one another and to look upon one another with an open heart – without defensiveness, without judgement, simply to understand.

As we practise digesting the Word of God in our hearts, we become automatically habituated in real practical life to also digesting events that happen to us, to see the greater picture, to be aware of the divine forces that are quietly working around us, to connect to a larger rhythm of life. This helps us to instantly cope with difficult people and situations. One of the distinct features of this Dispensation is that the divine civilization it promises will appear not only through Bahá'u'lláh's teachings but through an organic process in which the individual believer's *understanding* of the teachings creates new habits and builds new character that will ultimately lead to that new civilization.

Elimination

Once the body identifies toxins, it contains this toxic waste until it pushes it out of the body. This is done through the skin, through exhaling, or through the kidneys and the bowels. While the toxins await release they bunch up and become more potent. In reflecting on this, I have come to believe that this biological process parallels the tendency of spiritual attachments to grow stronger just before they are released.

When the mind chooses nutritional spiritual food, fewer attachments are created and there will be less need for elimination. Daily elimination is required for the heart to be free of attachments and the mind directed towards God. Practically, this translates into paying attention to the ideas, beliefs, expectations, people, and things we are attached to.

I've seen with my clients that an open heart allows easy elimination, and doesn't stifle past grievances or strong emotions. When strong emotions arise and need to be eliminated, and attachments have taken over the heart, we may need help. One tool, shown in Table 12.3, starts with breathing deeply.

Table 12.3 Processing strong emotions through the heart centre

1. Fling open the heart door, and visualize the breath going in and out. With each deep breath try to reach down to your belly.
2. Make the intent to connect with your true self and disengage from the thoughts that are spinning in your head.
3. Focus your attention by shifting down into the body, sense what the strong emotion is, identify it, and describe it as best as possible. Acknowledge what you are feeling and validate it with compassion.
4. Continue to breathe into your strong emotions. Notice the energy transform and dissipate through the heart centre as you do this.
5. You can cross your ankles and wrists as you do this to process it faster.
6. Recognize negative automatic thoughts; these equate to 'spiritual bleeding'. Release this toxic habit – it just doesn't serve you in any way.

I've witnessed clients transform their own empowerment and relationships with this small tool. For example, one young lady was so afraid of not getting her needs met that she became paranoid and started fights with her husband. We explored the strong fears she was having and discovered that they were related to past occurrences in her life with her father and other men. As she practised this breathing and visualization exercise, she called more and more on her spirit and processed the strong feelings when they came up. In a matter of a few weeks of practice, she was able to better handle herself in the thick of an argument and feel more connected to the greater; she felt confident and didn't believe any more that her needs would not be met. She connected with a strength she had only known for a few moments of her life. Her confidence led her to express her needs openly to her husband, which changed the dynamic of their relationship. Her attachment to not getting her needs met was processed and she spent time nourishing the parts of her that were suffering.

When we immerse ourselves in the Bahá'í teachings, we learn that one of the remedies Bahá'u'lláh gave us was to detach ourselves from all things save God. 'Abdu'l-Bahá comments:

> God has given man a heart and the heart must have some attachment.

> We have proved that nothing is completely worthy of our heart's devotion save reality, for all else is destined to perish. Therefore the heart is never at rest and never finds real joy and happiness until it attaches itself to the eternal.⁶⁵

The human heart is prone to attachment. Like the body's impulse to overeat, so our hearts have the impulse to collect and hold on to things. I wonder if these attachments actually result from the search for our Beloved. Our ego believes we can find Him in food, drugs and other material pleasures. Therefore, we must continually re-habituate our heart to attach to the eternal, and not the material, and realize what we truly are searching for. A helpful way to know if we have attachments in a particular situation is when we cannot control our emotions in the moment. When we feel as though we're sliding, spinning or going out of control, there is an attachment revealing itself and needing to be released.

In volume 2 of his series of books *The Revelation of Bahá'u'lláh*, Adib Taherzadeh discusses three levels of attachment described by Bahá'u'lláh in a Tablet called the Tablet of the City of Radiant Acquiescence (Lawḥ-i Madinatu'r-Riḍá).⁶⁶ The first is attachment to this mortal world and everything enveloped within it. The second is attachment to the next world and 'all that is destined for man in the life hereafter'. God created us to worship Him alone and not for His rewards. The Bahá'í Writings do however address the rewards of a true believer in the next life, and herein lies the motive for this kind of attachment. Are you serving for the rewards? Are you fasting to draw nearer to God, out of obedience, or for the illimitable bounty bestowed in the energies of the Fast?

The third type of attachment is to the 'Kingdom of Names'. The Bahá'í texts state that everything in creation reflects an attribute of God, but that humanity has the ability to reflect all attributes.

> In the spiritual world, these attributes are manifest with such intensity that man will never be able to comprehend them in this life. In the human world, however, these attributes appear within the 'Kingdom of Names' and man often becomes attached to these names . . . For instance, generosity is an attribute of God, and it manifests itself in human beings. However, a person who has this attribute often becomes proud of it and loves to be referred to as generous. When his generosity is acknowledged by other people, he becomes happy,

and when it is ignored, unhappy. This is one form of attachment to the Kingdom of Names. Although this example concerns the name 'generosity', the same is true of all the names and attributes of God manifested within the individual. Usually, man ascribes these attributes to his own person rather than to God and employs them to exalt his own ego. For instance, a learned man uses the attribute of knowledge to become famous and feels gratified and uplifted when his name is publicized far and wide. Or there is the individual whose heart leaps with feelings of pride and satisfaction when he hears his name mentioned and finds himself admired. These are examples of attachment to the Kingdom of Names.[67]

Tests and difficulties help crystallize our 'soul lessons'. Our attachments lead us to feel victimized, irritated, resistance, struggle, anxiety, hurt, grief, jealousy, hate and anger. Recognizing our 'stuff' and knowing we can handle it allows us to release these worldly attachments and provides opportunities to draw nearer to God through obedience to His commands. Our spiritual development is incumbent upon releasing attachments. It's easy to obey the commands we agree with, but more difficult to obey those that challenge our habitual ways of thinking. This dichotomy tests our faith and steadfastness. When engineers design a ship, they test its ability to cut through the water at great speeds and to withstand torrential rains and waves. They check the resistance of the wind as it moves through the air. The faster the ship goes the more resistance it experiences because of its speed. This process is similar to strengthening one's faith and certitude.

Protection

Just as our bodies require protection from the elements through clothing, so the heart requires protection if we are to ensure that its door remains open and the soul is free to express itself through the body. The soul expresses courage, even when the body is afraid. Many situations and people will present themselves to us and our ego will respond in fear. It's normal for the body and lower heart to instinctually feel fear. However, courage allows us to access the higher heart, the soul, and keep us open enough to connect to our clarity and discernment to get through the situation with diplomacy and wisdom.

When fear seizes the heart and we feel protective of ourselves, we must first ask ourselves if the threat is real or illusory. There are real threats to our safety and well-being, and there are illusions that bring up past thoughts, hurts and memories and can lead us to perceive our world incorrectly. If we meet a large bear on a path, our lower instinct and body will respond with fear. This is appropriate, and if we articulate the fear in depth, we may find a sense of awe mixed in with it. But if a co-worker is criticizing a job we have done, our body may be seized with as much fear as it is with the bear! When we keep the heart open, we can discern a false response from a true one, and work through the intense feelings without personalizing the criticism.

In those moments when we feel defensive and the need for protection, we can call on the power of Bahá'u'lláh, at the same time chanting repeatedly in our minds the reminder to 'stay open'. 'Open' or 'soften' seem to be the best words I have found to help our body and mind to stay connected to wisdom and clarity. When I hear a client speak, I see how we usually know when we need to stand up and fight for what we believe, or to set a boundary and say no. We know when to call on courage to be patient and compassionate. We can discern the situation and take the right action. This gives us courage to not personalize what others do or say. The need for protection is really the call for the release from the prison of self on a deeper level.

I see many clients going through extremely stressful and survival-type situations. Legal battles, for example, can bring out the worst in people and become very stressful. I had a client who would have a panic attack and be out of commission for two days every time she received an email from her attorney. A phone call would put her 'into orbit' and she'd be breathless with heart palpitations for hours. Her sleep was fitful. Through consultation, we created her authentic self to be her 'secretary'. Every time there was a call, she would work on opening her heart, connecting to her true self and having it take a message for her or negotiate on her behalf. Her true self would also answer emails and reassure her that everything was being taken care of, remind her to have faith in her attorney and know that she could handle and accept whatever the outcome would be. While it wasn't an easy process, this helped her to feel tremendously more grounded and centred. The challenge was to rewrite her old habits of the body responding with fear and feeling out of control, to regain balance by acknowledging her fear and yet act with courage. After several mindful attempts at allowing her authentic self the reins, something clicked and she was able to feel only 20 per cent of her previous amount of fear.

'Abdu'l-Bahá is reported to have said that radiant acquiescence keeps the door open, allowing the fluidity of the spirit. One is released from the prison of self: 'Unless one accepts dire vicissitudes, not with dull resignation, but with radiant acquiescence, one cannot attain this freedom.'[68]

Meditating on radiant acquiescence, we may see how it works with the body; I have found that resistance creates toxic substances in the body and closes the door of the heart, creating rigidity and cutting us off from the soul's power. The paradox is that resisting something actually brings it closer. A trusting heart is a heart that feels safe within the protection of God, that knows He gives us what is best for us, that He closes one door to open another. In an attitude of trust, we focus our attention on finding that opening rather than standing frustrated at the closed door. Over and over again in my practice I see that God always gives us what we need, although not always what we want. Again, turning to the Bahá'í Writings we see that 'Abdu'l-Bahá expounds on this theme:

> The afflictions which come to humanity sometimes tend to centre the consciousness upon the limitations. This is a veritable prison. Release comes by making of the will a door through which the confirmations of the spirit come. They come to a man or woman who accepts his life with radiant acquiescence.[69]

Acquiescence requires knowledge of the spiritual teachings for today and the laws of God. Obedience to these laws is an integral part of acquiescing to God's will. In the body, all cells acquiesce to the good of the whole organ. If one cell should decide that it has its own ideas and wishes to fulfil its own marching orders, disease begins. In the metaphor of the ship, after engineers design, test and create the ship, those who are to sail it are trained in its technology so as to keep it safe. They learn to read the gauges that show the overall situation – navigational, temperature, speed, etc. They also learn the wisdom of obeying the commands of the coastguard. When in danger, they must have faith in the captain or the central command, which informs them of the direction to steer and when they are given permission to dock. They *unhesitatingly* obey orders. From this example, it's easier to see the danger of attachment to one's own self and ideas. Following one's own promptings instead of relying on the gauges (one's state of mind and emotions) can endanger one's spiritual life. Bahá'u'lláh demonstrates this in the Tablet of the Branch, when referring to 'Abdu'l-Bahá:

> They who deprive themselves of the shadow of the Branch, are lost in the wilderness of error, are consumed by the heat of worldly desires, and are of those who will assuredly perish.[70]

This is how obedience and radiant acquiescence can work together to safeguard our journey.

Fear of God

The best protective clothing for the heart is the fear of God: its 'raiment is the fear of God'. Bahá'u'lláh writes: 'Adorn . . . your hearts with the attire of the fear of God.'[71] The Bahá'í texts emphasize the supreme ability of the fear of God to protect the inhabitants of the world; it is likened to a weapon against wrongdoing, a shield from the onslaught of self, the greatest commander in the attainment of victory. It is, writes Bahá'u'lláh,

> a sure defence and a safe stronghold for all the peoples of the world. It is the chief cause of the protection of mankind, and the supreme instrument for its preservation. Indeed, there existeth in man a faculty which deterreth him from, and guardeth him against, whatever is unworthy and unseemly, and which is known as his sense of shame. This, however, is confined to but a few; all have not possessed and do not possess it.[72]

> He should cleanse his heart from all evil passions and corrupt desires, for the fear of God is the weapon that can render him victorious, the primary instrument whereby he can achieve his purpose. The fear of God is the shield that defendeth His Cause, the buckler that enableth His people to attain to victory.[73]

The fear of God can help us differentiate between the higher and lower influences of the heart. A heart possessed by fear does not possess love, but, Bahá'u'lláh tells us, a heart possessed by the fear of God cannot fear anything else:

> he that feareth God shall be afraid of no one except Him, though the powers of the whole earth rise up and be arrayed against him.[74]

The fear of God is a sign that we are drawing nearer to Him. The closer we approach, the more aware of our inabilities and powerlessness we become

Contentment

Another aspect of protection for the heart is contentment. 'Abdu'l-Bahá is reported to have said:

> Contentment is real wealth. If one develops within himself the quality of contentment he will become independent. Contentment is the creator of happiness.[75]

It helps protect us from mental states which can cause ill-health, as Bahá'u'lláh confirms:

> Verily the most necessary thing is contentment under all circumstances; by this one is preserved from morbid conditions and from lassitude. Yield not to grief and sorrow: they cause the greatest misery. Jealousy consumeth the body and anger doth burn the liver: avoid these two as you would a lion.[76]

In the Tablet of the City of Radiant Acquiescence (Lawḥ-i-Madinatu'r-Riḍá),[77] Bahá'u'lláh mentions there are infinite levels of contentment, but reveals only three aspects of it.

The first is contentment with the will of God and to accept radiantly what He has destined.

The second is being contented with oneself. In order to succeed at this level we must detach ourselves from both the material world and the things of the next world. We also will never be content with ourselves as long as we act outside the laws of God.

The third level is being content with our fellow believers and showing humility before them. Elevating the self over the believers is the same as showing pride towards God. We show contentment when we seek the believers' good pleasure.

We must also protect our soul from dangerous influences – just as we protect our eyes from UV rays. Being around gossip or backbiting endangers our spiritual life, and should be regarded as life-threatening. Certain spiritual diseases can be spread like leprosy. We must eschew the company of the ungodly, and associate with people who are firm in the Covenant. 'Abdu'l-Bahá tells us:

> Bad associates bring about infection of bad qualities. It is like leprosy; it is impossible for a man to associate and befriend a leper and not be infected. This command is for the sake of protection and to safeguard . . . In short, the point is this: . . . Just as in bodily diseases we must prevent intermingling and infection and put into effect sanitary laws, because the infectious physical diseases uproot the foundation of humanity; likewise one must protect and safeguard the blessed souls from the breaths and fatal spiritual diseases; otherwise violation, like the plague, will become a contagion and all will perish.[78]

This concept may also be related to an internal spiritual power, the imagination. We must protect our mind from the dangers of this power, as explained by 'Abdu'l-Bahá:

> Imagination is one of our greatest powers and a most difficult one to rule. Imagination is the father of superstition . . . It is a great power of the soul but without value unless rightly controlled and guided.[79]

Bahá'u'lláh has revealed many prayers giving us an indication of the importance of protection against both internal and external forces. In the following example, Bahá'u'lláh indicates that His imprisonment was not to protect Him from the world, but to provide the world with the evidence of His greatness in sustaining tribulations. The prayer indicates that there's a time for protection, and a time to be exposed to tests:

> Thy bondage is not for my protection, but to enable me to sustain successive tribulations, and to prepare me for the trials that must needs repeatedly assail me. Perish that lover who discerneth between

the pleasant and the poisonous in his love for his beloved! Be thou satisfied with what God hath destined for thee. He, verily, ruleth over thee as He willeth and pleaseth. No God is there but Him, the Inaccessible, the Most High.[80]

Movement

The human temple requires more than just ingesting, digesting, transforming and eliminating its food. If one leads a sedentary life but eats all day, the muscles will eventually atrophy and sag; one becomes constipated and puts on a lot of weight. The body requires movement. So does the soul. Exercise and movement for the spirit consist in our ability to move the Writings into action, in spiritual transformation, building character, serving humanity and teaching the Cause.

If our hearts are not open, we cannot receive the breaths of the Holy Spirit or connect to higher guidance and insight. Nor can we give the love and guidance offered by the teachings to our fellow human beings. I am often consulted by clients who are exhausted and fatigued because they are giving so much of themselves to their work, their families and their faith. When we are overtired and our bodies undernourished, our mind and heart 'close down'. This is our signal to change – but we are such a resilient species that most of us continue to do and think right through it. After some conversation and exploration, I talk to these clients about letting God's love flow through them. When the heart is open, we have free access to limitless energy flowing in and out. How else can we explain how the Master in His later years travelled so far and engaged so many people for so long, even at times with a fever?

Bahá'u'lláh reminds us:

> It is incumbent upon every man of insight and understanding to strive to translate that which hath been written into reality and action . . . That one indeed is a man who, today, dedicateth himself to the service of the entire human race.[81]

'Abdu'l-Bahá explained that under certain conditions action is counted as prayer:

Table 12.4 Knowledge into action

	Apathy	Ignorance	Disobedience	Actions without intention (mindless)	Striving	Obedience
Form	Non-action, non-thought	Not knowing what to do or how to do it. Devoid of knowledge, awareness, or education	Choice involved: refusal to obey, or neglect	Choice without the powers of the intellect, not paying attention	Devoting serious effort or energy, struggle in opposition	Submitting and choosing to align
Motivation	Lack of interest, feeling or caring	May want to change, or may not know change is necessary	Selfish desires, attachments, stubbornness	Doing things to just do them – going through the motions	Trying to submit and align one's actions to God's will	Love, fear or hope of bounty
Results	Not interested, not connected, stagnation	Common belief that ignorance is bliss, unaware that it's really oppression and imprisonment	Self-importance, I don't belong, don't have to, it doesn't apply to me	Illusion of not having a choice, or of unthinking obligation, perhaps to tradition (a type of prison)	In failure, subject to loss of enthusiasm, but victory ingrains new habit	Attaining true liberty, ultimately helping the true self

All effort and exertion put forth by man from the fullness of his heart is worship, if it is prompted by the highest motives and the will to do service to humanity. This is worship: to serve mankind and to minister to the needs of the people. Service is prayer.[82]

There are numerous levels of translating what has been written into action. Table 12.4 shows a sample scale that I created to delineate a wide range of actions and the motivations behind them. How many times have we been stuck by our inability to take action when action is needed? Or take the right action in a situation? We can be very attracted to the teachings of Bahá'u'lláh in theory, but it is when they are reflected in our actions that the spirit gets its exercise, creating spiritual health. At one end of the spectrum, apathy is like a spiritual death. The more we strive to align our actions with the teachings, the more confusion and ignorance will dissipate.

'Abdu'l-Bahá said that ignorance is a type of torment, and the Universal House of Justice wrote in its Riḍván message of 2012, 'Ignorance is the most grievous form of oppression.' Many actions stem from a type of ignorance; for example, disobedience is a type of ignorance, for even when it's intentional stubbornness, the disobedient person doesn't truly have knowledge and understanding of why an action would benefit them. Going through the motions, or doing the same thing over and over again, was also questioned by Bahá'u'lláh. He likened unquestioning obedience to tradition to a prison, especially accepting things without the investigation of truth.

The place that divides one from habit and a newly acquired spiritual skill is the attribute of ***striving***. On the one hand our actions are still aligned with past habits (ignorance) and on the other our will is connected to the Will of God, wanting change, as Shoghi Effendi and 'Abdu'l-Bahá have told us:

> Effort is an inseparable part of man's life . . . Life is after all a struggle. Progress is attained through struggle, and without such a struggle life ceases to have a meaning; it becomes even extinct.[83]

> Man must be tireless in his effort. Once his effort is directed in the proper channel if he does not succeed today he will succeed tomorrow. Effort in itself is one of the noblest traits of human character.[84]

The very act of striving with pure intention helps us to attain an attribute more quickly. I think of striving as comparable to strength training for the body, for instance by lifting weights. Here's how it can play out in practical terms: we may be in a chasm between seeing what we should do, and not wanting to do it. For example, I ask many clients to pray for the forgiveness of someone who has hurt them. The clients don't feel like doing it, so they don't, but they know it's the right thing. It's acceptable to stimulate your will to do the action until you attain the attraction or desire to do it. It comes down to a choice between what is right, and what is easy. We must supplicate to the Blessed Beauty through prayer to be able to overcome our own failings while at the same time exerting our efforts to obey the teachings. Pretty soon we will cross into the territory of being attracted to that action, and wholly reflect the teaching through desire and action.

God accepts actions performed out of obedience, fear of retribution, or wanting His bounties; but actions performed *out of love* yield the most fruits and are most pleasing to God. Even in our careers, being mindful of purpose towards the betterment of the world will contribute to our well-being. **Servitude** is the highest station we can attain in this day. It's the individual's efforts towards laying the foundation of the new spiritual order in the world that makes the greatest change.

Since our true purpose in this earthly life lies in carrying forward 'an ever-advancing civilization' – building the new world order in this age, the quickest and best way of doing this is by teaching the Message of Bahá'u'lláh, in obedience to His injunction: 'Open, O people, the city of the human heart with the key of your utterance. Thus have We, according to a pre-ordained measure, prescribed unto you your duty.'[85] It is a command He gave without any exemptions, including age, status, health or culture.

When we serve and teach we lose all sense of 'self'. Problems move to the background. This is the ultimate expression of a human – selflessness. The prayer revealed by 'Abdu'l-Bahá as the Tablet of Visitation reveals His greatest wish:

> Give me to drink from the chalice of selflessness; with its robe clothe me, and in its ocean immerse me. Make me as dust in the pathway of Thy loved ones . . . [86]

Catalysts

As we have seen earlier in this book, the human body requires catalysts to transform and absorb nutrition and to differentiate nutrition from toxins, moving these out of the body. Enzymes fill this role. The changes in the body at puberty leading to transformation and maturity are caused by hormones. Without these chemical agencies, processes cannot take place.

In our spiritual progress too, catalysts are an integral part of the journey. Without a catalyst such as faith, prayer is like trying to run your boat without wind. We must give our sails the 'gentle winds of the Dawn of Thy Manifestation'. To change the metaphor, we must select the right channel on our communication radio systems to begin talking. We must establish a relationship with the One to whom we are praying.

It is recommended that Bahá'ís pray to Bahá'u'lláh to intercede on our behalf. It's perfectly acceptable to pray directly to God, but since God is unknowable it can be difficult. When we choose to pray through Bahá'u'lláh, the Master, or even an ancestor, we know and love them. It can be easier to feel love, faith and submission in prayer because we trust they will do everything to help us. We must trust that our prayers will be heard and answered in God's infinite wisdom and mercy.

Yearning, faith and sacrifice are the catalysts that open the door of the heart, the portals to the next world. Among the many people I work with, those who cling to faith, who yearn to grow and sacrifice their old patterns and habits, make the fastest progress and have the best results in working their way back to health. In our daily battles, this world drains our spirit and can overwhelm us. When we are drained, we are vulnerable to egoistic habits such as judging or criticizing. As we make mistakes, our faith and yearning to do better will encourage us and keep us connected to hope, being aware of our needs and tending to our own garden. It's at these times that we take the opportunity to make peace, rebalance our lives.

Faith

The ascent of our soul depends upon the health of our two wings: one wing representing knowledge and the other faith. Faith isn't defined as our ability to believe in things unseen, but as the love that flows from our heart to God – our attraction to the Kingdom. Faith implies action, because we must have knowledge first and then be attracted to following through with action. This action will be guided by God when it is conscious and loving. No-one can steer a parked car. God cannot direct our actions if we are not moving. When we are, He can gently guide us.

Faith is the very quality our souls are meant to manifest – to give birth to the 'spirit of faith'. So powerful is the animating force of faith, 'Abdu'l-Bahá said, that 'Nothing shall be impossible to you if you have faith . . . As ye have faith so shall your powers and blessings be.'[87] It is the divine rod that attracts divine confirmations, like a magnet. 'Abdu'l-Bahá is reported to have said, 'A man of faith bears every trial, every hardship, with self-control and patience. One without faith is always wailing, lamenting, carrying on.'[88]

Yearning

In our ship analogy, communications are sent via radio waves, and communication is instant. Anything in our mind is transmitted into waves. If we have a weak connection, or no response on the line, we may need electricity. The spiritual parallel to this might be great yearning. We must pray with desire and longing for nearness: 'Thou disappointest no one who hath sought Thee, nor dost Thou keep back from Thee any one who hath desired Thee.'[89] When we wish and long to be nearer to our Lord, the door is always open.

Yearning also affects the way we read and listen. We can read the Writings as an intellectual exercise, or with yearning which opens the heart. When we stand at the shore of this great Ocean, like a diver we prepare our mind and hearts to plunge into the depths, seeking the treasures enshrined therein. The more the diver yearns to find treasure, the more joyful and zealous the journey. As we dive, our senses are heightened and feel more alive. Bahá'u'lláh writes:

> It is the duty of every seeker to bestir himself and strive to attain the shores of this ocean, so that he may, in proportion to the eagerness of his search and the efforts he hath exerted, partake of such benefits as have been pre-ordained in God's irrevocable and hidden Tablets.[90]

The efforts we make to understand must be in proportion to our thirst for understanding. Desire then culminates in certitude. Bahá'u'lláh eloquently writes,

> Only when the lamp of search, of earnest striving, of longing desire, of passionate devotion, of fervid love, of rapture, and ecstasy, is kindled within the seeker's heart, and the breeze of His loving-kindness is wafted upon his soul, will the darkness of error be dispelled, the mists of doubts and misgivings be dissipated, and the lights of knowledge and certitude envelop his being.[91]

Sacrifice

I think of the mystery of sacrifice as the catalytic converter of all deeds. 'Abdu'l-Bahá gives a clear description:

> Until a being setteth his foot in the plane of sacrifice, he is bereft of every favour and grace; and this plane of sacrifice is the realm of dying to the self, that the radiance of the living God may then shine forth.[92]

Sacrifice is giving up something lower for something higher, as Shoghi Effendi writes:

> Self-sacrifice means to subordinate this lower nature and its desires to the more godly and noble side of ourselves. Ultimately, in its highest sense, self-sacrifice means to give our will and our all to God to do with as He pleases. Then He purifies and glorifies our true self until it becomes a shining and wonderful reality.[93]

Sacrifice is expressed in different ways. Our spiritual growth benefits even when the sacrifice is a physical one, if the deed is done in love. Another example is when one form is sacrificed and transformed into another, as when a tiny seed is planted and gives up its current form (a shell) to break open for a shoot to grow into a plant. The Master explains that when pain or suffering is endured for a higher cause it takes on a special significance:

> Sacrificial love is the love shown by the moth towards the candle, by the parched wayfarer towards the living fountain, by the true lover towards his beloved, by the yearning heart towards the goal of its desire.[94]

Third, the sacrifice of our own characteristics can sometimes appear on the surface as self-denial, or repression of our right to take offence – a kind of inauthenticity – for example, if someone treats us unkindly but we return kindness as the Master asked us to. But Shoghi Effendi explained the results of self-sacrifice in this manner:

> It is only through suffering that the nobility of character can make itself manifest. The energy we expend in enduring the intolerance of some individuals of our community is not lost. It is transformed into fortitude, steadfastness and magnanimity . . . Sacrifices in the path of one's religion produce always immortal results . . [95]

Yearning, faith and self-sacrifice are catalysts in spiritual development and necessary ingredients for spiritual health. They propel the heart to stay open, hopeful and to keep going. The Fast offers an opportunity to reflect upon our development of these attributes, and strengthen these qualities into a more habitual way of living.

Cleanliness

Any ship owner understands the necessity of keeping the decks, instruments and hull clean. In the same way, the fasting period offers us a time of retrospection to cleanse our hearts of the dust of this world and to polish our mirrors to better reflect the rays of the 'Sun of Truth'. We can think of this as putting our ship 'in dock' during this period. Purity, sanctity, holiness and orderliness are all aspects of spiritual cleanliness, as 'Abdu'l-Bahá explained:

> As soon as the mirror is cleaned and purified, the sun will manifest itself. The more pure and sanctified the heart of man becomes, the nearer it draws to God, and the light of the Sun of Reality is revealed within it.[96]

The clarity that comes from keeping ourselves clean, truthful and authentic becomes more prevalent. We see our lives, our interactions with others, our bodies, our words, actions and thoughts as holy sites. We can treat these as we would when walking through the holy gardens and visiting the holy places. Most pilgrims wish to clean themselves inside and out before entering the holy places; the cleanliness and sanctity of the gardens invite us in and we feel that we never want to leave. In the same way, we need to sanctify our thoughts, make our words truthful and holy so that our spirit feels invited to stay. When we live in truth and fearless to see what is, our work is clear. Keep your environment orderly, your thoughts and words orderly, so that your spirit will desire to stay with you, energizing you and guiding you.

I help many clients who are very sick to cleanse their homes and create an orderly outer environment. Simultaneously, we work on purifying their inner environment. We work together to find the negative thought patterns, the unsupportive dialogue, the lies. We work to open the heart and find how the ego is always trying to close the door by feeling defensive or using avoidance techniques.

In one case, we frequently examined the avoidance techniques that kept coming up. Every time there was a deadline, this client would avoid looking at her emails and stop cleaning her house. When we looked deeper into this habit and what it was doing for her, she found a defensive part of herself that closed off others and the world, believing she would be safe. This illusion provided a buffer between her and the world; however, it was preventing her from accomplishing some very important daily tasks. Cleaning up her environment – and the beliefs within herself – helped her to better recognize and understand her inner dynamic. An orderly physical environment provided the structure and safety she was craving and allowed her to work with the inner part of herself and address the issues she was facing.

In the Bahá'í teachings the metaphors of dust, rust or dress of this world on the mirror of the heart can signify egotism, natural emotions, chains of habits, earthly defilements, sins, remoteness, doubts, pride, vainglory, backbiting, and acquired knowledge, to name a few. Bahá'u'lláh encourages us: 'Wash your hearts from all earthly defilements, and hasten to enter the Kingdom of your Lord, the Creator of earth and heaven.'[97] He also tells us:

It behoveth thee to consecrate thyself to the Will of God. Whatsoever hath been revealed in His Tablets is but a reflection of His Will. So complete must be thy consecration, that every trace of worldly desire will be washed from thine heart. This is the meaning of true unity.[98]

'Abdu'l-Bahá has written that cleanliness of the heart denotes nearness, and gives the example of rust as an impediment:

Consequently, it hath been proven that nearness and remoteness signify smoothness, clearness and fineness; or rust, impurity and roughness, respectively.[99]

The natural emotions are blameworthy and are like rust which deprives the heart of the bounties of God. But sincerity, justice, humility, severance, and love for the believers of God will purify the mirror and make it radiant with reflected rays from the Sun of Truth.[100]

Cleansing the body during the Fast has its counterpart on the spiritual level in cleansing the heart of things of this world. There are many means by which to cleanse the heart. Bahá'u'lláh attests that the rust from our hearts has been cleansed through a 'twofold distinction':

All praise and glory be to God Who, through the power of His might, hath delivered His creation from the nakedness of non-existence, and clothed it with the mantle of life. From among all created things He hath singled out for His special favour the pure, the gem-like reality of man, and invested it with a unique capacity of knowing Him and of reflecting the greatness of His glory. This twofold distinction conferred upon him hath cleansed away from his heart the rust of every vain desire, and made him worthy of the vesture with which his Creator hath deigned to clothe him. It hath served to rescue his soul from the wretchedness of ignorance.[101]

Fire and water. Elements found in the material world used for purification are mentioned in the Bahá'í Writings for spiritual purification as well. Fire and water are mystical metaphors that reveal the highest forms of spirituality. Fire purifies, while water is used for bathing, cleansing the body as well as the spirit.

Water is related to Revelation, the Word of God itself, as in these words of the Báb:

> The waters of that river flow forth from my tongue and pen with that which God willeth, imperishable and everlasting. This water is the well-spring of the Elixir . . . [102]

However, the water which cleanses the heart has distinct qualities. The Writings of Bahá'u'lláh are replete with references to these:

> . . . wash me thoroughly with the waters of Thy graciousness and mercy, and attire me with the raiment of wholesomeness, through Thy forgiveness and bounty.[103]

> . . . and mayest wash away the dust of ignorance, and cleanse the darkened self with the waters of mercy flowing from the Source of divine Knowledge . . . [104]

> Purify your ears that they may hearken unto the Voice of God. By God! It is even as fire that consumeth the veils, and as water that washeth the souls of all who are in the universe.[105]

And 'Abdu'l-Bahá writes, 'you have been attracted by the perfumes of God and . . . you have bathed in the sea of knowledge.'[106]

Scrubbing. Besides elements like fire and water, action is required to cleanse ourselves. One could simply sit in clear water and consider it bathing, or simply stand under the shower, but a good scrub is usually required. God's mercy and forgiveness wash away sins, giving us a fresh start, but it is incumbent on us to *ask* for forgiveness daily in order to bathe in the love and mercy of our Lord, as Bahá'u'lláh clarifies:

> Wherefore, hearken ye unto My speech, and return ye to God and repent, that He, through His grace, may have mercy upon you, may wash away your sins, and forgive your trespasses.[107]

Adib Taherzadeh writes that in a Tablet to one of His hand-maidens Bahá'u'lláh affirms that the heart is the dawning-place of light of His Countenance, and the treasure-house of the pearls of His love. He urges her to bathe her heart with the waters of certitude, so that it may be cleansed from the remembrance of anyone save Him.[108]

Bounty. Did you ever think of tests as a form of washing? 'Abdu'l-Bahá writes:

> These tests ... do but cleanse the spotting of self from off the mirror of the heart, till the Sun of Truth can cast its rays thereon; for there is no veil more obstructive than the self, and however tenuous that veil may be, at the last it will completely shut a person out, and deprive him of his portion of eternal grace.[109]

Earlier in the same Tablet, he explains the meaning of tests:

> Thou didst write of afflictive tests that have assailed thee. To the loyal soul, a test is but God's grace and favour; for the valiant doth joyously press forward to furious battle on the field of anguish, when the coward, whimpering with fright, will tremble and shake. So too, the proficient student, who hath with great competence mastered his subjects and committed them to memory, will happily exhibit his skills before his examiners on the day of his tests. So too will solid gold wondrously gleam and shine out in the assayer's fire.
>
> It is clear, then, that test and trial are, for sanctified souls, but God's bounty and grace, while to the weak, they are a calamity, unexpected and sudden.[110]

And Shoghi Effendi writes of the cleansing power of tests for an entire community:

> The ten years which followed (1903–1913), so full of the tests and trials which agitated, cleansed and energized the body of the earliest pioneers of the Faith in that land, had as their happy climax 'Abdu'l-Bahá's memorable visit to America.[111]

The importance of spiritual cleanliness

The importance of cleanliness is conveyed by performing ablutions prior to prayer. Here is the symbol of simultaneously washing the body as we prepare to use the Word of God to symbolically wash our hearts and minds. Once the mind and heart are cleansed, we can understand the prayer we are reciting better, as 'Abdu'l-Bahá reminds us:

> It is easy to read the Holy Scriptures, but it is only with a clean heart and a pure mind that one may understand their true meaning. Let us ask God's help to enable us to understand the Holy Books. Let us pray for eyes to see and ears to hear, and for hearts that long for peace.[112]

When the early believers came on pilgrimage to meet Bahá'u'lláh, the Master would prepare them for attaining His presence. Outward and inward cleanliness was one of the most important objectives in preparation for this most important meeting of their lives. Similarly, in His writings 'Abdu'l-Bahá offers us a simple method to use if we wish to attain God's presence in 'the world of vision':

> When thou desirest and yearnest for meeting in the world of vision; at the time when thou art in perfect fragrance and spirituality, wash thy hands and face, clothe thyself in clean robes, turn toward the court of the Peerless One, offer prayer to Him and lay thy head upon the pillow. When sleep cometh, the doors of revelation shall be opened and all thy desires shall become revealed.[113]

And in another instance:

> Arise and wash thy body, wear a pure gown, and, directing thyself to the Kingdom of God, supplicate and pray to Him. Sleep in a clean, well prepared and ventilated place, and ask for appearance (or display) in the world of vision. Thou wilt have visions which will cause the doors of doubts to be closed, which will give you new joy, wonderful dilation, brilliant glory. Thou wilt comprehend realities and meanings.[114]

13

RECOMMENDATIONS FOR THE FAST

As before, this chapter mainly presents a selection of assignments I often give to my clients; they are in no way 'official' Bahá'í teachings, but simply provide some ideas for applying the principles of spiritual health to our daily life during the Fast, with the aim of cleansing our spirit of old habits, recreating new habits for a healthy, connected spirit and maintaining these efforts so as to stay in balance. New habits take time and patience to integrate into one's lifestyle.

Cleansing and balancing the spirit

Giving the heart a 'fast' from attachments

Wash and purify your heart from attachments during the Fast, using the fire of attraction and the water of His words. Attachments to the self can lead us to estrangement, and the fasting period offers us a time to cleanse our spirits of these. 'Abdu'l-Bahá tells us that

> Everything which conduces to separation and estrangement is satanic because it emanates from the purposes of self.[1]

and that

> Souls are inclined to estrangement. Steps should first be taken to do away with this estrangement, for only then will the Word take effect.[2]

Attachments and desires are harmful to our soul. Here is an example I sometimes use: Why would a bird build a nest where a landowner continually cuts the grass when sheltered tall grass is nearby? Answer:

Because that's where the bird *wants* to build it. Bahá'u'lláh says we ask for things that are harmful to us:

> Consider the pettiness of men's minds. They ask for that which injureth them, and cast away the thing that profiteth them.³

The Fast allows time for reflection on what we are attached to that may cause separation, apathy or estrangement. The following questions may inspire you to search deeply into your heart to find your attachments:

- With whom am I not my authentic self? With whom do I lose my centre? What exactly about being with them causes me to lose centre? What are my expectations with that person? Which persons draw me closer to God, and which persons lead me to remoteness from God? Can I help myself in that process?
- Do I take time for contemplation, reflection or meditation? What are the obstacles I allow to distract me?
- What things in my life will I *not* throw away? What items am I ready to release? What is it about the things I'm unwilling to throw away? Is this thing important to keep? Does it promote nearness to or remoteness from God?
- What beliefs or ideas am I unwilling to give up? What opinions cause me to feel defensive? What am I afraid of losing? Are they in alignment with the teachings? Do they draw me nearer to God?
- What habits do I love the most? Which ones cause the most comfort? Do those habits contribute to my spiritual progress? Do any of them interfere with my job, my relationships, etc.? Do I have to defend those habits?
- How do I use music?
- What takes my attention away from the Divine? What distractions in this world do I cling to?
- What or who takes up most of my time and attention?
- Where in my life do yearning desire, faith and sacrifice play out?
- What am I resisting, and what am I acquiescing to?

Table 13.1 Opening the heart

1. Breathe deeply. Focus on the heart centre, breathing in and out. Breathe from low down.
2. Love yourself and others in a true sense of the word.
3. Connect to your body. Observe sounds around you, the colours, the bottom of your feet on the floor, your feelings, the taste in your mouth, the smells that surround you.
4. Know your true self and what it loves, what brings it joy.
5. Surround yourself with those who validate, support and strengthen your true self.
6. Keep clear boundaries between yourself and others while holding the understanding that we are all the leaves of one tree and so interconnected that the healing of one is the healing of all.
7. Face the tests and misfortunes of life with an open attitude, faith and patience. Embrace strong emotions with compassion and understanding.
8. Have the courage to stand up for what is just.

The Fast gives us the opportunity to solidify spiritual practices to achieve optimal health during the rest of the year. In a letter dated 6 December 1983 the Universal House of Justice wrote about the spiritual practices which strengthen the soul:

> Bahá'u'lláh has stated quite clearly in His Writings the essential requisites for our spiritual growth, and these are stressed again and again by 'Abdu'l-Bahá in His Talks and Tablets. One can summarise them briefly in this way:
>
> 1. The recital each day of one of the Obligatory Prayers with pure-hearted devotion.
>
> 2. The regular reading of the Sacred Scriptures, specifically at least each morning and evening, with reverence, attention and thought.
>
> 3. Prayerful meditation on the teachings, so that we may understand them more deeply, fulfil them more faithfully, and convey them more accurately to others.

4. Striving every day to bring our behaviour more into accordance with the high standard that are set forth in the Teachings.

5. Teaching the Cause of God.

6. Selfless service in the work of the Cause and in the carrying on of our trade or profession.[4]

This list represents *core actions* collected from the Baháʼí teachings to maintain our spiritual health and growth. Therefore, I would give these the most consideration during the Fast. Find ways of incorporating these practices into your life as a newly acquired habit. Ask yourself: When is the best time to say my obligatory prayer? Meditation? Try out different times of day. You will have various methods of applying these healthy habits, depending on your specific rhythms and routines – for example, during the week, the weekends, or travelling. After the Fast, they will feel like a natural rhythm to your daily routine. If you forget to carry out one of these practices once the new habit is established, you will notice how you start to feel hungry, or as though 'something is missing', and you will soon remember.

The following provides some ideas of how to connect with your spirit during the Fast. I commonly recommend these for basic healthy living.

Before sunrise

- Reenter the world with the remembrance of your Lord. Welcome your spirit and breathe in love.
- Would listening to quiet, meditative music while you prepare breakfast help connect to spiritual energies? This is a great time to hear chanting of the Holy Writings.
- While eating, would activating the feelings of gratitude help connect you to the present moment?
- When you recite the Writings, take some minutes to listen. Where is your mind? How do you feel? What are you experiencing?
- It's commonly recommended that meditation before sunrise is a heightened time of awareness. Does this work in your schedule?

- I often recommend Yoga or Tai Chi to integrate the soul with the body and calm the mind.

During the day

- Check your breathing: how deeply are you breathing? Is your heart open or closed?
- How aware are you of attachments? Practise placing God before you and put His face on everyone you meet. Does this make a difference to your interactions?
- If it feels appropriate, say your noonday prayer.
- Try using the Long Obligatory Prayer during the Fast, or memorizing it.
- Take a walk and practise listening. Appreciate the outdoor environment on the walk, the splendour of nature. Try to experience what the concept of 'absorption' means.
- Are there opportunities to serve? Does someone need a helping hand? Write a letter of encouragement or praise.
- Take time to reflect on the meaning of a specific teaching and how it can be translated into action.
- How are your teaching efforts?
- Try to encourage and support others' inspirations and positive actions. Believe in those around you. Do you trust God's confirmations?

After sunset

- How does it feel to give thanks while preparing food and sitting down to eat?
- When you feel spiritually 'hungry' again, have your spiritual dinner by reading the evening Bahá'í Writings.
- Take 15–30 minutes to meditate and train the mind. Does evening meditation suit you?
- Spend time with those closest to you. What is your level of unity?

Before bed

- Take account for your actions today. Start from this present moment and go backwards through your day.
- During this meditation, can you find your heart's attachments to this world and reattach it to the eternal?
- What do you want to manifest this year? Visualize and imagine yourself achieving a goal you have made. Feel the feelings of carrying out that goal, all the sensational experiences of that goal. Feel the love in the heart centre when you visualize this and give thanks, as though you already have it. Put the belief in your heart that the universe is a friendly place of abundance and all your needs will be anticipated and met. Feel how you are surrounded by this nurturing, loving energy.

Healing crisis

As with the body and mind, I see clients experiencing resistance from the ego when attachments are addressed and challenged. Observe your reactions to fasting from your usual habits, creature comforts, people, etc. The resistance will manifest itself in the various forms already discussed in the chapters on the body and mind. When we go searching for God, there will be a tug of war for the reins of the horse, and egotism often resorts to bashing the horse. Gentleness to oneself, steadfastness, faith in God's mercy, and patience are critical to our capacity to endure the crises of spiritual healing. Perseverance will act as a magnet to divine blessings.

I always tell my clients that the most distinct and painful part of a healing crisis in spirituality lies in the awareness of being remote from God. In a healthy state the mind knows that after joy comes sorrow, and after sorrow comes joy, and this too shall pass. This is the wisdom in the Christian teaching, 'Be in the world, but not of the world.' This resembles our awareness of the pain of this world, yet remaining connected in faith to the Kingdom.

In the case of apathy, try the remedy of prayer. I sometimes recommend that clients say a few short 'warm-up prayers' to get their mind focused and their hearts attracted. Try invoking the Greatest Name. It is your best helper, a most powerful weapon against the healing crisis. Pray until celestial feelings develop, no matter how small.

Rebuilding spiritual health

Our spiritual capacity depends on both our 'pre-ordained measure' and the direct result of our efforts. The exertion we make to understand the Writings and apply them to our action in daily living affects the rate of our spiritual progress.

Integrate new habits

'Abdu'l-Bahá said:

> The attainment of any object is conditioned upon knowledge, volition and action. Unless these three conditions are forthcoming, there is no execution or accomplishment.⁵

Although our reading of the Writings provides knowledge, there must be attraction (heart) to the goal and a strong will (mind) to follow through. When we begin to integrate these habits into our beings, resistance naturally crops up. This can reveal the heart's attachments.

Working with the concept of two

- *Intention vs. impulse.* These two forces can feel similar to each other. Did you just perform an action out of impulse or intention? Intention implies thought and consideration while keeping your centre. Impulse can send us a sense that 'If I don't do or have this, I won't be well.' There is more of an urgent sensation to impulse, like an animalistic response. It's usually reflected in our first urge to action. Take a moment before speaking or acting to identify a specific intention, then follow through with action.
- *Pain vs. despair.* In my experience, daily living and relationships present problematic situations, difficulties and stress. Pain and suffering are a condition of life on earth. Sometimes acutely felt needs cannot be satisfied. Pain from relationships, as discussed previously, affects the soul, while the soul is exempt from any physical pain. Pain is simply an indication of direction. When we experience pain, we need to find a different path, belief, or

way of doing something. Often, pain flips into despair. If pain is out of balance it can transform us into being a victim. Pain is simply something we must endure; and if we do, the pain may dissipate. If it leads to despair, we hang on to the pain instead of releasing it. Despair comes whenever a soul dwells upon the pain and indulges in the painful feelings.

- *Trust vs. fear.* Do you trust God to care for you and your loved ones? If you believe this to be true, do your actions reflect that belief? Bahá'u'lláh writes that 'the source of all good is trust in God, submission unto His command, and contentment with His holy will and pleasure'.[6] Our actions stem out of a heart filled with either trust or fear: they cannot be both, as fear and trust cannot reside in the same place. We can say to ourselves: 'I trust I can handle whatever lies ahead. God will not give a soul more than it can bear. I trust that others can handle the truth. I trust that others will take care of their own lives and circumstances, allowing for mistakes.' Keeping an open mind/open heart policy when life gets scary is a skill. This skill is mastered when we look towards God, ourselves, and others through the eyes of trust.

Spiritual 'supplements'

Why not choose a daily 'supplement' for the spirit? I playfully refer to the following as supplements to help balance out our lives and make them meaningful and more connected to spirit. Examples might include music, being in delightful places, writing, arts (including the performing arts) and sciences. Your heart will be specifically attracted to different avenues of creativity. This may change with your life experiences, depending on circumstances, time and friends.

An area I find all too often lacking in a client's lifestyle assessment is the section on joy and creativity. But creativity and joy fill the heart, as in the saying 'my cup runneth over'. Spiritual practices will fill the cup, but other forms of spiritual food are necessary to create a balanced life. Typically, such a food will be an activity we are so immersed in that we forget all sense of self, time and place. It is a time when we are flowing with our inner faculties, allowing whatever is inside to come out. Each day the spirit longs for 'flow', for uninterrupted time to play.

Bahá'u'lláh celebrated the arts and sciences. He

> proclaimed before the face of all the peoples of the world that which will serve as the key for unlocking the doors of sciences, of arts, of knowledge, of well-being, of prosperity and wealth.[7]

In this divine period the doors of arts and sciences have been unlocked! Take advantage of the spiritual springtime! 'Abdu'l-Bahá wrote:

> Arts and industries have been reborn, there are new discoveries in science, and there are new inventions; even the details of human affairs, such as dress and personal effects – even weapons – all these have likewise been renewed.[8]

He discusses how these bring beauty into our lives from the invisible world:

> All sciences, knowledge, arts, wonders, institutions, discoveries and enterprises come from the exercised intelligence of the rational soul. There was a time when they were unknown, preserved mysteries and hidden secrets; the rational soul gradually discovered them and brought them out from the plane of the invisible and the hidden into the realm of the visible.[9]

In a contemplative moment, write a list of things that bring you joy and what you love to do. Think about all the things you love. I love to hear birds sing, I love to work with children, I love to taste something freshly baked. I love praying. This list can be a freeing experience. Many of my clients say, 'I want to find my purpose in life.' This purpose is of course related to the soul's journey towards God, and it is very connected to what you love. When you've created a healthy list, make sure you maintain it once in a while and do something from it often.

Music

Music is a chief instrument in creating a state of joy. The Bahá'í Writings tell us that our souls may ascend through uplifting spiritual music. Music is such a delicate and powerful instrument that we must be careful not to allow it to lead us into desire and passion, or into doing things which are make us heedless. 'Abdu'l-Bahá reminds us that in this new age, Bahá'u'lláh

> hath, in His holy Tablets, specifically proclaimed that music, sung or played, in spiritual food for soul and heart.
>
> The musician's art is among those arts worthy of the highest praise, and it moveth the hearts of all who grieve.[10]

Arts and sciences

So wondrous are the gifts of humanity that the arts, sciences and crafts have been elevated to the station of worship, especially when carried out with a pure motive and to benefit mankind. 'Abdu'l-Bahá said:

> In the Bahá'í Cause arts, sciences and all crafts are (counted as) worship. The man who makes a piece of notepaper to the best of his ability, conscientiously, concentrating all his forces on perfecting it, is giving praise to God. Briefly, all effort and exertion put forth by man from the fullness of his heart is worship, if it is prompted by the highest motives and the will to do service to humanity.[11]

There are innumerable creative crafts that can be a source of rejuvenation: working with textiles, wood, metal, clay, paper, canvas, plants, glass, nature or fashion are just a few. Working and developing our skill in a craft is a time to connect with the soul.

Writing

'Abdu'l-Bahá likened the heart to a box, of which language is the key:

> the function of language is to portray the mysteries and secrets of human hearts. The heart is like a box, and language is the key. Only by using the key can we open the box and observe the gems it contains.[12]

And Bahá'u'lláh reiterates in several important passages in His Writings the importance of how we choose our words, as for instance:

Utterance must needs possess penetrating power. For if bereft of this quality it would fail to exert influence. And this penetrating influence dependeth on the spirit being pure and the heart stainless. Likewise it needeth moderation . . . And moderation will be obtained by blending utterance with the tokens of divine wisdom which are recorded in the sacred Books and Tablets. Thus when the essence of one's utterance is endowed with these two requisites it will prove highly effective and will be the prime factor in transforming the souls of men.[13]

Delightful places

Spending time in places where we feel a sense of awe, wonder, delight and inner joy can nourish our spirits like nothing else. Such places are usually found in nature. These special spots allow us to unwind, relax, connect with and ground our energies. Spaces that cause delight often include the sound of the wind, birds or water, or the sound of silence. Spiritual delight comes from visual stimulation in colour and movement, from trees of varying heights and textures, and gardens with varying shades of colours and sizes. These places invoke a sense of wonder and connection to history, to oneself and each other.[14] Bahá'u'lláh is reported to have said, 'The country is the world of the soul, the city is the world of bodies.'[15]

PART V

WHERE DO I GO FROM HERE?

14

ALTERNATIVES FOR THOSE WHO CANNOT FAST

> Everyone has a physician inside him or her; we just have to help it in its work. The natural healing force within each one of us is the greatest force in getting well.
>
> *Hippocrates*

Many who cannot physically participate in the Fast feel loss during this time. Remembering the purpose of fasting, however, is helpful in giving us a sense of renewal. Can I participate in the Fast even if I cannot physically fast this year? The answer, I believe, is yes.

Bahá'u'lláh explains, 'There are various stages and stations for the Fast and innumerable effects and benefits are concealed therein. Well is it with those who have attained unto them.'[1] This chapter sets out to explore some of the options for those not fasting, but wanting to attain some of its bounties.

Conditions in which one should not fast

Bahá'u'lláh states:

> The law of the Fast is ordained for those who are sound and healthy; as to those who are ill or debilitated, this law hath never been nor is now applicable.[2]

> In clear cases of weakness, illness, or injury the law of the Fast is not binding. This injunction is in conformity with the precepts of God, eternal in the past, eternal in the future. Well is it with them who act accordingly.[3]

Bahá'u'lláh has clearly laid out the wisdom of NOT fasting when conditions are not propitious.[4] From a naturopathic standpoint, fasting during any of the following conditions would be harmful to the body, not helpful:

- Becoming ill during the Fast
- Menstruation
- Being undernourished (overweight individuals can also be undernourished)
- Recovering from surgery
- Mental/emotional or physical severe injury
- Mental/emotional or physical weakness (very low vitality)
- Mental/emotional or physical exhaustion

If you become ill during the Fast, or start menstruating but recover before the end, you can start to Fast again. For those with questionable conditions or poor health, or who are inexperienced, it would be wise to have a healthcare provider supervise your fast. 'Abdu'l-Bahá advised that those with any questions about their health and fasting should consult an expert doctor, and that if the doctor says that fasting would be injurious to the health, then you should not fast.

Another question concerned fasting in a family where difficulties may arise if one keeps the Fast. 'Abdu'l-Bahá answered that just because there may be difficulties, this would not prevent one from fasting. However, 'if fasting gives rise to inharmony it is injurious'.[5]

Many take prescription drugs and must have food with them during the day. Ask your pharmacist what amount of food would suffice with the medication. Some require only a glass of milk. In the spirit of the Fast, you can take your medications, follow any directions from the pharmacist, and reduce other food.

Exploring the bounties of the Fast while not fasting

A letter from the Universal House of Justice points out the significance of this time and encourages us to make use of the spiritual energies available to us:

> The House of Justice is confident that the friends will also want to pray for the believers in Iran during the Fast, *particularly at dawn,*

and it would be useful for National Spiritual Assemblies to remind the friends of the *privilege of joining universally in prayers during this period about which Bahá'u'lláh has written, 'Thou hast endowed every hour of these days with a special virtue, inscrutable to all except Thee . . .'*[6] [emphasis added]

This letter addresses everyone, not just those who are physically fasting, which would indicate to me that every human being can partake of the bounties offered from the Kingdom during the Fast.

This sentiment is also reflected in the prayer for Naw-Rúz, where Bahá'u'lláh acknowledges that whether one has fasted or not is dependent on God's acceptance:

> Since thou hast adorned them, O my Lord, with the ornament of the fast prescribed by Thee, do Thou adorn them also with the ornament of Thine acceptance, through Thy grace and bountiful favour. For the doings of men are all dependent upon Thy good-pleasure, and are conditioned by Thy behest. *Shouldst Thou regard him who hath broken the fast as one who hath observed it,* such a man would be reckoned among them who from eternity had been keeping the fast. And *shouldst Thou decree that he who hath observed the fast hath broken it,* that person would be numbered with such as have caused the Robe of Thy Revelation to be stained with dust, and been far removed from the crystal waters of this living Fountain.[7] [emphasis added]

We cannot underestimate the power of intention. When we beseech God and ask Him to accept our efforts, it is in His good pleasure to accept them or not. This is why we pray to God to accept our efforts and to be pleasing unto Him.

Bahá'u'lláh says, 'Every act ye meditate is as clear to Him as is that act when already accomplished.'[8] Even those who cannot wholly participate can imagine themselves as participating and follow some of the recommendations below.

A major purpose of the Fast is to achieve true unity – within ourselves and ultimately with God. This involves self-sacrifice. The Fast:

- allows us to connect with our Beloved;
- prepares us for the New Year and gives us spiritual recuperation;

- helps us practise choice and moderation;
- balances and purifies us;
- cleanses our hearts of attachments; and
- preserves us from tests.

Bahá'u'lláh exempts some people from fasting for wise reasons, so if you are severely ill or injured, it's imperative to follow the advice of a competent doctor. Strive towards true health: freedom from bodily ailments, freedom of mind from the insistent self, and to become selfless and fully creative in life. If you are well enough, you can consider some of the following options.

Options for participation

The suggestions in this section stem from working with those who wish to Fast but cannot physically fast They come purely from my perspective as a practitioner and personal thoughts about the spiritual energies behind the Fast.

Bahá'u'lláh asks us to observe the Fast, 'which is to protect one's eye from beholding whatever is forbidden and to withhold one's self from food, drink and whatever is not of Him.'[9] If you cannot participate in the material fast, then participate spiritually and partake of the bounties flowing from the eternal Fountain. This time of year contains a special potency and offers bounties. Take time to reflect, meditate on your life, where you need to clean up, what is distracting you from service and nearness to God, and what you want to bring into the New Year. Even if we cannot participate fully in the material fast, we can plan New Year reflections, study the sacred texts and take account of our actions during the past year. Staying in this rhythm helps us to feel part of the community – a worldwide movement and celebration. The main factor is to identify patterns of behaviour needing change. Determine what sacrifices we can make to contribute to the betterment of our lives and to the world.

Health ensures that the spirit is fine-tuned and can freely animate the body. Bahá'u'lláh writes, 'That a sick person showeth signs of weakness is due to the hindrances that interpose themselves between his soul and his body . . .'[10] Any efforts you make during the Fast that would benefit, heighten and retune your energy will reduce such hindrances and enhance your life's experience.

The recommendations and suggestions given in earlier chapters of this book in Parts III and IV on the mind and soul may enable you to participate in the spirit of the Fast. Focus on what will draw you nearer to God, and what constitutes 'whatever is not of Him': 'just as a person abstains from physical appetites, he is to abstain from self-appetites and self-desires.'[11]

From Part II on the body, you may wish to determine how much of it applies to your situation. Among the themes explored there are some of the ways to regain balance and health in your life through diet choices. Perhaps you can choose to give up your luxury foods or going to restaurants. Spiritually, you can get up at dawn, eat, pray and join others in doing so. Maybe, as a service you could even prepare the meal for those fasting, ensuring they are properly nurturing their bodies, and offering plenty of encouragement and positive talk.

If it is determined that you cannot physically fast, consider the following options and temper them with wisdom according to your particular situation:

- Eat only what you need to sustain your energy and nourish your body.
- Eat in private.
- Eat modestly and refrain from snacking.
- Eat nourishing foods.
- Refrain from forms of eating and drinking for entertainment.
- Refrain from extravagant foods/drinks, or comfort foods/drinks.
- Move your body daily, unless ill or injury prevents it.
- Chew your food at least 15 times prior to swallowing.
- Pay attention to urges and impulses to eat – what are your body's addictions? Are you eating out of hunger, boredom, or emotional pain?
- Before eating, try to let your stomach growl before eating again. One of the wonderful parts of the Fast is to give the digestive system a rest. Thoroughly emptying the contents of the stomach is conducive to health.
- Take a short walk after eating to stimulate the digestion.
- Drink teas or tisanes to sooth the digestive system (peppermint, ginger, fennel, chamomile).

Table 14.1 A sample diet plan when you must eat during the Fast

Time	Amount	Example	Notes
Breakfast (before dawn if desired)	1–2 cups	Distilled/ Spring water	Add lemon to warm water.
	1–2 cups	Wholegrain meal such as oatmeal	
Lunch	Salad plate	Protein plus vegetable	Eat the protein at lunch to sustain energy into the afternoon.
Dinner	Salad plate	Complex carbo-hydrate plus vegetable	Starches at night feel more comforting.
Snacks (between meals and after the last meal has been fully digested)	1 piece 1 handful 1 cup	Fruit Nuts, seeds, raw vegetables Tea	

Through the power of intention and modifying impulses and urges, taking part in the Fast's energies is possible! The suggestions listed above are merely a starting point to inspire reflection and contemplation about your level of participation. Just because circumstances exempt full participation in the physical aspect of fasting does not imply that the spirit of the Fast needs to be forgotten. In fact, fasting in the mind and soul would provide ample opportunities to feast from the banquet of bounties offered by God during the Fast.

A note on children

The education of children, says Bahá'u'lláh, is the most meritorious of all deeds. In today's society of excess and indulgence, teaching children self-sacrifice will be a key to the health of our future. Our fasting gives the children an example of:

- *Self-discipline.* The highest station one can attain in this day is servitude.

- *Obedience.* Each Manifestation of God has taught that after obedience to God comes obedience to one's parents. If a child does not obey its parents, it will grow up to disobey God's Will. That child will not receive the protection one receives from conforming to the laws of God.
- *Attitude.* Fasting in front of the children with a positive attitude will instil confidence in them to do the same. It creates an awareness of the mystery and wonder of the Fast. The Fast should be carried out with the utmost love and yearning to please God. As the child grows older, earning privileges, such as fasting, is a natural part of becoming a responsible adult. Be mindful of your dialogue in front of children while fasting, such as making excuses or complaining.
- *Education.* Talk to children about the significance of fasting, and how to properly fast. Let them know and see the benefits on the mind, body and soul. Humanity has always used fasting as a means to reach a higher purpose.

Training children to joyfully sacrifice is paramount. No one likes chores, obligations and doing things they don't look forward to. People commit themselves to activities when they find joy in doing them, not necessarily for the outcomes. Three elements will help you and your children in sacrifice: knowledge, will and attraction. Firstly, you can build willpower by saying yes to some things, but denying impulses. Too often busy parents give in to demands and impulses, creating a challenge with self-discipline. (And we give in to our own impulses too much.)

Secondly, knowledge helps a child comply. Explaining to a child in a language they can understand helps them commit to a decision. Sometimes it's necessary to use stories, visuals and examples from nature to help them understand. Relate more difficult concepts to things they understand already, like their favourite things.

The power of attraction, or love, is contagious. When we love something, we are drawn to it. Gravity has been likened to the power of love. Create a desire in the children to sacrifice. If fasting appears to the child as laborious or cumbersome, they may grow to do it out of obedience, but not experience the joy.

* * *

You will come to find you can participate in the spirit of the Fast just as well as anyone. And you can make simple modifications in your daily routines to participate physically as much as possible. The results can be marvellous!

15

RE-ENTRY: LIFE AFTER THE FAST

> Fasting will bring spiritual rebirth to those of you who cleanse and purify your bodies. The light of the world will illuminate within you when you fast and purify yourself. More caution and perhaps more restraint are necessary in breaking a fast than in keeping it.
>
> **Attributed to Mahatma Gandhi**

Congratulations! God willing, your efforts for the last 19 days will be accepted and pleasing in the sight of God. It's time to celebrate Naw-Rúz, or the 'new year', 'new day'. It's most befitting that the new year should start on the spring equinox while nature is in its time of renewal – at least in the northern hemisphere.

Naw-Rúz festivities – our first act in the new year

During the Naw-Rúz festivities, we can practise the new habits we have worked so hard to integrate. Sundown on the last day opens a strong temptation to fulfil impulses and forget the efforts and discipline already accomplished. Each night when the Fast breaks the desire to graze and snack all night looms over us, but the potential for losing ground during Naw-Rúz and the following ten days is even greater; it is so easy to fall into old habits and patterns. It often starts with the Naw-Rúz feast itself – everywhere I've travelled in the world, I find a festivity with too many foods, the combination of the wrong foods and abundant temptation!

A letter from the Universal House of Justice clarifies the distinction between celebration and frivolity:

> One of the signs of a decadent society, a sign which is very evident in the world today, is an almost frenetic devotion to pleasure

and diversion, an insatiable thirst for amusement, a fanatical devotion to games and sport, a reluctance to treat any matter seriously, and a scornful, derisory attitude towards virtue and solid worth. Abandonment of 'a frivolous conduct' does not imply that a Bahá'í must be sour-faced or perpetually solemn. Humour, happiness, joy are characteristics of a true Bahá'í life. Frivolity palls and eventually leads to boredom and emptiness, but true happiness and joy and humour that are parts of a balanced life that includes serious thought, compassion and humble servitude to God are characteristics that enrich life and add to its radiance.[1]

In preparation for Naw-Rúz we can explore how celebrations can manifest the qualities of humour, happiness and joy without the influence of amusement, frivolity and empty pleasure. Just think of a celebration focused on and infused with the appetite for beauty, for the arts, for the spirit, rather than the food. From the quotation above it would seem that moderation may remain the best remedy. Since the Fast creates an opportunity to abandon addictions of all kinds, the virtue of moderation fits perfectly, as it protects us from the power of addiction. Perhaps the Fast has brought out our addiction to specific emotions, such as feeling powerless or stimulated. Perhaps it has brought our attention to a specific way of thinking that needs changing, like always needing control over situations or criticizing.

The opposite of addiction could be deprivation. Celebration in the middle way does not imply deprivation or suppression, but just what is needed and perfect for this moment. Moderation maintains the balance that the nineteen-day Fast strives to help us attain. Children and youth often have amazing celebratory ideas and should be included in the consultation.

The transition back to 'reality'

Once you experience a few Fasts, some of its 'stations and innumerable effects' will come to light. Each Fast will have its own unique potentiality for you as well as for the community. As a practitioner, having many clients during the Fast has given me the distinct impression of certain themes in different years. For example, some years I find that many report the Fast as being especially difficult. In other years many say it has been unusually easy, or emotional. I've seen a 'collective' theme across the board at times. This is interesting What is going on that many are experiencing the same phenomena? – not that every single person does, but that a large percentage do. I have the impression that there exists a collective mind and sense of unity, without individual conscious realization, which confirms our oneness.

As before in this book, the suggestions that follow are simply the result of my personal and professional experience; they are not part of any official Bahá'í teachings, although I have drawn on the Bahá'í Writings in putting them together.

Taking time to reflect during the first week following Naw-Rúz on our efforts and results enables us to understand and raise the quality of our future actions. It helps us to gain perspective more quickly. Approaching the Fast in this systematic pattern creates a closer relationship to our Lord and enhances understanding of the self.

Questions for reflection:

- How did the self emerge?
- How did the 'heat' of the Fast manifest itself internally and externally?
- Do I feel closer to God? More occupied with serving Him and praising Him?
- In what ways am I more detached?
- What am I bringing into the new year, and what would I like to leave behind?
- What are the ways the insistent self hooks me?
- Are my mind, body and soul more balanced?
- Am I more aware of my emotions? Do I understand better how to validate and redirect them?
- Can I maintain my heart open in the throes of the ego's cries for attention?
- Have my tastes changed? Do I think about eating to nourish rather than entertain?
- Are my self-appetites and self-desires more apparent? What distracted me from drawing near to God during the Fast?
- What confirmations were manifested?

When the Fast ends, attunement to an inner compass enables healthier choices, choices that are tempered with wisdom and discernment. This transitional period parallels how astronauts experience and manoeuvre their 're-entry' when coming back to Earth. While a space mission is dangerous enough, it is the risks involved in re-entering the Earth's atmosphere that present the most peril. The shuttle must be guided through the turbulent and heat-filled atmosphere. When an object enters our atmosphere it's met with instant resistance, specifically with the forces of gravity and drag. We understand from the Baháʼí teachings that the insistent self acts like gravity, pulling us down in the clutches of the ego. Gravity alone would cause the shuttle to fall naturally back to earth, but at tremendously fast speeds. But Earth's atmosphere contains particles in the air which cause friction when an object falls, so that it experiences air resistance, or drag. This friction causes the object's fall to slow down, but it also causes extreme heat. In order to overcome these tests, space programmes have designed their shuttles so as to block out the heat and keep it away from the vehicle as well as aerodynamically slowing the fall. Any wrong choice endangers the crew, causing instant death or incineration.

Space missions deal with the issues of transition not only in the re-entry phase, but in returning to daily life on Earth. NASA even addresses the spiritual and emotional effects on astronauts in their personal lives if re-entry is not handled properly.[2] Astronauts have trained for their mission and simulated it so when the required time comes to actually perform the transition, handling it would feel natural.

These experiences can provide an analogy for us. The nineteen days of the Fast provide time to train ourselves and 'simulate' our re-entry moment when 'You are clear to enter.' The 'heat' of the Fast Baháʼu'lláh refers to can especially be felt in the transition. Any slip in our training can end in a fiery ordeal – perhaps physically by heartburn! The friction felt by the space shuttle is very much like the desires and impulses that crop up during the Naw-Rúz feast and the days following: 'I get to eat anything I want, anytime!' For some, food becomes what the mind focuses on. The ease of choices to stay within the bounds of moderation is indicative of the training period during the Fast. If you've been following some of the recommendations in this book you will have created an aerodynamic strength of the soul over the body which slows its fall, while enabling it to arrive safely at its landing site.

At the end of the Fast, sensitivities may arise that weren't noticed before, such as to certain environments, foods, people and thought patterns. If your diet was changed to a more natural one during the Fast, your palate will have changed as well. The body will be attuned to more natural tastes, being less prone to crave sugary, high-calorie snacks. If you still have these cravings, they may represent emotional needs rather than a true physical demand for nutrition.

Cleanliness and sanctity have an exalted station in the Baháʼí Writings because they are the essential qualities of a free soul. Baháʼuʼlláh exhorts His followers to become the embodiments of purity among the peoples of the world. The first condition for this exists in the soul, where we purify our defects during the Fast. Purification allows us to reflect the perfect Divine Light.

Purity and sanctity will help the transition into a regular diet for the mind and body. It must be gradual. The sun does not come out into its daytime splendour instantly! It rises gradually and allows us time to get used to its vibrancy, power and light.

The body

Let's first investigate a re-entry plan for the body. Many experts suggest taking half of our total cleansing time to move back into our regular living; in this instance approximately ten days. Planning your meals for the days following the Fast is vital to prevent sickness and imbalance. Study the list of foods in the next chapter and eat accordingly for the first ten days. Remember, your digestive system has rested and been cleansed. The following recommendations will protect you from instant 'incineration' in your re-entry:

- Help your body adjust by eating small portions for lunch.
- Move your protein meal for the day to lunch, as it will help you sustain energy throughout the late afternoon. Keep your carbohydrate meal for comfort and renewed energy in the evening (see Table 15.1 below).
- Prepare simple foods; do not mix too many types of foods together. Lightly steamed vegetables and vegetable proteins, or soups, are great choices. Introduce fish at the protein meal if you choose to eat it. Emphasize high fibre and cultured foods to maintain cellular health.

- Focus on hydration. Drink water between meals and when you feel hungry or like snacking.
- Take probiotics on an empty stomach to stimulate the colon. The body will have to transition into eating more foods again when it isn't used to it and some are prone to constipation (or the opposite) when this happens.
- Take notes on how your body reacts to certain foods. If it reacts strongly to a food, remove it from your diet and try to introduce it again after a week.
- Pay attention to digestive function, sleep patterns and cravings.
- Enjoy food and be thankful, remembering God at the beginning of every meal.

The mind

The first ten days invite feelings of relief. It's amazing how quickly reintegration occurs. Be mindful of how easy it is to fall into the same routines, the same thought patterns, the same outlooks as before. Our autopilot-driven life is comforting, yet doesn't leave room for flexibility and creativity and reinforces old habits. Shoghi Effendi reminds us:

> Life is a constant struggle, not only against forces around us, but above all against our own 'ego'. We can never afford to rest on our oars, for if we do, we soon see ourselves carried down stream again.[3]

Just as the physical body has experienced a rest, the mind has acquired more 'space'. Build choices which include moderation, cleanliness and sanctity in nurturing the mind. The following recommendations will help you avoid a crash re-entry!

- Regulate what enters the mind.
- Continue to refrain from harmful habits of the mind.
- Take ownership of your circumstances.
- Build knowledge and intellect.
- Integrate the ego through healing, education and discipline.
- Try to incorporate regular changes in routines or patterns of living to encourage neural plasticity and challenge the establishment of permanent neural pathways.

The spirit

A natural tendency arises to stop the spiritual practices carried out during the Fast. Remember that the rule of 'eating until full' applies also to reading and studying the sacred texts. Appetites may change; it's a natural time to pay attention to how hungry the spirit is. Nature has times when the flowers open for the morning sun and close at sunset to rest for the evening. The spirit has similar cycles where we feel nearer and some times farther away. 'O Son of Man! Sorrow not save that thou art far from Us. Rejoice not save that thou art drawing near and returning unto Us', writes Bahá'u'lláh.[4] Learn to recognize the relativity of closeness and separateness as a natural cycle, so that you can feel comfortable and content wherever you are on the path today. While acquiring balance for the body and mind will have meant experiencing a rest, the spirit will probably have been more active than usual – it has filled up to reach a balanced state during the Fast.

- Continue being mindful of attachments.
- Maintain the systematic structure set up in drawing closer to God through prayer, reciting the sacred texts morning and evening, meditation, study, taking account of yourself and teaching.
- Practise 'flipping' the heart into faith and trust under all circumstances.
- Practise putting God's face on all people and remaining in His presence at all times.
- See the oneness of all of God's creation.

Rebalancing the body throughout the year

After the first ten days, reintegrate back into a regular diet for the rest of the year. Add in 1–2 foods every couple of days, noticing your body's reaction to them. Keep up the habits you've already established. The following table, repeated from Chapter 14, will help you identify healthy eating patterns.

Figure 15.1 Daily eating guide

Time	Amount	Example	Notes
Breakfast	1–2 cups	Distilled/ spring water	Add lemon to warmed water.
	1–2 cups	Wholegrain meal such as oatmeal	
Lunch	Salad plate	Protein plus vegetable	Eat the protein at lunch to sustain energy into the afternoon
Dinner	Salad plate	Complex carbohydrate plus vegetable	Starches at night feel more comforting.
Snacks (between meals and after the last meal has been fully digested.)	1 piece 1 handful 1 cup	Fruit Nuts, seeds, raw vegetables Tea	

- Slowly incorporate other foods, including animal products if you desire.
- If desired, incorporate a light snack between breakfast and lunch, such as a handful of nuts. Another snack time, if needed, would be between lunch and dinner, again, equalling a handful of single foods. Remember to use the size of your palm as a general guide to proportions that are proper to you.
- **Use foods to nourish the body, not for entertainment or comfort**. Remember that empty stomach feeling while fasting? When your stomach rumbled? That is the feeling you should have prior to eating. Relearn your body's signals of hunger, and distinguish between emotional eating and the body needing nourishment. In the Tablet to a Physican, Bahá'u'lláh writes, 'The taking of food before that which you have already eaten is digested is dangerous . . .'[5] We also find this in the science of natural healing, where putting food into your stomach when the past meal has not yet been digested is considered harmful to your health. The average digestion time can vary with the

individual, but on average, a meal with red meats can take up to two hours, while fruit on an empty stomach averages 20 minutes.

Mini-fasts throughout the year to maintain balance

While the nineteen-day Fast enjoined on us by Bahá'u'lláh will be our main source of cleansing, I often recommend mini-fasts lasting one day or three days to enhance this process throughout the year. A short fast should be simple, such as drinking fresh juices or soups for the body during the day. Follow the recommendations on refraining for the mind, and make sure to enhance the spiritual practices for the soul. There are many helpful guides on juice-fasting or three-day cleanses. Sometimes if I've been at a celebration or have overeaten, I'll skip the next meal while hydrating with water to regain balance. I do not recommend this as a habit though – giving yourself permission to continually overeat and skip the next meal – because the body's metabolism will be harmfully affected.

A change in the season is a perfect time to carry out a short cleanse; the fall equinox is recommended, or when the weather becomes temperate again. Cleanses can prepare the body for the coming winter and help avoid colds and flu, which are a way the body readjusts itself to the temperature.

A short fast can also be helpful in the following circumstances (and this is by no means a definitive list):

Body: After travelling, overeating, holidays, lethargy, indigestion, some surgeries, bloating, fatigue.
Mind: After a shocking event, grief, high anxiety, great anger.
Soul: Hurt by a loved one, apathy, estrangement.

Systematically taking account of oneself at the end of each day helps us understand the communications within. Reflect on daily habits, consult your spirit about better alternatives, and take better action the next day. Adding prayer to this plan engenders true progress.

Forbearance enables our mind to avoid a place of judgement. Since in this world we are immersed in the sea of excess in appetites of all kinds, acknowledging that temptation is everywhere can be vital to survival. We should enjoy the things God created in this material world – but be mindful of when the body and mind are indulging impulses. This is the balance I have found.

Joyous Naw-Rúz and blessings throughout the year!

A prayer for Naw-Rúz revealed by Bahá'u'lláh

Praised be Thou, O my God, that Thou hast ordained Naw-Rúz as a festival unto those who have observed the fast for love of Thee and abstained from all that is abhorrent unto thee. Grant, O my Lord, that the fire of Thy love and the heat produced by the fast enjoined by Thee may inflame them in Thy Cause, and make them to be occupied with Thy praise and with remembrance of Thee.

Since thou hast adorned them, O my Lord, with the ornament of the fast prescribed by Thee, do Thou adorn them also with the ornament of Thine acceptance, through Thy grace and bountiful favour. For the doings of men are all dependent upon Thy good-pleasure, and are conditioned by Thy behest. Shouldst Thou regard him who hath broken the fast as one who hath observed it, such a man would be reckoned among them who from eternity had been keeping the fast. And shouldst Thou decree that he who hath observed the fast hath broken it, that person would be numbered with such as have caused the Robe of Thy Revelation to be stained with dust, and been far removed from the crystal waters of this living Fountain.

Thou art He through Whom the ensign 'Praiseworthy art Thou in Thy works' hath been lifted up, and the standard 'Obeyed art Thou in thy behest' hath been unfurled. Make known this Thy station, O my God, unto Thy servants, that they may be made aware that the excellence of all things is dependent upon Thy bidding and Thy word, and the virtue of every act is conditioned by Thy leave and the good-pleasure of Thy will, and may recognize that the reins of men's doings are within the grasp of Thine acceptance and Thy commandment. Make this known unto them, that nothing whatsoever may shut them out from Thy Beauty, in these days whereon the Christ exclaimeth: 'All dominion is Thine, O Thou the Begetter of the Spirit (Jesus)'; and Thy Friend (Muḥammad) crieth out: 'Glory be to Thee, O Thou the Best-Beloved, for that thou hast uncovered thy Beauty, and written down for Thy chosen ones what will cause them to attain unto the seat of the revelation of Thy Most Great Name, through which all the peoples have lamented excepted such as have detached themselves from all else except Thee, and set themselves towards Him Who is the Revealer of Thyself and the Manifestation of Thine attributes.'

He Who is Thy Branch and all Thy company, O my Lord, have broken this day their fast, after having observed it within the precincts of Thy court, and in their eagerness to please Thee. Do Thou ordain for Him, and for them, and for all such as have entered Thy presence in those days all the good Thou didst destine in Thy Book. Supply them, then, with that which will profit them, in both this life and in the life beyond.

Thou, in truth, art the All-Knowing, the All-Wise.[6]

16

RECIPES

This chapter offers recipes for healthy eating during the Fast (and to continue year round if you wish). Before we get started, here is a grocery list of ingredients used in the recipes. The items in bold are ideal for the first five days of the Fast, when it is best to have a very simple diet subsisting of deep-healing foods such as cruciferous vegetables, sea vegetables, alliums (garlic, onions), nuts and seeds, sprouts, yogurt and teas.

A grocery list for the Fast

Organic vegetables

Sprouts
Artichokes
Asparagus
Beets
Bok choy
Broccoli
Brussels sprouts
Cabbages
Carrots
Cauliflower
Celery
Collards
Corn
Cucumbers
Dandelion greens
Eggplant
Garlic
Green peas
Herbs
Kale
Kohlrabi

Leeks
Lettuce
Mustard greens
Okra
Onions
Parsley
Parsnips
Peppers
Potatoes
Radishes
Scallions
Spinach
String beans
Squashes
Swiss chard
Tomatoes
Turnips
Watercress
Wheatgrass
Yams

Fruits*
Apples
Apricots
Avocados
Bananas
Berries
Cantaloupes
Cherries
Cranberries
Dates
Figs
Grapefruits
Grapes
Honeydew melon
Kiwi
Lemon
Limes
Mangos
Nectarines
Oranges
Papayas
Peaches

Pears
Pineapples
Plums
Prunes
Strawberries
Watermelon

Dried fruits should be unsulphured

Whole grains
Amaranth
Barley
Basmati rice
Brown rice
Buckwheat
Bulgur
Couscous
Corn meal
Millet
Oats (steel-cut)
Oat bran
Flax
Quinoa
Rye
Wheat berries
Wild rice

Breads
Ezekiel
Essene
7-sprouted Grain
Tortillas

Vegetable protein
Fungi
Quorn™ (fungi)
Tempeh
Seitan
Tofu
Textured vegetable protein (TVP) (beans, nuts and seeds)

Veggieburger

Oils*
Canola oil
Coconut oil
Olive oil
Flax oil
Safflower oil
Sesame seed oil

Buy cold-pressed or expeller-pressed oils

Dairy & Alternatives
Greek yogurt (NOT non-fat)
Feta cheese
Soy milk
Almond milk
Rice milk

Pasta
Rice noodles
Udon noodles
Soba noodles
Semolina

Sweeteners
Honey, raw uncooked
100% maple syrup
Stevia
Date sugar
Blackstrap molasses
Agave nectar

Teas
Peppermint
Chamomile
Herbal non-caffeine
Green

Mushrooms*
Shiitake
Enokidake
Maitake
Oyster
Wild
Bella
Crimini
Portobello (button)

Cook mushrooms, never eat raw

Beans and legumes
Anasazi
Adzuki
Black
Pinto
Garbanzo
Lentils
Lima beans
Mung
Split peas
Soybeans

Seasonings
Ginger
Herbs
Spicy/dry mustard
Yeast flakes
Garlic
Peppers
Citrus juice
Miso
Tamari
Horseradish
Apple cider vinegar

Nuts and seeds
Almonds
Brazils
Cashews
Hazelnuts
Macadamias

Pecans	**Sea vegetables**	**Optional additions**
Pine nuts	**Nori**	**for protein shakes**
Pumpkin seeds	**Korubu**	Spirulina powder
Sesame seeds	**Wakame**	Raw wheat germ
Sunflower seeds	**Hiziki**	Raw honey
Walnuts		Vitamin C powder
	↯	Psyllium husk powder
Buy whole or unshelled. Store in fridge or freezer		Rice bran
		Lecithin granules
↯		Chlorophyll

Eat simply. Use up to 7 ingredients to create each meal. Gradually integrate a few more foods each day, and pay attention to your body's reaction to them. Foods can be used to reduce cravings during the Fast. Use bitter herbs like dandelion root, collard greens, almonds and kale in cravings for coffee and cigarettes. Sweet cravings can be helped by eating sour-tasting foods like citrus, cranberries and rhubarb.

My favourite fasting recipes are deliberately simple, with limited directions. This is to encourage you to be creative and intuitive when you prepare food, and get a sense of tastes you like, as well as proportions. If you come to a point in the directions where you have doubts, experiment. Feel free to adjust the proportions according to your tastes and preferences, such as more shredded carrots than cabbage. Think then about how these changes may affect the other ingredients, such as the oil and seasoning ratios.

For the most part, these recipes leave out sugars and salt to accustom your tongue to natural tastes. The Fast offers us the bounty of resetting the palate. Most of us are accustomed to the refined foods which contain taste enhancers. Taste enhancers excite the brain and access the addiction centre – that's why it's difficult to eat just a handful of chips, or just one scoop of ice cream.

In creating the recipes, proportions are difficult to judge and I usually advise people to eat according to their hand sizes, i.e. a handful of nuts or fruit for snacks, or meat the size of their palm for the day. We have to take into consideration a person's lifestyle, age, amount of energy expended in a day, their size, the speed of their metabolism, etc. . . . there are many factors that determine the size of a meal one person can eat. In general, the amounts given in the recipe will serve at least two adults. Some recipes, such as the salads and dinners, feed up to four. It's good to have leftovers, too, during the Fast so that you are not constantly preparing and cooking. I purposely mean you to eat less than you normally would, because it's the Fast. At least you have here the combination of ingredients and their proportion to each other to achieve the desired tastes if you want to double or triple the recipes. In my own cookbooks I always write the number of portions on the side (double/triple) of each recipe for future use and quick reference.

The recipes are divided into cycles:
- Cleansing (Days 1–5)
- Rebuilding (Days 6–12)
- Integrating (Days 13–19)

and according to the following headings:

Drinks

Fruits

Morning

    Protein Shake (Days 1–5)
    Vegetable Protein Breakfasts (Days 6–12)
    Protein Dishes (Days 13–19)

Breaking the Fast

    'Street Sweeper' Salads (Days 1–12)
    Salads (Days 13–19)
    Sauces and Dressings

Dinner

    Brown Rice and Steamed Veggies (Days 1–5)
    Soups, Grains and Veggies (Days 6–12)
    Carbohydrate Dinners (Days 13–19)

Evening Snacks

Naw-Rúz Dessert

The following abbreviations are used:		
T=tablespoon	tsp=teaspoon	oz=ounces

Drinks

These drinks are fabulous for breaking the Fast, whether it's in the morning (break-fast) or after a day of fasting. They are refreshing and soothing to the digestive tract. Dehydration is the most difficult during the Fast, so use distilled spring water liberally first thing in the morning, when breaking the Fast after sunset, and then liberally in the evening at least an hour after eating dinner.

Basic Liver Tonic

8 oz [1 cup] hot water or room temperature water mixed with squeezed fresh lemon juice or 1 oz [2 T] apple cider vinegar.

Master Cleanser

1 oz [2 T] fresh lemon juice
½ oz [1 T] pure maple syrup
1/10 tsp red cayenne pepper
8 oz [1 cup] water

Basic Juice

Organic produce: 3 carrots, 2 cups dark greens, 1 pear and 1 apple
Use a juicer, and add any additional ingredients as desired.

Haifa Lemon Mint Toner

8 oz [1 cup] water
1 oz [2 T] fresh lemon juice (or to taste)
Touch of stevia or agave
Fresh mint leaves bruised (smash leaves and immediately put in glass)
Stir and enjoy chilled but not cold.

Aloe Soother

Aloe vera juice, cold pressed, 4 oz [1/2 cup] chilled

Organic Apple Juice

Cranberry Juice

RECIPES

Fruits

Eat a cup of fruit before sunrise or for evening snacks, about 1½ hours after dinner. Try eating fruit after drinking water, or while serving dinner. Try to eat fruit that is more in season where you live. Frozen organic fruits are a great option if you'd like to blend them together to make a smoothie. Eat melons by themselves.

Tropical salad

Cut mango, pineapple, kiwi, papaya.
Squirt lime juice over and toss together.
Cut up some mint leaves and toss together.

Fruit Smoothie Option: put cut-up fruit in blender with 6 oz orange juice and some crushed ice if using fresh mango, otherwise use frozen mango. A banana is good to add. Adjust liquids to desired consistency and blend until smooth.

The Blues

4 oz [½ cup] blueberries
4 oz [½ cup] blackberries
1 banana, sliced

Fruit Smoothie Option: Blend with cranberry or cherry juice and crushed ice (or frozen fruit instead of crushed ice). Adjust liquid to desired consistency.

The Red Rose

4 oz [½ cup] raspberries
2 oz [¼ cup] pomegranate seeds
4 oz [½ cup] strawberries

Fruit Smoothie Option: Blend with pear juice and 1 T lemon until smooth.

Orange Sunset

1 tangerine, peeled and sliced
1 apricot or nectarine, sliced

1 peach, sliced
Squirt lemon juice over and toss together.

Fruit Smoothie Option: Blend with coconut milk kefir, 1 T lime juice, and a little crushed ice. Adjust liquid to desired consistency.

Prune Dessert

1 package pitted prunes **½ oz [1 T] vanilla** **2 oz [¼ cup] natural cane sugar**	Place in large pan and fill with water to just cover prunes. Turn heat to medium high and bring to boil, stirring until sugar dissolves. Turn heat down to medium low for 15 minutes.
1 cinnamon stick **Peel of 1 orange** **Star anise if desired**	Add cinnamon sticks, peel, and star anise. Cook until desired tenderness. Take off heat and immediately put in refrigerator to stop further cooking. Serve over Greek yogurt with a little syrup.

Morning

Protein Shake (Days 1–5)
Basic Protein Shake

8 oz [1 cup] almond, rice, coconut or soy milk (men should not overconsume soy milk)
Protein powder (per instructions for 8 oz of liquids)
4 oz–8 oz [½–1 cup] yogurt with live cultures
1 banana
½–1oz [1–3 T] flax oil
Mix together in blender. Adjust liquids to desired consistency.

Optional additions
Spirulina powder
Raw honey
Psyllium husk powder
Lecithin granules

Raw wheat germ
Vitamin C powder
Rice bran
Chlorophyll

Vegetable Protein Breakfasts (Days 6–12)

Tofu Scrambles

Don't like tofu? Substitute scrambled eggs or brown rice instead. Try a non-meat product resembling ground meat or sausage, usually found in the natural foods freezer section or the produce section in the grocery store.

Southern Scramble

½ oz [1 T] olive oil
½ onion chopped,
½ oz [1 T] minced garlic

Put olive oil in pan and smear thoroughly with paper towel. Heat pan to medium heat. Cook onions and garlic until translucent.

½ –1 package firm tofu
Seasonings: sprinkle of cumin, chili powder and a touch of oregano

Push aside onion mix and add tofu, smashing it with spatula until it resembles scrambled eggs. Sprinkle in seasonings and mix well.

4 oz [½ cup] black beans
1 T salsa
3 T coloured peppers

Add rest of ingredients at once until heated.

Veggie Wrap

3 T olive oil
1 portobello mushroom, sliced long
Leftover roasted veggies from dinner, or onions and peppers

Place oil in medium frying pan over medium-high heat. Cook portobello mushroom until shiny and cooked through. Mix in roasted veggies and heat.

½ package tofu, tempeh or seitan, chopped
1 t ground cumin
½ oz [1 T] lime juice

Add tofu, tempeh or seitan to mushroom mix. Smash tofu with spatula until it resembles scrambled eggs. If using tempeh or seitan, cut in pieces and stir-fry with the mushrooms.

Add desired sauce
2 multigrain tortillas or corn tortillas

See recipes in *Sauces* section.
Heat tortillas in oven or on stove top. Wrap ingredients.

Italian Sausages

½ oz [1 T] olive oil 3 cloves garlic ½ purple onion, diced 1 handful spinach 2 artichoke hearts, chopped ½ pepper, chopped	Place oil in medium frying pan over medium heat. Cook onion and garlic until opaque. Mix in artichoke hearts and red peppers. Sauté for 1 minute. Add spinach and heat until wilted. Set aside on separate plate.
2–3 Italian tofu 'sausages'	Cut sausage links to desired size. Sauté in the pan until heated through.
½–1 oz [1–2 T] diced tomatoes or pesto	Add all ingredients in pan and mix.

Mediterranean Scramble

½ oz [1 T] olive oil 2 cloves garlic, minced ½ yellow onion, diced 1 zucchini, chopped 1 tomato, chopped and seeds taken out (blood type AB or O)	Place oil in medium frying pan over medium heat. Cook onion and garlic until opaque. Add zucchini, cook 2 minutes. Mix in tomato.
½–1 package firm tofu	Push ingredients to one side of pan while adding tofu, smashing it with spatula until it resembles scrambled eggs.
Sprinkle with tahini dressing if desired	See recipe in *Sauces* section.

Thai Scramble

½ oz [1 T] olive oil ½ onion, chopped ½ cup broccoli or spinach 2 oz [4 T] coloured peppers	Place oil in medium frying pan over medium heat. Cook onion until opaque. Add peppers and broccoli. Sauté 2 minutes.
½–1 package firm Tofu 1 T Thai chili paste Curry paste (optional)	Mix chili paste with vegetables in pan. Push aside vegetables into one corner of the pan and add tofu, smashing it with spatula until it resembles scrambled eggs.
1 T chopped nuts	Sprinkle nuts and serve.

Protein Dishes (Days 13–19)

Protein Porridge

16 oz [2 cups] leftover rice, kashi, or other grains. If using oatmeal, use whole or steel-cut oats
4 oz [½ cup] Greek yogurt
Pinch of cinnamon
4 oz [½ cup] almond milk

If using leftover grains, stir together and heat (if desired) until warm. If using oats, cook per instructions on package until just tender and then mix in the remaining ingredients.

2 oz [¼ cup] chopped or ground walnuts

Sprinkle on top or mix in.

Veggie Omelettes

Use any of the ingredients for the tofu scrambles to create a unique omelette.

1 clove garlic, crushed and chopped
2 eggs, dash of milk or water whipped together

Rub a coat of canola oil onto a very small frying pan and heat on medium heat. Fry garlic until soft, not browned. Place beaten eggs in pan. When eggs start to set on sides, slowly pour ¼ cup boiling water into the side of the pan and quickly cover for 1 minute.

Greek Omelette
Handful fresh spinach, wilted
½ oz [1 T] feta or goat cheese

Add spinach and feta onto egg mixture and cover until done. Fold one side of omelette over the spinach and slide it onto a plate.

Asparagus & Mushroom Omelette
½ oz [1 T] olive oil
4 stalks fresh asparagus, chopped
4 oz [½ cup] shiitake mushrooms, chopped
½ onion diced

Stir-fry vegetables in olive oil with garlic. Follow the direction for the eggs above. Cover until fully cooked on top. Fold one side over the other.

Creamy Portobello Breakfast Stroganoff

1 package egg noodles or udon noodles	Cook according to directions on package.
1 oz [2 T] olive oil 1 yellow onion, chopped 2 cloves garlic, minced 2 large heads portobello (button) mushrooms, chopped, (or 2 cups mushrooms in grocery list)	Fry onion in pan until opaque. Add garlic and mushrooms until browned and softened.
1 oz [2 T cup] non-alcoholic red wine (not sparkling) 2 oz [¼ cup] vegetable broth 1 tsp lime zest 4 oz [½ cup] PLAIN almond milk	Stir red wine into onion mixture and cook until almost evaporated. Add vegetable broth, lime zest and almond milk. If desired, add a little heavy cream. Change liquid proportions to desired consistency.
4 oz [½ cup] tofu, sour cream or plain Greek yogurt (add until desired consistency)	Mix in until smooth. Gently fold in noodles, mixing well.
Parsley, chopped	Sprinkle with chopped parsley

Veggie Frittata

1 clove garlic, crushed and chopped 2 scallions, chopped 1 Roma tomato, thinly sliced (blood type AB or O) 1 oz [2 T] various chopped fresh herbs 3 eggs, dash of milk or water whipped together	Brush a small frying pan with canola oil, let pan heat up on medium heat. Sauté garlic until soft. Place beaten eggs in pan. Cover and cook 5 minutes, or until bottom is cooked and top is almost set. Place tomato slices on top. Transfer pan to oven and broil/grill until top is set. Check after 2 minutes. Do not brown!
Feta, kefir or farmer's cheese	Sprinkle with cheese before serving. Cut into pie wedges to serve.

Mushroom Delight

½ oz [1 T] olive oil
3 large cloves garlic, smashed & chopped
1 onion, sliced

8 oz [1 cup] shiitake mushrooms
8 oz [1 cup] oyster or maiitake mushrooms
1 oz fresh herbs
1 T black pepper

½ cup vegetable broth
1 tsp miso paste
1 oz [1 T] apple cider vinegar
Dash of soy sauce
7 handfuls fresh spinach

Additional option:
Add 1 cup chopped vegetable protein if desired.
1 tsp horseradish instead of soy sauce

Put olive oil in a large skillet on medium high heat (don't let the olive oil smoke). Sauté onion and garlic until translucent, about 4 minutes.

Add mushrooms and herbs and sauté, covering the pan. Cook until soft by stirring occasionally.

Ensure miso paste is dispersed evenly by adding to a little warmed broth, breaking up the paste with a fork. Add all of broth, miso paste and vinegar to pan. Add spinach by the handful, stirring in each one. The dish is done when the spinach just wilts.

If adding protein, sauté it with the onions and garlic.

Lentil Spread

½ oz [1 T] olive oil
½ white onion, diced
6 oz [¾ cup] red lentils
10 oz [1¼ cup] vegetable broth

2 tsp curry powder
1 tsp cumin
½ tsp coriander
1 oz [2 T] lemon juice
1 egg

Wholegrain pitas, 1 slice multigrain bread, oven toasted, or fresh veggies

Stir-fry onion in olive oil over medium heat.

Bring lentils to boil in vegetable broth in a saucepan, simmer for 20 minutes or until tender (don't overdo!). Cool.

Add all ingredients to blender. Heat oven to 400°F (200°C). Spread lentil mixture in oiled bread pan. Smooth top. Cook about 40 minutes, until it springs back when touched. Cool on rack then place in refrigerator over night.

Slice and serve warm if desired.

Breaking the Fast

'Street Sweeper' Salads (Days 1–12)

Eat these salads after breaking the Fast with water (and fruit if desired). They act as a cleanser, going through your intestines and sweeping out old debris, ultimately sweeping the bowels. Find any vegetables that are hard and shred them, mix with an oil-based dressing and enjoy. Adjust the dressing amount to your preferences – I like my salads just wet with dressing, not drenched.

Red, Orange and White Salad

1½ oz [3½ T] olive oil 2 tsp spicy mustard 1 oz [2 T] apple cider vinegar 1 oz [2 T] freshly squeezed lemon juice	Whisk together in a serving bowl.
2 beets and 2 turnips (about the same size), peeled and shredded (or ½ cup each) 2 carrots, peeled and shredded 1 kohlrabi, peeled and shredded (optional)	Place beets on dressing, then put carrots, then turnips. Gently toss in dressing. (Beets bleed, so don't over mix, to maintain the colours.)

Asian Salad

2 oz [5 T] sesame oil 1½ oz [3T] rice vinegar Dash of chili paste 1 tsp freshly grated ginger	Whisk together dressing in serving bowl.
8 oz [1 cup] shredded red cabbage 8 oz [1 cup] green cabbage or 8 oz [1 cup] broccoli slaw 3 large carrots, shredded, or ¾ cup matchstick cut carrots 2 oz [¼ cup] cut green onions	Place ingredients on top of dressing and toss together. Use broccoli slaw instead of cabbage if desired.
4 oz [½ cup] peanuts	Gently mix in.
1 oz [2T] sesame seeds	Sprinkle over the top.

Cruciferous Salad

2 oz [¼ cup] safflower oil
1½ oz [3 T] apple cider vinegar
½ oz [1 T] liquid amino acids
¼ tsp dried mustard
Freshly cut basil

Mix dressing in serving bowl.

1 head of broccoli
1 head of cauliflower
1 red pepper

Cut veggies into desired bite sizes, but uniform. Place in the serving bowl over the dressing. Mix together and return to refrigerator. Allow one hour to marry the flavours.

Sprout Salad

1 oz [2 T] sesame oil
1 tsp lime juice
1 tsp freshly minced ginger (if desired)
½ oz [1 T] tamari sauce

Whisk together in a serving bowl.

8 oz [1 cup] mung bean sprouts
½ chopped cucumber (small slices are best)
1½ oz [3 T] sesame seeds

Toss together with dressing and sprinkle seeds on top.

Kickin' Slaw

3 oz [5 T] olive oil
1 oz [2 T] apple cider vinegar
½ lemon, juiced
2 tsp black pepper

Stir dressing together in serving bowl. Toss juice with apples so they don't brown.

8 oz [1 cup] shredded green cabbage
4 oz [½ cup] shredded purple cabbage
8 oz [1 cup] shredded carrots or celery, chopped
8 oz [1 cup] chopped nuts
8 oz [1 cup] diced apple (leave peel on if organic) or raisins

Mix ingredients together.

Wheat Berry Crunch

16 oz [2 cups] cooked wheat berries	Mix ingredients together.
½ chopped 'English' cucumber (less bitter than other varieties)	
½ cup chopped cherry tomatoes (blood type AB or O)	
½ diced red onion	
1 oz [2 T] chopped flatleaf parsley	
2 oz [¼ cup] toasted pine nuts	
3 oz [5 T] olive oil	Stir dressing together in separate bowl.
1½ oz [3 T] lemon juice	Pour dressing on salad while stirring.
Dash of cinnamon	

Salads (Days 12–19)

Basic Green Salad

8 oz [1 cup] spinach leaves	Mix in any measurements. Remove or add coloured veggies as desired.
16 oz [2 cups] mixed greens	
Herbs: mint, parsley, tarragon, chives	
2 oz [4 T] coloured peppers	
1 chopped avocado	
Cucumbers	
Celery	
Tomatoes (if AB or O blood type)	
Mix with dressing	See section on *Sauces and Dressings*.

Kale & Beet Salad

3 cups kale	Remove stems. Chop kale into ¼ inch (6mm) strips. Toss lemon juice with kale strips until softened.
1 lemon, juiced	
4 beets, peeled	Chop beets into match sized strips. Gently toss together kale, shallot and beets.
1 shallot, finely chopped	
2 T olive oil	Whisk together dressing ingredients. Toss with beet mixture and let flavours marry for 15 minutes.
1.5 T Balsamic vinegar	
1 T Dijon mustard	
Black pepper (to taste)	

Squash Delight

1 tsp olive oil
1 acorn squash

Preheat oven to 400°F (200°C). Peel acorn squash and chop into similar sized pieces. Toss with 1 tsp olive oil, or until coated. Lay pieces on cookie sheet and roast until just softened and browned.

16 oz [2 cups] arugula leaves
Herbs: tarragon and chives
1 chopped avocado
4 oz [½ cup] toasted pumpkin or sunflower seeds
4 oz [½ cup] goat cheese

While squash is roasting, place arugula leaves on a plate. Sprinkle herbs to desired taste. Put equal amounts of avocado, seeds and cheese on each plate. Sprinkle warm squash on top.

4 oz [¼ cup] olive oil
1 oz [2 T] balsamic vinegar

Whisk ingredients together and drizzle over salad before serving.

Middle Eastern Cucumber Salad

2 cucumbers cut into chunks
2 Roma tomatoes cut into chunks (AB or O blood type)
½ small red onion, chopped

Cut veggies to desired size. Chunky sizes usually work best.

Dressing 1: 8 oz [1 cup] Greek yogurt, dill and parsley. 1 oz [2 T] lemon juice

Mix with one of the dressings.

Dressing 2: 2 oz [¼ cup] olive oil, 2 oz [¼ cup] fresh lemon juice, chopped mint leaves

Beet Salad

4 beets

Steam beets covered or wrapped in foil (or roast at 400°F, 200°C) until tender. Allow to cool completely. Peel and chop in large chunks.

4 oz [½ cup] goat cheese

Break into clumps.

4 oz [½ cup] walnuts, chopped

1 oz [2 T] olive oil
2 oz [¼ cup] rice vinegar
½ tsp agave nectar
Salt and pepper if needed

Mix dressing. Toss all ingredients gently together. Serve on greens if desired. Arugula adds a spicy crunch.

Black Bean Salad

Black beans, 1 can, rinsed
8 oz [1 cup] frozen corn, thawed
4 oz [½ cup] diced red onion
2 Roma tomatoes, diced and deseeded
Flatleaf parsley, chopped (or cilantro)

Mix ingredients.

2 oz [¼ cup] olive oil
1½ oz [3 T] lime juice
½ oz [1 T] chili powder
1 tsp cumin
Salt/pepper to taste

Whisk together and toss with ingredients.

Serve on a bed of greens if desired. Spinach is especially delicious with this salad.

Sauces and Dressings

These can be substituted for the dressings listed with the salads above. Be flexible with the measurements, creating new tastes according to your preferences.

Thai Dressing

½ oz [1 T] fresh grated ginger
1 tsp garlic, minced finely
1½ oz [3 oz] lime juice
2 oz [¼ cup] olive oil
1 tsp honey

Stir ingredients together. Use for cold green salads.

Vegan Dressing

4 oz [½ cup] vegan mayonnaise; plain yogurt
2 oz [¼ cup] apple cider vinegar

Whisk ingredients together. Use for cold salads.

Tahini Sauce

1 clove garlic
4 oz [½ cup] tahini
4 oz [½ cup] water
4 oz [½ cup] lemon juice

Adjust water/lemon juice to desired consistency

Mix ingredients in food processor or with whisk.

Use in pita sandwiches, falafel, salads, or a sauce over a dinner dish or kebabs.

Garlic Sauce

5 cloves garlic
4 oz [½ cup] olive oil
2 oz [¼ cup] lemon juice
Black pepper
1 T goat cheese/feta cheese

Place in blender or small food processor. Blend until smooth, making sure the cloves are fully blended.

Sprinkle on top of salad.
Use as a salad dressing, dip, over kebabs, or extra flavouring in dishes.

Yogurt Sauce

2 cloves garlic, smashed and minced
2 oz [¼ cup] fresh chopped mint
1 quart [4 cups] yogurt
8 oz [1 cup] water mixed with 1 T cornstarch

Mix ingredients in food processor or whip with whisk. Use with pita sandwiches, cold salads, or a sauce over a dinner dish.

Pesto

1 bunch fresh basil leaves plucked off their stems
3 garlic cloves
4 oz [½ cup] walnuts (or pine nuts or almonds)
2 oz [¼ cup] olive oil
1 T parmesan cheese, or miso paste (optional)

Place in food processor and blend together to desired thickness by using more or less olive oil.

Uses: Serve over noodles and roasted veggies tossed together. Use as a spread. Put 1 T into roasted veggie soup for extra flavour.

Dinner

After your 'Street sweeper' salads, enjoy this simple dinner to cleanse the palate and body in the first few days at least. You can continue with this the rest of the Fast if desired.

Brown Rice and Steamed Veggies (Days 1–5)

Basic Brown Rice

4 oz [½ cup] brown rice

2 cooked vegetables, e.g. yams, beets or broccoli. Cut into chunks and steam until tender.

Herbed Brown Rice

8 oz [1 cup] basic brown rice recipe

Freshly cut herbs (dill, basil, oregano, tarragon, thyme, parsley)
½ oz [1 T] rice vinegar
Sea salt, lightly sprinkled

Toss rice with herbs, vinegar and seasonings.

Soups, Grains and Veggies (Days 6–12)

Soups

Keep your portion to 1– 1½ cups.

Roasted Vegetable Soup

1 quart [3–4 cups] vegetable or mushroom broth
1 quart leftover roasted veggies (from recipes in next section)
1 tsp black pepper
1 T olive oil

Chop vegetables, add to the broth and blend. Heat and season.

Miso Soup

1 quart [4 cups] vegetable or mushroom broth
1 tsp sesame oil
1 tsp grated fresh ginger
1 tsp minced garlic
Bok choy (tops and partial white portion, thinly sliced)
1 oz [2 T] sea vegetables, chopped
3 green onions, chopped into rings
1 oz [2 T] miso paste

Bring broth to a rolling boil.

Stir-fry ginger and garlic until tender but not browned. Cut green onions thinly until you get to where the green tops become limp. Use the crispest part. Add all ingredients to the broth and stir. Add miso paste 1 T at a time into a small bowl of warm water and thoroughly dissolve while mixing with a fork.

Add rice udon noodles if desired.

Vegetable Soup

1 T olive oil
3 large garlic cloves, smashed and finely minced
1 yellow onion, chopped
2 leeks, chopped and well washed
1 cup cabbage, chopped

1 cup yellow waxy potatoes (such as Yukon Gold), chopped to bite size
2 cups carrots, chopped
1 cup celery, chopped
1 cup green beans, fresh or frozen

2 quarts vegetable or mushroom stock
1 tsp saffron
2 T freshly cut herbs

Additional options:
1 T olive oil
10 oz can drained diced tomatoes

In large stockpot heat oil on medium heat. Add the onions and leeks and sauté until translucent. Add garlic and heat 1 minute.

Add vegetables to pot and sauté 5 more minutes.

Add stock and seasoning and bring to boil. Simmer until vegetables are tender.

Adjust amount of stock depending upon whether you like a chunkier soup or more broth.

Grains and Veggies

Try these grains in addition to brown rice with roasted veggies.

- Quinoa
- Wheat berries
- Millet
- Amaranth
- Buckwheat
- Bulgur
- Any whole grains listed in the grocery list

Cook the grains according to the package instructions. Try substituting vegetable broth or mushroom broth for water in cooking. Add beans, cumin, or herbs as well. Dried fruit and a sprinkling of fresh toasted nuts make a great 'pilaf'.

Roasted veggies can be made in larger quantities than needed for just one recipe. Leftovers make a great soup the next day: add enough vegetable broth to blend a smooth, delicious fast soup.

Mediterranean Roasted Veggies

1 bulb fennel, sliced (cut off bottom and innermost core) **1 zucchini, sliced** **1 yellow squash, sliced** **2 Roma tomatoes** **2 cloves garlic, minced** **1 red onion, sliced** **Coloured peppers**	Cut into similar-sized chunks.
1 oz [2 T] olive oil **½ oz [1 T] balsamic vinegar** **Dried oregano and marjoram** **Seasoned salt/pepper**	Preheat oven to 425°F, 220°C. Toss veggies with olive oil and herbs until just coated. Spread evenly in one layer on baking sheet. Bake until tender, about 35 minutes. Stir veggies once, about halfway through baking time.

Root Vegetable Spread

2 parsnips, peeled and chopped
3 carrots, peeled and chopped
2 yellow potatoes, chopped and rinsed
1 yellow onion, chopped in large chunks
1 rutabaga, peeled and chopped
2 beets, peeled and chopped

2 oz [¼ cup] olive oil
Fresh herbs, bruised and minced

Cut veggies about the same size so they will cook in the same time. The small end of the parsnips will cook more rapidly than the rest, so add them in 10 minutes before the dish is finished cooking.

Preheat oven to 425°F, 220°C. Toss veggies with olive oil and herbs until just coated. Spread evenly in one layer on baking sheet. Bake until veggies are tender, about 35 minutes. Stir veggies once about halfway through baking time.

Green Roasted Veggies

½ bunch asparagus, chopped and hard ends cut off
Handful green beans & yellow wax beans
1 red onion, chopped in similar size as beans and asparagus
1 oz [2 T] olive oil

Toss veggies with enough olive oil to coat. Lay single layer on pan and roast at 400°F, 200°C until desired. Check at 20 minutes and stir.

Pan-cooked Veggies

12 Brussels sprouts
2 parsnips
3 carrots

Cut Brussels sprouts in half, trim off the bottoms and pull any yellowing leaves off. Make them about the same size. Chop the parsnips and carrots about the same size. Steam until a fork can just poke through the surface (firm, but NOT soft). Set aside on plate.

1 leek, sliced (thoroughly wash & drain)
1 chopped onion
4 T olive oil
Fresh thyme, hint of nutmeg, or dash of cayenne pepper

Toss leeks and onion in the pan with warmed olive oil over medium heat. Cook until opaque. Add steamed veggies, herbs and seasoning. Cook until tender over low heat, covered, about 5 minutes.

Basic Roasted Potatoes

16 oz new potatoes, yellow potatoes, or sweet potatoes	Cut into 2-inch cubes.
1 oz [2 T] olive oil (enough to coat) *Add to olive oil for flavour:* **Squirt of spicy mustard** **Kosher salt/pepper**	For potato coating, mix seasoning together and toss potatoes until just coated, not soaked. Place single layer on pan and roast at 425°F, 220°C for about 45 minutes, or until golden brown.
Flatleaf parsley, chopped	Sprinkle and toss in when cooking is finished.

Carbohydrate Dinners (Days 13–19)

You can now gradually add more ingredients. Enjoy the taste, and pay attention to any physical reactions. The gentle adding of ingredients will prepare the body to integrate back into a normal diet.

Peanut Soup

1 oz [2 T] olive oil 1 large white onion, chopped 4 large cloves garlic, 1 oz [2 T] curry powder 1 tsp cayenne pepper	Heat oil in stockpot over medium heat. Take the blade of a butcher knife and lay it flat over the garlic clove. Pound it with your fist so it smashes the clove flat. This releases the healing juices inside. Take the knife and finely chop. Sauté onion and garlic until translucent. Tip: add garlic after the onion has cooked a few minutes, otherwise, the smaller garlic will turn brown or burn. Add spices and cook until fragrant.
1 quart vegetable broth [4 cups] 14 oz can diced tomatoes 14 oz coconut milk ⅔ cup organic peanut butter	Add broth, tomatoes, coconut milk and peanut butter. Stir well and parboil. Simmer for 15 minutes.
Additional options: **Cooked diced squash** **Minced ginger** **Chopped cooked asparagus** **Chopped cooked potatoes**	If desired, serve over bed of brown rice in bowl.

RECIPES

Stuffed Brown Rice Peppers

16 oz [2 cups] cooked brown rice 1 onion, diced 3 cloves garlic	Preheat oven to 350°F, 175°C Take the blade of a butcher knife and lay it flat over the garlic clove. Pound it with your fist so it smashes the clove flat. This releases the healing juices inside. Take the knife and finely chop. Stir-fry onion and garlic until translucent, not brown. Tip: add garlic after the onion has cooked a few minutes, otherwise, the smaller garlic will turn brown or burn.
Option 1: Southern Chopped parsley ½ oz [1 T] cumin 1 oz [2 T] chili pepper ½ oz [1 T] lime juice 4 oz [½ cup] corn 2 Roma tomatoes, diced and deseeded ½ cup cooked pinto beans	Add spices and mix together. Cook until fragrant. Add tomato and beans. Toss all ingredients together.
Option 2: Middle Eastern 4 oz [½ cup] pine nuts 8 oz [1 cup] garbanzo beans ½ oz [1 T] cinnamon	Add pine nuts and spices to rice and onion mix, cooking until fragrant.
2 green peppers Olive oil to coat pan	Cut tops off and cut in half, taking out any seeds. Oil a roasting pan and place peppers in. Fill peppers with mix, don't be afraid of filling to overflow a bit.
1 cup crushed tomatoes	Add ¼ cup parboiled water to crushed tomato in separate bowl and whisk until blended. Pour over peppers. Cover pan and bake for 30 minutes, or desired tenderness.

Risotto and Butternut Squash Casserole

2 butternut squash, diced 1 oz [2 T] olive oil	Toss squash with oil and roast 400°F, 200°C until soft.
1 onion, diced	Fry onion in olive oil
1 tsp turmeric 1 tsp cinnamon	Add when onions become opaque.

(continued on next page)

8 oz [1 cup] prunes without pits, cut in half 8 oz [1 cup] walnuts 12 oz [1½ cups] risotto rice	Mix these ingredients over medium-high heat until risotto is moist.
1 quart [4 cups] vegetable broth	Add one cup of broth at a time and stir. Cook until the broth is absorbed, stirring frequently.

Moroccan Couscous and Vegetables

1 oz [2 T] olive oil 1 white onion, sliced 2 garlic cloves, minced 8 oz [1 cup] carrots, cut into matchsticks	Put olive oil in large frying pan and heat to medium heat. Cook onion until opaque. Add garlic and carrots.
½ oz [1 T] each curry powder, cinnamon 1 tsp each turmeric, coriander	Add spices and mix, cooking until fragrant.
4 oz [½ cup] currants or raisins 8 oz [1 cup] swiss chard (if desired) or 1 roasted sweet potato, chopped	Mix in currants and swiss chard.
12 oz [1½ cups] vegetable broth 8 oz [1 cup] couscous	Add vegetable broth and bring to boil. Add couscous, stir and take pan off heat. Cover and allow liquids to fully absorb.
Chopped flatleaf parsley	Toss in parsley and serve immediately.

Roasted Portobello Mushrooms

1 head roasted garlic	Take entire garlic head, coat with olive oil and put in covered at 400°F (200°C) oven for 30 minutes, or when garlic is soft depending upon the size. Let cool and squeeze out the cloves to create a spread.
2 large portobello mushrooms, washed and thickly sliced	Brush with olive oil. Broil (grill) or fry in pan until cooked through. Add olive oil as needed to keep surface moist.
½ onion, cut to desired size (I prefer long strings) Sliced avocado (optional) Seasoned salt/pepper	Fry in olive oil until soft.

Multi-grain bread, thickly sliced

On multi-grain bread, spread roasted garlic. Cover with fried onions. Place avocado slices and then portobello mushrooms. Serve with a salad or side serving of roasted veggies.

Side serving of Kale

8 oz kale	Rinse thoroughly in bowl of cold water. If a lot of grit comes off, use another fresh bowl of water. Shake off and place in colander.
2 T olive oil	Heat oil over medium heat. Toss the kale until leaves just wilt (or until heated through).
Lemon juice (from at least 1 lemon)	Toss in lemon juice to desired taste. The lemon juice will soften the kale.

Option 1: add fried onions and pine nuts with a hint of nutmeg instead of lemon juice.

Option 2: Chop kale into ¼ inch (6 mm) strips, dip in lemon juice until softened, and add to salads, soups or rice.

Roasted Cloves Pasta

12 oz wide egg noodles 6 oz [¾ cup] ground walnuts 2 heads roasted garlic 4oz [½ cup] olive oil (or less if desired)	Cook al dente. Set aside to cool. Place garlic in roasting pan, drizzling a little olive oil over it and bake at 400°F (200°C) for 30 minutes or until tender, depending upon size. When finished, squeeze out soft garlic cloves into food processor. Add walnuts and olive oil. Blend until smooth for sauce.
2 cups spinach 1 colored pepper, chopped 4oz [½ cup] vegetable stock 1/8 tsp cayenne red pepper Flatleaf parsley and basil, chopped	Stir-fry pepper for 2 minutes. Add spinach until just wilted. Combine noodles, vegetable stock mix, and walnut sauce. Add olive oil if you wish. Sprinkle parsley and serve immediately.

Pad Thai

1 oz [2T] lime juice 4 tsp fish sauce or soy sauce 1 tsp red pepper chili paste 1 tsp grated ginger 1 tsp white pepper	Mix sauce and set aside.
12 oz rice noodles	Heat water to almost a rolling boil. Immediately immerse noodles in water for 5 minutes (al dente), then strain them in colander.
2 cloves minced garlic 1 package firm tofu diced 2 tsp sesame oil	Stir-fry garlic and tofu for 1 min in oil. Add softened noodles. Add the sauce and stir. Keep heat on high.
Carrots, diced	Add carrots and cook until tender, constantly stirring.
3 spring onions, sliced in rings	Toss in and mix until heated.
Toppers: Mung bean sprouts Pea shoots Fresh basil, chopped Chopped peanuts	Add bean sprouts, basil, pea shoots and mix well. Put entire contents on serving platter and sprinkle chopped peanuts on top.

Mexican Stuffed Squash

2 large squash cut in half (yellow summer squash or zucchini)	Cut in half and scrape out seeds with spoon. Bake in 400°F (200°C) degree oven until soft, about 25 minutes. Brush tops lightly with olive oil if desired.
4 oz [½ cup] quinoa or amaranth	Cook according to directions on label.
4 oz [½ cup] corn 4 oz [½ cup] cooked black beans 4 oz [½ cup] coloured peppers, chopped ½ small red onion, finely chopped ¼ cup cilantro leaves, chopped	Toss these ingredients together with warm cooked quinoa in bowl. Remove squash from oven and let it cool for 5 minutes.
¼ cup lime juice 1 tsp chili powder ½ tsp cumin Herbal salt alternative	Toss warmed quinoa and veggie mixture with juice mix. Spoon mixture into warm squash bases. If desired, place in oven until warmed through.

RECIPES

Acorn Squash with Wild Rice Stuffing

2 acorn squash cut in half (2 servings per squash)	Cut acorn squash in half, take out the seeds. Roast in oven uncovered 400°F (200°C) until tender. Or, steam in oven by placing filling the bottom of a baking pan with water, cover and bake for 40 minutes, depending upon size (check for tenderness).
1 oz [2 T] olive oil ½ onion, diced 4 oz [½ cup] crimini mushrooms	Fry onion and mushrooms until tender.
2 cloves garlic, minced 2 stalks celery, chopped	Add garlic and celery.
5 dried unsulphured apricots, diced ½ oz [1 T] raisins Seasonings: oregano, thyme, sage 8 oz [1 cup] cooked wild rice	Toss in dried fruit, herbs and rice.
24 oz [3 cups] corn bread stuffing 3 oz [1/3 cup] vegetable broth (add more if you like your stuffing wet)	Mix in corn bread stuffing and soak in vegetable broth. If you don't have stuffing available, you can bake your own corn bread, or take any dried, hardened whole grain bread and break it into small pieces. Fill acorn squash with stuffing and bake at 350°F (175°C) until heated through: 20 minutes.

Evening Snacks

You may be surprised how little you need to eat after sunset, but the impulse to snack may remain. Instead, focus on rehydrating in the evening through teas and broths. If you have exerted yourself during the day and feel the stomach growling (empty), but not wanting to eat out of boredom, try some of the following suggestions.

- Herbal non-caffeinated tea
- Medjool dates (filled with ½ tsp almond butter)
- ½ cup veggies dipped in 1 T hummus
- Apple slices dipped in 1 T peanut butter

- Air-popped popcorn
- 1 piece of fruit
- Rice or nut crackers
- 1 cup of soup

Naw-Rúz Dessert

You've made it this far, now celebrate your efforts by gradually adding a sweeter taste with these healthy treats.

Apple Tartlet

8 oz [1 cup] wholewheat pastry flour
1 oz [2 T] date sugar
½ tsp salt
2 oz [¼ cup] non-dairy shortening (non-hydrogenated fat)
½ tsp apple cider vinegar
4 oz [½ cup] ice water

2 golden apples, peeled, thinly sliced and cored
½ oz [1 T] dark brown sugar
1 tsp vanilla
1 tsp flour
½ tsp cinnamon

Set aside a small glass of ice water. Mix together flour, sugar and salt in food processor. Pulse in shortening until it resembles breadcrumbs. Measure water (without ice) and mix with vinegar. Gradually add to flour mixture while pulsing until it reaches a dough-like consistency. (Add more water if too dry.) Rest dough in fridge for at least 20 minutes.

Heat small frying pan to medium heat. Gently heat apples, adding sugar and vanilla. When warm, drop onto a plate and sprinkle with flour and cinnamon. Allow to cool while working with the dough.

Lightly oil a cookie sheet. Preheat oven to 400° (200°C). Roll dough on clean surface into a square shape, about ½ inch thick. Cut out desired serving size and shapes – 4 diamonds, 4 circles, or 6 small shapes. Place dough on cookie sheet, and raise up the edges by pushing them in a bit so the apple juices won't spill over the sides. Place at least 4 apple slices on larger sizes. Drizzle the leftover juices over each tartlet. Bake about 12 minutes, or until golden brown.

Bruised Pear Crumble

4 sliced pears (if organic, leave skin on)
1 oz [2 T] lemon juice
8 oz [1 cup] blackberries, fresh or frozen
4 oz [½ cup] chopped raisins
1 oz [2 T] arrowroot powder
1 ½ oz [3 T] maple syrup
½ oz [1 T] cinnamon
1 tsp nutmeg
8 oz [1 cup] oats (not quick oats)
1½ oz [3 T] brown sugar or agave
1 tsp cinnamon
4 oz [½ cup] wholewheat pastry flour
2 oz [¼ cup] butter or vegan shortening, or canola oil

Slice pears and toss with lemon juice. Mix in blackberries, raisins, arrowroot, maple syrup and spices.

Let the mixture sit while you make the topping.

Preheat oven to 375° (190°C). Mix together all ingredients except shortening. Cut shortening into oat mixture. Pour fruit mix into medium cake pan and sprinkle oat mixture on top. (Don't pat topping.) Bake until golden brown, about 30–40 minutes.

17

PRAYERS FOR THE FAST: A SELECTION

Beginning the Fast

This is, O my God, the first of the days on which Thou hast bidden Thy loved ones to observe the Fast. I ask of Thee by Thy Self and by him who hath fasted out of love for Thee and for Thy good-pleasure – and not out of self and desire, nor out of fear of Thy wrath – and by Thy most excellent names and august attributes, to purify Thy servants from the love of aught except Thee and to draw them nigh unto the Dawning-Place of the lights of Thy countenance and the Seat of the throne of Thy oneness. Illumine their hearts, O my God, with the light of Thy knowledge and brighten their faces with the rays of the Daystar that shineth from the horizon of Thy Will. Potent art Thou to do what pleaseth Thee. No God is there but Thee, the All-Glorious, Whose help is implored by all men.

Assist them, O my God, to render Thee victorious and to exalt Thy Word. Suffer them, then, to become as hands of Thy Cause amongst Thy servants, and make them to be revealers of Thy religion and Thy signs amongst mankind, in such wise that the whole world may be filled with Thy remembrance and praise and with Thy proofs and evidences. Thou art, verily, the All-Bountiful, the Most Exalted, the Powerful, the Mighty, and the Merciful.

Bahá'u'lláh [1]

Praised be Thou, O God, my God! These are the days whereon Thou hast enjoined Thy chosen ones, Thy loved ones and Thy servants to observe the Fast, which Thou hast made a light unto the people of Thy kingdom, even as Thou didst make obligatory prayer a ladder of ascent unto those who acknowledge Thy unity. I beg of Thee, O my God, by these two mighty pillars, which Thou hast ordained as a glory and honour for all mankind, to keep Thy religion safe from the mischief of the ungodly and the plotting of every wicked doer. O Lord, conceal not the light which Thou hast revealed through Thy strength and Thine omnipotence. Assist, then, those who truly believe in Thee with the hosts of the seen and the unseen by Thy command and Thy sovereignty. No God is there but Thee, the Almighty, the Most Powerful. *Bahá'u'lláh*[2]

Before breaking the Fast

Praise be unto Thee, O Lord my God! We have observed the Fast in conformity with Thy bidding and break it now through Thy love and Thy good-pleasure. Deign to accept, O My God, the deeds that we have performed in Thy path wholly for the sake of Thy beauty with our faces set towards Thy Cause, free from aught else but Thee. Bestow, then, Thy forgiveness upon us, upon our forefathers, and upon all such as have believed in Thee and in Thy mighty signs in this most great, this most glorious Revelation. Potent art Thou to do what Thou choosest. Thou art, verily, the Most Exalted, the Almighty, the Unconstrained. *Bahá'u'lláh*[3]

O God! As I am fasting from the appetites of the body and not occupied with eating and drinking, even so purify and make holy my heart and my life from aught else save Thy Love, and protect and preserve my soul from self-passions and animal traits. Thus may the spirit associate with the Fragrances of Holiness and fast from everything else save Thy mention. *'Abdu'l-Bahá*[4]

Prayers for meditation

In the Name of Him Who hath been promised in the Books of God, the All-Knowing, the All-Informed! The days of fasting have arrived wherein those servants who circle round Thy throne and have attained Thy presence have fasted. Say: O God of names and creator of heaven and earth! I beg of Thee by Thy Name, the All-Glorious, to accept the fast of those who have fasted for love of Thee and for the sake of Thy good-pleasure and have carried out what Thou hast bidden them in Thy Books and Tablets. I beseech Thee by them to assist me in the promotion of Thy Cause and to make me steadfast in Thy love, that my footsteps may not slip on account of the clamour of Thy creatures. Verily, Thou art powerful over whatsoever Thou willest. No God is there but Thee, the Quickener, the All-Powerful, the Most Bountiful, the Ancient of Days.

Bahá'u'lláh[5]

I beseech Thee, O my God, by Thy mighty Sign, and by the revelation of Thy grace amongst men, to cast me not away from the gate of the city of Thy presence, and to disappoint not the hopes I have set on the manifestations of Thy grace amidst Thy creatures. Thou seest me, O my God, holding to Thy Name, the Most Holy, the Most Luminous, the Most Mighty, the Most Great, the Most Exalted, the Most Glorious, and clinging to the hem of the robe to which have clung all in this world and in the world to come.

I beseech Thee, O my God, by Thy most sweet Voice and by Thy most exalted Word, to draw me ever nearer to the threshold of Thy door, and to suffer me not to be far removed from the shadow of Thy mercy and the canopy of Thy bounty. Thou seest me, O my God, holding to Thy Name, the Most Holy, the Most Luminous, the Most Mighty, the Most Great, the Most Exalted, the Most Glorious, and clinging to the hem of the robe to which have clung all in this world and in the world to come.

I beseech Thee, O my God, by the splendour of Thy luminous brow and the brightness of the light of Thy countenance, which shineth from the all-highest horizon, to attract me by the fragrance of Thy raiment, and make me drink of the choice wine of Thine utterance. Thou seest me, O my God, holding to Thy Name, the Most Holy, the Most Luminous, the Most Mighty, the Most Great, the Most Exalted, the Most Glorious, and clinging to the hem of the robe to which have clung all in this world and in the world to come.

I beseech Thee, O my God, by Thy hair which moveth across Thy face, even as Thy most exalted pen moveth across the pages of Thy Tablets, shedding the musk of hidden meanings over the kingdom of Thy creation, so to raise me up to serve Thy Cause that I shall not fall back, nor be hindered by the suggestions of them who have cavilled at Thy signs and turned away from Thy face. Thou seest me, O my God, holding to Thy Name, the Most Holy, the Most Luminous, the Most Mighty, the Most Great, the Most Exalted, the Most

Glorious, and clinging to the hem of the robe to which have clung all in this world and in the world to come.

I beseech Thee, O my God, by Thy Name which Thou hast made the King of Names, by which all who are in heaven and all who are on earth have been enraptured, to enable me to gaze on the Daystar of Thy Beauty, and to supply me with the wine of Thine utterance. Thou seest me, O my God, holding to Thy Name, the Most Holy, the Most Luminous, the Most Mighty, the Most Great, the Most Exalted, the Most Glorious, and clinging to the hem of the robe to which have clung all in this world and in the world to come.

I beseech Thee, O my God, by the Tabernacle of Thy majesty upon the loftiest summits, and the Canopy of Thy Revelation on the highest hills, to graciously aid me to do what Thy will hath desired and Thy purpose hath manifested. Thou seest me, O my God, holding to Thy Name, the Most Holy, the Most Luminous, the Most Mighty, the Most Great, the Most Exalted, the Most Glorious, and clinging to the hem of the robe to which have clung all in this world and in the world to come.

I beseech Thee, O my God, by Thy Beauty that shineth forth above the horizon of eternity, a Beauty before which as soon as it revealeth itself the kingdom of beauty boweth down in worship, magnifying it in ringing tones, to grant that I may die to all that I possess and live to whatsoever belongeth unto Thee. Thou seest me, O my God, holding to Thy Name, the Most Holy, the Most Luminous, the Most Mighty, the Most Great, the Most Exalted, the Most Glorious, and clinging to the hem of the robe to which have clung all in this world and in the world to come.

I beseech Thee, O my God, by the Manifestation of Thy Name, the Well-Beloved, through Whom the hearts of Thy lovers were consumed and the souls of all that dwell on earth have soared aloft, to aid me to remember Thee amongst Thy creatures, and to extol Thee amidst Thy people. Thou seest me, O my God, holding to Thy Name, the Most Holy, the Most Luminous, the Most Mighty, the Most Great, the Most Exalted, the Most Glorious, and clinging to the hem of the robe to which have clung all in this world and in the world to come.

I beseech Thee, O my God, by the rustling of the Divine Lote-Tree and the murmur of the breezes of Thine utterance in the kingdom of Thy names, to remove me far from whatsoever Thy will abhorreth, and draw me nigh unto the station wherein He Who is the Dayspring of Thy signs hath shone forth. Thou seest me, O my God, holding to Thy Name, the Most Holy, the Most Luminous, the Most Mighty, the Most Great, the Most Exalted, the Most Glorious, and clinging to the hem of the robe to which have clung all in this world and in the world to come.

I beseech Thee, O my God, by that Letter which, as soon as it proceeded out of the mouth of Thy will, hath caused the oceans to surge, and the winds to blow, and the fruits to be revealed, and the trees to spring forth, and all past traces to vanish, and all veils to be rent asunder, and them who are devoted to Thee to hasten unto the light of the countenance of their Lord, the Unconstrained, to make known unto me what lay hid in the treasuries of Thy knowledge and concealed within the repositories of Thy wisdom. Thou seest me, O my God, holding to Thy Name, the Most Holy, the Most Luminous, the Most Mighty, the Most Great, the Most Exalted, the Most Glorious, and clinging to the hem of the robe to which have clung all in this world and in the world to come.

I beseech Thee, O my God, by the fire of Thy love which drove sleep from the eyes of Thy chosen ones and Thy loved ones, and by their remembrance and praise of Thee at the hour of dawn, to number me with such as have attained unto that which Thou hast sent down in Thy Book and manifested through Thy will. Thou seest me, O my God, holding to Thy Name, the Most Holy, the Most Luminous, the Most Mighty, the Most Great, the Most Exalted, the Most Glorious, and clinging to the hem of the robe to which have clung all in this world and in the world to come.

I beseech Thee, O my God, by the light of Thy countenance which impelled them who are nigh unto Thee to meet the darts of Thy decree, and such as are devoted to Thee to face the swords of Thine enemies in Thy path, to write down for me with Thy most exalted Pen what Thou hast written down for Thy trusted ones and Thy chosen ones. Thou seest me, O my God, holding to Thy Name, the Most Holy, the Most Luminous, the Most Mighty, the Most Great, the Most Exalted, the Most Glorious, and clinging to the hem of the robe to which have clung all in this world and in the world to come.

I beseech Thee, O my God, by Thy Name through which Thou hast hearkened unto the call of Thy lovers, and the sighs of them that long for Thee, and the cry of them that enjoy near access to Thee, and the groaning of them that are devoted to Thee, and through which Thou hast fulfilled the wishes of them that have set their hopes on Thee, and hast granted them their desires, through Thy grace and Thy favours, and by Thy Name through which the ocean of forgiveness surged before Thy face, and the clouds of Thy generosity rained upon Thy servants, to write down for everyone who hath turned unto Thee, and observed the fast prescribed by Thee, the recompense decreed for such as speak not except by Thy leave, and who forsook all that they possessed in Thy path and for love of Thee.

I beseech Thee, O my Lord, by Thyself, and by Thy signs, and Thy clear tokens, and the shining light of the Daystar of Thy Beauty, and Thy Branches, to cancel the trespasses of those who have held fast to Thy laws, and have observed what Thou hast prescribed unto them in Thy Book. Thou seest me, O my God, holding to Thy Name, the Most Holy, the Most Luminous, the Most Mighty, the Most Great, the Most Exalted, the Most Glorious, and clinging to the hem of the robe to which have clung all in this world and in the world to come. *Bahá'u'lláh*[6]

Praise be to Thee, O Lord my God! I beseech Thee by this Revelation whereby darkness hath been turned into light, through which the Frequented Fane hath been built, and the Written Tablet revealed, and the Outspread Roll uncovered, to send down upon me and upon them who are in my company that which will enable us to soar into the heavens of Thy transcendent glory, and will wash us from the stain of such doubts as have hindered the suspicious from entering into the tabernacle of Thy unity.

I am the one, O my Lord, who hath held fast the cord of Thy loving-kindness, and clung to the hem of Thy mercy and favours. Do Thou ordain for me and for my loved ones the good of this world and of the world to come. Supply them, then, with the Hidden Gift Thou didst ordain for the choicest among Thy creatures.

These are, O my Lord, the days in which Thou hast bidden Thy servants to observe the fast. Blessed is he that observeth the fast wholly for Thy sake and with absolute detachment from all things except Thee. Assist me and assist them. O my Lord, to obey Thee and to keep Thy precepts. Thou, verily, hast power to do what Thou choosest.

There is no God but Thee, the All-Knowing, the All-Wise. All praise be to God, the Lord of all worlds. *Bahá'u'lláh*[7]

These are, O my God, the days whereon Thou didst enjoin Thy servants to observe the fast. With it Thou didst adorn the preamble of the Book of Thy Laws revealed unto Thy creatures, and didst deck forth the Repositories of Thy commandments in the sight of all who are in Thy heaven and all who are on Thy earth. Thou hast endowed every hour of these days with a special virtue, inscrutable to all except Thee, Whose knowledge embraceth all created things. Thou hast, also, assigned unto every soul a portion of this virtue in accordance with the Tablet of Thy decree and the Scriptures of Thine irrevocable judgment. Every leaf of these Books and Scriptures Thou hast, moreover, alloted to each one of the peoples and kindreds of the earth.

For Thine ardent lovers Thou hast, according to Thy decree, reserved, at each daybreak, the cup of Thy remembrance, O Thou Who art the Ruler of rulers! These are they who have been so inebriated with the wine of Thy manifold wisdom that they forsake their couches in their longing to celebrate Thy praise and extol Thy virtues, and flee from sleep in their eagerness to approach Thy presence and partake of Thy bounty. Their eyes have, at all times, been bent upon the Day-Spring of Thy loving-kindness, and their faces set towards the Fountain-Head of Thine inspiration. Rain down, then, upon us and upon them from the clouds of Thy mercy what beseemeth the heaven of Thy bounteousness and grace.

Lauded be Thy name, O My God! This is the hour when Thou hast unlocked the doors of Thy bounty before the faces of Thy creatures, and opened wide the portals of Thy tender mercy unto all the dwellers of Thine earth. I beseech Thee, by all them whose blood was shed in Thy path, who, in their yearning over Thee, rid themselves from all attachment to any of Thy creatures, and who were so carried away by the sweet savours of Thine inspiration that every single member of their bodies intoned Thy praise and vibrated to

Thy remembrance, not to withhold from us the things Thou hast irrevocably ordained in this Revelation – a Revelation the potency of which hath caused every tree to cry out what the Burning Bush had foretime proclaimed unto Moses, Who conversed with Thee, a Revelation that hath enabled every least pebble to resound again with Thy praise, as the stones glorified Thee in the days of Muḥammad, Thy Friend.

These are the ones, O my God, whom Thou hast graciously enabled to have fellowship with Thee and to commune with Him Who is the Revealer of Thyself. The winds of Thy will have scattered them abroad until Thou didst gather them together beneath Thy shadow, and didst cause them to enter into the precincts of Thy court. Now that Thou hast made them to abide under the shade of the canopy of Thy mercy, do Thou assist them to attain what must befit so august a station. Suffer them not, O my Lord, to be numbered with them who, though enjoying near access to Thee, have been kept back from recognizing Thy face, and who, though meeting with Thee, are deprived of Thy presence.

These are Thy servants, O my Lord, who have entered with Thee in this, the Most Great Prison, who have kept the fast within its walls according to what Thou hast commanded them in the Tablets of Thy decree and the Books of Thy behest. Send down, therefore, upon them what will thoroughly purge them of all that Thou abhorrest, that they may be wholly devoted to Thee, and may detach themselves entirely from all except Thyself.

Rain down, then, upon us. O my God, that which beseemeth Thy grace and befitteth Thy bounty. Enable us, then, O my God, to live in remembrance of Thee and to die in love of Thee, and supply us with the gift of Thy presence in Thy worlds hereafter – worlds which are inscrutable to all except Thee. Thou art our Lord and the Lord of all worlds, and the God of all that are in heaven and all that are on earth.

Thou beholdest, O my God, what hath befallen Thy dear ones in Thy days. Thy glory beareth me witness! The voice of the lamentations of Thy chosen ones hath been lifted up throughout Thy realm. Some were ensnared by the infidels in Thy land, and were hindered by them from having near access to Thee and from attaining the court of Thy glory. Others were able to approach Thee, but were kept back from beholding Thy face. Still others were permitted, in their eagerness to look upon Thee, to enter the precincts of Thy court, but they allowed the veils of the imaginations of Thy creatures and the wrongs inflicted by the oppressors among Thy people to come in between them and Thee.

This is the hour, O my Lord, which Thou hast caused to excel every other hour, and hast related to the choicest among Thy creatures. I beseech Thee, O my God, by Thy Self and by them, to ordain in the course of this year what shall exalt Thy loved ones. Do Thou, moreover, decree within this year what will enable the Daystar of Thy power to shine brightly above the horizon of Thy glory, and to illuminate by Thy sovereign might, the whole world.

Render Thy Cause victorious, O my Lord, and abase Thou Thine enemies. Write down, then, for us the good of this life and of the life to come. Thou art the Truth, Who knoweth the secret things. No God is there but Thee, the Ever-Forgiving, the All-Bountiful.

Bahá'u'lláh[8]

Glory be to Thee, O Lord my God! These are the days whereon Thou hast bidden all men to observe the fast, that through it they may purify their souls and rid themselves of all attachment to anyone but Thee, and that out of their hearts may ascend that which will be worthy of the court of Thy majesty and may well beseem the seat of the revelation of Thy oneness. Grant, O my Lord, that this fast may become a river of life-giving waters and may yield the virtue wherewith Thou hast endowed it. Cleanse Thou by its means the hearts of Thy servants whom the evils of the world have failed to hinder from turning towards Thy all-glorious Name, and who have remained unmoved by the noise and tumult of such as have repudiated Thy most resplendent signs which have accompanied the advent of Thy Manifestation Whom Thou hast invested with Thy sovereignty, Thy power, Thy majesty and glory. These are the servants who, as soon as Thy call reached them, hastened in the direction of Thy mercy and were not kept back from Thee by the changes and chances of this world or by any human limitations.

I am he, O my God, who testifieth to Thy unity, who acknowledgeth Thy oneness, who boweth humbly before the revelations of Thy majesty, and who recognizeth with downcast countenance the splendours of the light of Thy transcendent glory. I have believed in Thee after Thou didst enable me to know Thy Self, Whom Thou hast revealed to men's eyes through the power of Thy sovereignty and might. Unto Him I have turned, wholly detached from all things, and cleaving steadfastly unto the cord of Thy gifts and favours. I have embraced His truth, and the truth of all the wondrous laws and precepts that have been sent down unto Him. I have fasted for love of Thee and in pursuance of Thine injunction, and have broken my fast with Thy praise on my tongue and in conformity with Thy pleasure. Suffer me not, O my Lord, to be reckoned among them who have fasted in the daytime, who in the night-season have prostrated themselves before Thy face, and who have repudiated Thy truth, disbelieved in Thy signs, gainsaid Thy testimony, and perverted Thine utterances.

Open Thou, O my Lord, mine eyes and the eyes of all them that have sought Thee, that we may recognize Thee with Thine own eyes. This is Thy bidding given us in the Book sent down by Thee unto Him Whom Thou hast chosen by Thy behest, Whom Thou hast singled out for Thy favour above all Thy creatures, Whom Thou hast been pleased to invest with Thy sovereignty, and Whom Thou hast specially favoured and entrusted with Thy Message unto Thy people. Praised be Thou, therefore, O my God, inasmuch as Thou hast graciously enabled us to recognize Him and to acknowledge whatsoever hath been sent down unto Him, and conferred upon us the honour of attaining the presence of the One Whom Thou didst promise in Thy Book and in Thy Tablets.

Thou seest me then, O my God, with my face turned towards Thee, cleaving steadfastly to the cord of Thy gracious providence and generosity, and clinging to the hem of Thy tender mercies and bountiful favours. Destroy not, I implore Thee, my hopes of attaining unto that which Thou didst ordain for Thy servants who have turned towards the precincts of Thy court and the sanctuary of Thy presence, and have observed the fast for love of Thee. I confess, O my God, that whatever proceedeth from me is wholly unworthy of Thy sovereignty and falleth short of Thy majesty. And yet I beseech Thee by Thy Name through which Thou hast revealed Thy Self, in the glory of Thy most excellent titles, unto all created things, in this Revelation whereby Thou hast, through Thy most resplendent

Name, manifested Thy beauty, to give me to drink of the wine of Thy mercy and of the pure beverage of Thy favour, which have streamed forth from the right hand of Thy will, that I may so fix my gaze upon Thee and be so detached from all else but Thee, that the world and all that hath been created therein may appear before me as a fleeting day which Thou hast not deigned to create.

I moreover entreat Thee, O my God, to rain down, from the heaven of Thy will and the clouds of Thy mercy, that which will cleanse us from the noisome savours of our transgressions, O Thou Who hast called Thyself the God of Mercy! Thou art, verily, the Most Powerful, the All-Glorious, the Beneficent.

Cast not away, O my Lord, him that hath turned towards Thee, nor suffer him who hath drawn nigh unto Thee to be removed far from Thy court. Dash not the hopes of the supplicant who hath longingly stretched out his hands to seek Thy grace and favours, and deprive not Thy sincere servants of the wonders of Thy tender mercies and loving-kindness. Forgiving and Most Bountiful art Thou, O my Lord! Power hast Thou to do what Thou pleasest. All else but Thee are impotent before the revelations of Thy might, are as lost in the face of the evidences of Thy wealth, are as nothing when compared with the manifestations of Thy transcendent sovereignty, and are destitute of all strength when face to face with the signs and tokens of Thy power. What refuge is there beside Thee, O my Lord, to which I can flee, and where is there a haven to which I can hasten? Nay, the power of Thy might beareth me witness! No protector is there but Thee, no place to flee to except Thee, no refuge to seek save Thee. Cause me to taste, O my Lord, the divine sweetness of Thy remembrance and praise. I swear by Thy might! Whosoever tasteth of its sweetness will rid himself of all attachment to the world and all that is therein, and will set his face towards Thee, cleaned from the remembrance of anyone except Thee.

Inspire then my soul, O my God, with Thy wondrous remembrance, that I may glorify Thy name. Number me not with them who read Thy words and fail to find Thy hidden gift which, as decreed by Thee, is contained therein, and which quickeneth the souls of Thy creatures and the hearts of Thy servants. Cause me, O my Lord, to be reckoned among them who have been so stirred up by the sweet savours that have been wafted in Thy days that they have laid down their lives for Thee and hastened to the scene of their death in their longing to gaze on Thy beauty and in their yearning to attain Thy presence. And were anyone to say unto them on their way, 'Whither go ye?' they would say, 'Unto God, the All-Possessing, the Help in Peril, the Self-Subsisting!'

The transgressions committed by such as have turned away from Thee and have borne themselves haughtily towards Thee have not availed to hinder them from loving Thee, and from setting their faces towards Thee, and from turning in the direction of Thy mercy. These are they who are blessed by the Concourse on high, who are glorified by the denizens of the everlasting Cities, and beyond them by those on whose foreheads Thy most exalted pen hath written: 'These! The people of Bahá. Through them have been shed the splendours of the light of guidance.' Thus hath it been ordained, at Thy behest and by Thy will, in the Tablet of Thine irrevocable decree.

Proclaim, therefore, O my God, their greatness and the greatness of those who while living or after death have circled round them. Supply them with that which Thou hast ordained for the righteous among Thy creatures. Potent art Thou to do all things. There is no God but Thee, the All-Powerful, the Help in Peril, the Almighty, the Most Bountiful.

Do not bring our fasts to an end with this fast, O my Lord, nor the covenants Thou hast made with this covenant. Do Thou accept all that we have done for love of Thee, and for the sake of Thy pleasure, and all that we have left undone as a result of our subjection to our evil and corrupt desires. Enable us, then, to cleave steadfastly to Thy love and Thy good pleasure, and preserve us from the mischief of such as have denied Thee and repudiated Thy most resplendent signs. Thou art, in truth, the Lord of this world and of the next. No God is there beside Thee, the Exalted, the Most High.

Magnify Thou, O Lord my God, Him Who is the Primal Point, the Divine Mystery, the Unseen Essence, the Dayspring of Divinity, and the Manifestation of Thy Lordship, through Whom all the knowledge of the past and all the knowledge of the future were made plain, through Whom the pearls of Thy hidden wisdom were uncovered, and the mystery of Thy treasured name disclosed, Whom Thou hast appointed as the Announcer of the One through Whose name the letter B and the letter E have been joined and united, through Whom Thy majesty, Thy sovereignty and Thy might were made known, through Whom Thy words have been sent down, and Thy laws set forth with clearness, and Thy signs spread abroad, and Thy Word established, through Whom the hearts of Thy chosen ones were laid bare, and all that were in the heavens and all that were on the earth were gathered together, Whom Thou has called 'Alí-Muḥammad in the kingdom of Thy names, and the Spirit of Spirits in the Tablets of Thine irrevocable decree, Whom Thou hast invested with Thine own title, unto Whose name all other names have, at Thy bidding and through the power of Thy might, been made to return, and in Whom Thou hast caused all Thine attributes and titles to attain their final consummation. To Him also belong such names as lay hid within Thy stainless tabernacles, in Thine invisible world and Thy sanctified cities.

Magnify Thou, moreover, such as have believed in Him and in His signs and have turned towards Him, from among those that have acknowledged Thy unity in His Latter Manifestation – a Manifestation whereof He hath made mention in His Tablets, and in His Books, and in His Scriptures, and in all the wondrous verses and gem-like utterances that have descended upon Him. It is this same Manifestation Whose covenant Thou hast bidden Him establish ere He had established His own covenant. He it is Whose praise the Bayán hath celebrated. In it His excellence hath been extolled, and His truth established, and His sovereignty proclaimed, and His Cause perfected. Blessed is the man that hath turned unto Him, and fulfilled the things He hath commanded, O Thou Who art the Lord of the words and the Desire of all them that have known Thee!

Praised be Thou, O my God, inasmuch as Thou hast aided us to recognize and love Him. I, therefore, beseech Thee by Him and by Them who are the Daysprings of Thy Divinity, and the Manifestations of Thy Lordship, and the Treasuries of Thy Revelation, and the Depositories of Thine inspiration, to enable us to serve and obey Him, and to empower us to become the helpers of His Cause and the dispersers of His adversaries. Powerful art Thou to do all that pleaseth Thee. No God is there beside Thee, the Almighty, the All-Glorious, the One Whose help is sought by all men!

Bahá'u'lláh[9]

ANNEX

REFLECTIONS ON THE BADÍ' CALENDAR

The calendar used by Bahá'ís today was introduced by the Báb and later confirmed by Bahá'u'lláh. The Báb based the new calendar on the structure of the Persian Bayán, which is made up of 19 sections each containing 19 'gates' or chapters, preparing the believers for Him Whom God Shall Make Manifest. The Báb also refers to the four traditional elements fire, air, water and earth as symbols of the four stages of spiritual creation. In his book *Gate of the Heart: Understanding the Writngs of the Báb*, Dr Nader Saiedi offers a luminous discourse on the spiritual significance of these elements: how they are integrated into the calendar and how they relate to the stages of divine creative action.[1] The following notes are based on Dr Saiedi's explanations.

Fire is the most crucial symbol; it refers to the Creative Word of God. The Báb often relates it to the symbol of water, representing their unity in opposites. Fire also represents joy and paradise, as experienced in attaining the presence of God. In nature, fire can burn and purify, but it can also destroy. This is symbolic in mystical terms of that fire which can either burn away veils or lead to smoke and more veils.

Air is symbolically the most exalted spiritual mystery and refers to various stations of the divine creative action or the 'Breath' of God. Things in nature inhale and exhale. A new life is breathed into us when we read the Word of God; we inhale the fragrances of the Almighty. Air is also what birds soar into, and send song upon its breezes.

Water refers to the Creative Force, the source of all life. It is essentially the Word of God, Revelation – the means by which all things come into existence. The natural creation has evolved through this life-giving substance. In the Writings of the Báb water is likened to the ink that flows from the pen, the Word of God streaming forth like a river through the Manifestation of God. It is the divine elixir that transforms all things.

Earth symbolizes the human body, which is also a symbol of the Word and should be considered a Temple. Earth is also likened to dust or soil, as in ploughing the fields of the heart, planting the seeds while encouraging them to grow. In this metaphor we can see the relationship and unity of these symbols: seeds grow only through the coordination of the oxygen in the air, the fire of the sun, and the living waters which rain down from the heavens.

Concerning these elements in relation to the calendar the Báb wrote:

> The first three months are the fire of God, the next four months, the air of eternity, and the subsequent six months are the water of divine unity which streameth forth upon all souls, descending from the atmosphere of eternity, which in turn is derived from the fire of God. The last six months pertain to earthly existence, whereby all that hath appeared from these three elements may be established within the element of dust, through which the fruit will be harvested.[2]

This gives us an amazing vision of how the months move through the stages of spiritual creative process to penetrate the world of being, offering it transformation and bringing it to fruition. In an individual's spiritual growth, these elements show how one's station is elevated throughout the course of the year in the finality of the Fast:

> For in the foremost station of the heart, the fire of love shineth forth; and in the second, the air of guardianship ascendeth; and in the third, the water of unity surgeth; and in the fourth, the dust of existence is elevated.[3]

The cycle of divine creative action in the Bahá'í calendar

The Bab has organized the calendar into a process of transformation and spiritual growth:

	Month	Arabic Name	Translation	First Days Naw-Rúz – 20 March	First Days Naw-Rúz – 21 March
Fire *Creative Word*	1st	Bahá	Splendour	20 March	21 March
	2nd	Jalál	Glory	8 April	9 April
	3rd	Jamál	Beauty	27 April	28 April
Air *Eternity*	4th	'Aẓamat	Grandeur	16 May	17 May
	5th	Núr	Light	4 June	5 June
	6th	Raḥmat	Mercy	23 June	24 June
	7th	Kalimát	Words	12 July	13 July
Water *Source of Life*	8th	Kamál	Perfection	31 July	1 August
	9th	Asmá'	Names	19 August	20 August
	10th	'Izzat	Might	7 September	8 September
	11th	Mashíyyat	Will	26 September	27 September
	12th	'Ilm	Knowledge	15 October	16 October
	13th	Qudrat	Power	3 November	4 November
Earth *Existence*	14th	Qawl	Speech	22 November	23 November
	15th	Masá'il	Questions	11 December	12 December
	16th	Sharaf	Honour	30 December	31 December
	17th	Sulṭán	Sovereignty	18 January	19 January
	18th	Mulk	Dominion	6 February	7 February
	19th	'Alá	Loftiness	(See note)	(See note)

Note: The month of 'Alá starts on 1 March when the upcoming Naw-Rúz is on 20 March and 2 March when the upcoming Naw-Rúz is on 21 March.

Therefore, during the first three months – the months of glorification – the fire of the hearts of existent beings is kindled. During the next four months – the months of the celebration of praise – the spirits of the contingent beings are created, during which time they are provided for. In the subsequent six months – the months of the exaltation of unity – God causeth the beings to expire, not as a physical death, but the death of negation and life in affirmation. Finally, in the last six months – which are the months of magnification – the Lord of the universe, glorified and exalted by He, quickeneth those souls who have died to the love of anyone other than Him and have remained steadfast in His love.[4]

The interaction of these elements can be compared to the seasons. Each year our individual spirituality is refreshed by the Fast and rejuvenated for the new year.

BIBLIOGRAPHY

'Abdu'l-Bahá. *'Abdu'l-Bahá in London* (1912). London: Bahá'í Publishing Trust, 1982.
— *Abdul Baha on Divine Philosophy.* Comp. I. F. Chamberlain. Boston: The Tudor Press, 1918.
— *Foundations of World Unity.* Wilmette, Ill: Bahá'í Publishing Trust, RP 1955.
— *Paris Talks: Addresses Given by 'Abdu'l-Bahá in 1911.* London: Bahá'í Publishing Trust, 12th ed. 1995.
— *The Promulgation of Universal Peace.* Wilmette, Ill: Bahá'í Publishing Trust, 2nd ed. 1982.
— *The Secret of Divine Civilization.* Wilmette, Ill: Bahá'í Publishing Trust, 1957.
— *Selections from the Writings of 'Abdu'l-Bahá.* Comp. Research Department of the Universal House of Justice. Haifa: Bahá'í World Centre, 1978.
— *Some Answered Questions* (1908). Comp. L. Clifford Barney. Wilmette, Ill: Bahá'í Publishing Trust, 3rd ed. 1981.
— *Tablets of Abdul-Baha Abbas.* 3 vols. Chicago: Bahá'í Publishing Society, 1909–1916.
— *The Tablets of the Divine Plan.* Wilmette, Ill: Bahá'í Publishing Trust, rev. ed. 1977.
— *Will and Testament.* Wilmette, Ill: Bahá'í Publishing Trust, RP 1990.
— *The Wisdom of the Master.* Los Angeles: Kalimát Press, 2002.
Amen, Daniel. *Change Your Brain, Change Your Life.* New York: Three Rivers Press, 1998.
Anderson, Eric; Siegel, Erika H.; Bliss-Moreau, Eliza; Feldman Barrett, Lisa. 'The visual impact of gossip', in *Science*, 19 May 2011; available at *Science DOI:* 10.1126/science.1201574.
Bahá'í Prayers: A Selection of Prayers revealed by Bahá'u'lláh, the Báb and 'Abdu'l-Bahá. Wilmette, Ill: Bahá'í Publishing Trust, 1991.
Bahá'í Readings: Selections from the Wiritings of the Báb, Bahá'u'llah and 'Abdu'l-Bahá for Daily Meditation. Toronto: National Spiritual Assembly of the Bahá'ís of Canada, 1984.
Bahá'í World Faith: Selected Writings of Bahá'u'lláh and 'Abdu'l-Bahá. Wilmette, Ill: Bahá'í Publishing Trust, rev. ed. 1956.

Bahá'u'lláh. *Gems of Divine Mysteries: Javáhiru'l-Asrár.* Haifa: Bahá'í World Centre, 2002.

— *Gleanings from the Writings of Baha'u'llah.* Wilmette, Ill: Bahá'í Publishing Trust, 1983.

— *The Hidden Words of Bahá'u'lláh.* Trans. Shoghi Effendi. Wilmette, Ill: Bahá'í Publishing Trust, 1970; New Delhi: Bahá'í Publishing Trust, 1987.

— *The Kitáb-i-Aqdas: The Most Holy Book.* Haifa: Bahá'í World Centre, 1992.

— *Kitáb-i-Íqán: The Book of Certitude.* Trans. Shoghi Effendi. Wilmette, Ill: Bahá'í Publishing Trust, 2nd ed. 1950.

— *Prayers and Meditations by Bahá'u'lláh.* Trans. Shoghi Effendi. Wilmette, Ill: Bahá'í Publishing Trust, 1938, 1987.

— *The Seven Valleys and the Four Valleys.* Trans. M. Gail with A-K.Khan. Wilmette, Ill: Bahá'í Publishing Trust, rev. ed. 1975.

— *The Summons of the Lord of Hosts: Tablets of Bahá'u'lláh.* Haifa: Bahá'í World Centre, 2002.

— *Tablets of Baha'u'llah Revealed after the Kitáb-i-Aqdas.* Haifa: Bahá'í World Centre, 1978.

Beinfield, Harriet; Korngold, Efrem. *Between Heaven and Earth: A Guide to Chinese Medicine.* New York: Ballantine Books, 1991.

Bhagavad Gita. *Bhagavad-Gita: As It Is.* Trans. A.C. Bhaktivedanta Swami Prabhupada. The Bhaktivedanta Book Trust, 1994.

Campbell, Don. *The Mozart Effect: Tapping the Power of Music to Heal the Body, Strengthen the Mind, and Unlock the Creative Spirit.* New York: HarperCollins, 1997.

The Compilation of Compilations. Prepared by the Universal House of Justice 1963–1990. 2 vols. Sydney: Bahá'í Publications Australia, 1991.

Carpenter, R. H. S. *Neurophysiology.* London: Arnold, 2003.

Chopra, Deepak. *Quantum Healing: Exploring the Frontiers of Mind/Body Medicine.* New York: Bantam Books, 1989.

Church, Dawson. *The Genie in your Genes.* Fulton, CA: Elite Books, 2007.

D'Adamo, Dr Peter J.; Whitney, Catherine. *Eat Right for Your Type: Complete Blood Type Encyclopedia.* New York: Riverhead Books, 2002.

Devries, Arnold. *Therapeutic Fasting.* Los Angeles: Chandler, 1963.

Esslemont, J. E. *Baha'u'llah and the New Era.* London: Bahá'í Publishing Trust, 1986.

Goleman, Daniel. *Emotional Intelligence.* New York: Bantam, 1995.

Grundy, Julia. *Ten Days in the Light of Acca.* Chicago: Bahai Publishing Society, 1907.

Hahnemann, Samuel. *Organon of the Medical Art*, ed. Wendy Brewster O'Reilly. Birdcage Books, 1996.

Hay, Louise L. *Heal Your Body.* Carlsbad, CA: Hay House, 1988.

Health and Healing. Comp. Research Department of the Universal House of Justice (1984, as *Selections from Bahá'í Writings on Some Aspects of Health, Healing, Nutrition and Related Matters*). New Delhi: Bahá'í Publishing Trust, 1986.

Hofman, Mark. *The Case for Free Will.* Bibliofiles, 2012.

Honnold, Annamarie. *Vignettes from the Life of 'Abdu'l-Bahá.* Oxford: George Ronald, rev. ed. 1991.

The Importance of Obligatory Prayer and Fasting. Comp. Research Department of the Universal House of Justice (2002), in *The Compilation of Compilations* (see above).

Kent, James Tyler. *Lectures on Homoeopathic Philosophy with Classroom Notes and Word Index.* New Delhi: B. Jain Ltd, 2009.

Kessler, David A. *The End of Overeating.* Emmaus, PA: Rodale Books, 2009.

Lample, Paul. *Revelation and Social Reality.* West Palm Beach: Palabra Publications, 2009.

Lights of Guidance: A Bahá'í Reference File. Comp. Helen Hornby. New Delhi: Bahá'í Publishing Trust, 3rd rev. ed. 1994.

Maxwell, May. *An Early Pilgrimage.* Oxford: George Ronald, 1987.

— and Mary Maxwell. *Haifa Notes of Shoghi Effendi's Words: Taken at Pilgrim House during the Pilgrimage of Mrs. May Maxwell and Miss Mary Maxwell. January, February, March.* 2 vols. Privately printed and distributed, 1937; available at: http://bahai-library.com.

Newberg, Andrew; Waldman, Mark Robert. *How God Changes your Brain.* New York: Ballantine Books, 2009.

Norretranders, Tor. *The User Illusion: Cutting Consciousness Down to Size.* Trans. Jonathan Sydenham. London: Penguin Press Science, 1998.

Prayer, Meditation, and the Devotional Attitude. Comp. Research Department of the Universal House of Justice. Melbourne: Bahá'í Publications Australia, 1980; Wilmette, Ill: Bahá'í Publishing Trust, 1980 (published as *Spiritual Foundations: Prayer, Meditation and the Devotional Attitude*). Also in *The Compilation of Compilations* (see above).

Pert, Candace B. *Molecules of Emotion: The Science Behind Mind–Body Medicine.* New York: Simon and Schuster, 1997.

Rabbani, Rúhíyyih. *The Guardian of the Bahá'í Faith.* London: Bahá'í Publishing Trust, 1988.

Rosenblum, Bruce; Kuttner, Fred. *Quantum Enigma: Physics Encounters Consciousness.* New York: Oxford University Press, 2nd ed. 2011.

Saiedi, Nader. *Gate of the Heart: Understanding the Writings of the Báb.* Association of Bahá'í Studies, Bahá'í Studies Series. Canada: Wilfred Laurier University Press, 2008.

Shoghi Effendi. *Arohanui: Letters from Shoghi Effendi to New Zealand.* Suva, Fiji: Bahá'í Publishing Trust, 1982.

— *Citadel of Faith: Messages to America, 1947–1957.* Wilmette, Ill: Bahá'í Publishing Trust, 1965.

— *Dawn of a New Day: Messages to India 1923–1957*. New Delhi: Bahá'í Publishing Trust, 1970.

— *Directives from the Guardian*. New Delhi: Bahá'í Publishing Trust, n.d.

— *The Promised Day is Come*. Wilmette, Ill: Bahá'í Publishing Trust, rev. ed. 1996.

— *Unfolding Destiny: The Messages from the Guardian of the Bahá'í Faith to the Bahá'í Community of the British Isles*. London: Bahá'í Publishing Trust, 1981.

Star of the West: The Bahai Magazine. Periodical, 25 vols. 1910–1935. Vols. 1–14 RP Oxford: George Ronald, 1978. Complete CD-ROM version: Talisman Educational Software/Special Ideas, 2001.

Taherzadeh, Adib. *The Revelation of Baha'u'llah*. Four vols. Oxford: George Ronald, 1974–1988.

Thich Nhat Hanh. *Anger: Buddhist Wisdom for Cooling the Flames*. New York: Riverhead Books, 2001.

Thompson, Juliet. *The Diary of Juliet Thompson*. Los Angeles: Kalimát Press, 1983.

True, Corinne. *Notes Taken at Acca: Table Talks by Abdul Baha Taken Down in Persian by Mirza Hadi at Acca, Feb. 1907*. Trans A. U. Fareed. Chicago: Bahai Publishing Society, 1907.

The Universal House of Justice. *Messages from the Universal House of Justice 1968–1973*. Wilmette, Ill: Bahá'í Publishing Trust, 1976.

— *Messages from the Universal House of Justice 1963–1986, The Third Epoch of the Formative Age*. Comp. Geoffry W. Marks, Wilmette, Ill: Bahá'í Publishing Trust, 1996.

Vithoulkas, George. *The Science of Homeopathy*. International Academy of Classical Homeopathy. New York: Grove Press, RP 1980.

Wallace, R. K.; Dillbeck, M.; Jacobe, E.; Harrington, B. 1982. 'The effects of the Transcendental Meditation and TM-Sidhi program on the aging process', in *International Journal of Neuroscience*, no. 16, pp. 53–8.

Wegner, Daniel M. *The Illusion of Conscious Will*. Cambridge, MA: MIT Press, 2002.

Weiss, Brian L. *Through Time into Healing*. New York: Fireside, 1992.

Whitman, Walt. *Leaves of Grass*. New York: Aventine Press, 1931.

Zajonc, Arthur. *Catching the Light: The Entwined History of Light and Mind*. New York: Oxford University Press, 1995.

REFERENCES

Introduction

1. 'Abdu'l-Bahá, *Promulgation of Universal Peace*, p. 28.
2. Bahá'u'lláh, in *The Importance of Obligatory Prayer and Fasting*, no. 3 (1: III).
3. 'Abdu'l-Bahá, ibid. no. 23 (2: II).
4. 'Abdu'l-Bahá, *Some Answered Questions*, no. 83, p. 297.
5. Bahá'u'lláh, in *Health and Healing*, p. 1; also in *Compilation of Compilations*, vol. 1, no. 1014, p. 458.
6. 'Abdu'l-Bahá, in *The Importance of Obligatory Prayer and Fasting*, no. 48 (2: XXVI).
7. 'Abdu'l-Bahá, *The Promulgation of Universal Peace*, p. 293.
8. Letter from Shoghi Effendi to an individual believer, 6 April 1928, in *Unfolding Destiny*, p. 423.
9. Letter from the Universal House of Justice to an individual believer, 31 January 1995, in *Questions on Scholarship*: 'The interpretations of 'Abdu'l-Bahá and the Guardian are divinely-guided statements of what the Word of God means and as such these interpretations are binding on the friends. However, the existence of authoritative interpretations in no way precludes the individual from engaging in his own study of the teachings and thereby arriving at his own interpretation or understanding. Indeed, Bahá'u'lláh invites the believers to "immerse" themselves in the "ocean" of His "words", that they "may unravel its secrets, and discover all the pearls of wisdom that lie hid in its depths".

    Far from being limited, Bahá'u'lláh asserts that "knowledge hath seventy meanings", and that the "meaning" of the Word of God "can never be exhausted" . . .

    Individual interpretations based on a person's understanding of the teachings constitute the fruit of man's rational power and may well contribute to a more complete understanding of the Faith. Such views, however, lack authority. The believers are, therefore, free to accept or disregard them. Further, the manner in which an individual presents his interpretation is important. For example, he must at no time deny or contend with the authoritative interpretation, but rather offer his idea as a contribution to knowledge, making it clear that his views are merely his own.'

Chapter 1: Transformation and Renewal

1. From a letter written on behalf of Shoghi Effendi to an individual believer, 18 February 1954, in *Lights of Guidance*, p. 114, no. 391.
2. Bahá'u'lláh, in *The Importance of Obligatory Prayer and Fasting*, no. 19.

3   Bahá'u'lláh, *Gleanings*, CLV, para. 2, p. 331.
4   Bahá'u'lláh, quoted by Shoghi Effendi, *God Passes By*, p. 214; also in Bahá'u'lláh, *The Kitáb-i-Aqdas*, quoted p. 16.
5   ibid. p. 16.
6   Bahá'u'lláh, in *The Importance of Obligatory Prayer and Fasting*, no. 14.
7   Bahá'u'lláh, *Kitáb-i-Aqdas*, para. 45, p. 36.
8   Bahá'u'lláh, in *The Importance of Obligatory Prayer and Fasting*, no. 3.
9   'Abdu'l-Bahá, *Selections*, no. 134, p. 152.
10 Bahá'u'lláh, Tablet to a Physician, provisional translation, available at http://bahai-library.com/bahaullah_lawh_tibb.

Chapter 2: A Brief History of Fasting

1   Attributed to Caliph Umar bin Abd al-Aziz (c. 682–720); often wrongly attributed to the Qur'án.
2   Hosea 6:6.
3   Leviticus 23:26.
4   Vendidad 3: 33.
5   Bahá'u'lláh, *Tablets*, pp. 149–50.
6   Matt. 6:16–18.
7   Matt. 9:15–17 ; Mark 3:19–22.
8   Mark 9:17–29.
9   Qur'án 2:183.
10 ibid 2:185.
11 Devries, *Therapeutic Fasting*, p. 9.
12 The Báb, Persian Bayán 8:18.
13 Bahá'u'lláh, Lawḥ-i-Maqṣúd, in *Tablets*, p. 167.

Chapter 3: Prescription for Today's World

1   Bahá'u'lláh, in *The Importance of Obligatory Prayer and Fasting*, no. 5 (1:V).
2   Bahá'u'lláh, *Kitáb-i-Aqdas*, paras. 2 and 3, p. 20.
3   Bahá'u'lláh, *Prayers and Meditations*, p. 142.
4   Bahá'u'lláh, *Kitáb-i-Aqdas*, para. 16, p. 25.
5   Bahá'u'lláh, in *The Importance of Obligatory Prayer and Fasting*, no. 54 (3:VI), para. 7.
6   ibid. no. 19 (1 :XIX).
7   Bahá'u'lláh, *Prayers and Meditations*, p. 65.
8   Bahá'u'lláh, *Kitáb-i-Aqdas*, para. 16, pp. 24–5.
9   Bahá'u'lláh, *Gleanings*, CLX, paras. 2–3, p. 338.
10 Bahá'u'lláh, Tablet of Maqṣúd, in *Tablets*, pp. 163–4.
11 'Abdu'l-Bahá, *Tablets*, p. 691.
12 Bahá'u'lláh, Lawḥ-i-Ḥikmat (Tablet of Wisdom), in *Tablets*, p. 142.
13 Shoghi Effendi, *Citadel of Faith*, p. 131.
14 Letter written on behalf of Shoghi Effendi to an individual believer, 12 July 1952, in *Lights of Guidance*, no. 405, p. 118.
15 Bahá'u'lláh, in *The Importance of Obligatory Prayer and Fasting*, no. 20 (1:XX).
16 Letter on behalf of the Universal House of Justice to an individual believer, 20 May 1991.
17 From 'Synopsis and Codification of the Laws and ordinances of the *Kitáb-i-Aqdas*',

in Bahá'u'lláh, *The Kitáb-i-Aqdas*, pp. 148–9.
18 'Questions and Answers', no. 71 in Bahá'u'lláh, *The Kitáb-i-Aqdas*, p. 128.
19 Bahá'u'lláh, *Kitáb-i-Aqdas*, para. 182, p. 85.
20 Bahá'u'lláh, *Kitáb-i-Íqán*, para. 8, p. 8.
21 ibid. para.233, p. 211.
22 Bahá'u'lláh, Tablet to Vafá, in *Tablets*, p. 183.
23 Bahá'u'lláh, *Gleanings*, LXXXIX, para. 1.
24 'Abdu'l-Bahá, *Paris Talks*, no. 30, p. 94.
25 Bahá'u'lláh, in *The Importance of Obligatory Prayer and Fasting*, no. 1 (1:I).
26 ibid. no. 2 (1 :II).
27 ibid. no. 3 (1 :III).
28 ibid. no. 4 (1 :IV).
29 ibid. no. 5 (1 :V).
30 ibid. no. 6 (1 :VI).
31 ibid. no. 12 (1:XII).
32 ibid. no. 14 (1 :XIV).
33 ibid. no. 15 (1 :XV).
34 ibid. no. 16 (1 :XVI).
35 ibid. no. 17 (1 :XVII).
36 ibid. no. 18 (1 : XVIII).
37 Bahá'u'lláh, *Kitáb-i-Íqán*, para. 40, pp. 39–40.
38 Bahá'u'lláh, *Gleanings*, CXXXVIII, para. 1.
39 Bahá'u'lláh, in *The Importance of Obligatory Prayer and Fasting*, no. 19 (1:XIX).
40 ibid. no. 20 (1 :XX).
41 ibid. no. 21 (1 :XXI).
42 'Abdu'l-Bahá, ibid. no. 22 (2 :I).
43 ibid. no. 23 (2 :II).
44 ibid. no. 47 (2 :XXVI).
45 ibid. no. 48 (2 :XXVII).
46 'Abdu'l-Bahá, as reported in Esslemont, *Bahá'u'lláh and the New Era*, p. 171.
47 'Abdu'l-Bahá, *Tablets*, p. 186.
48 'Abdu'l-Bahá, as reported in *'Abdu'l-Bahá in London*, p. 95.
49 'Abdu'l-Bahá, as reported in *Abdul Baha on Divine Philosophy*, pp. 98–9.
50 'Abdu'l-Bahá, *Tablets*, p. 56.
51 'Abdu'l-Bahá, as reported by Corinne True, *Table Talks*, reprinted in *Star of the West*, vol. IV, no. 18, p. 305, partially reprinted in *Lights of Guidance*, no. 779, p. 234.

Chapter 4: The Human Experience

1 Shoghi Effendi, *Arohanui*, p. 89.
2 Bahá'u'lláh, Súriy-i-Ra'ís, para. 35, in *Summons of the Lord of Hosts*, p. 154.
3 'Abdu'l-Bahá, Tablet to August Forel, in *The Bahá'í World*, vol. XV, pp. 17–43.
4 *The Importance of Obligatory Prayer and Fasting*, no. 19 (1:XIX).
5 'Abdu'l-Bahá, *Promulgation of Universal Peace*, p. 10.
6 Bahá'u'lláh, *Gleanings*, LXXXII, para. 5, p. 160.
7 Bahá'u'lláh, quoted in Shoghi Effendi, *Promised Day*, p. 115.
8 Bahá'u'lláh, *Gleanings*, LXXX, para. 2, pp. 153–4.
9 Letter from the Universal House of Justice to an individual, 12 November 1975, in *The Compilation of Compilations*, vol. 1, no. 1094, p. 486.

10 Kent, *Lectures on Homeopathic Philosophy*, p. 73.
11 George Vithoulkas is a professor of homeopathic medicine, and winner of the Alternative Nobel Prize.
12 Vithoulkas, *The Science of Homeopathy*, p. 104.
13 'Abdu'l-Bahá, *Selections*, no. 134, pp. 153–4.
14 'In lab, how life began', NPR radio, 8 January 2009.
15 'Abdu'l-Bahá, *Selections*, no. 134, p. 152.
16 ibid. no. 133, pp. 151–2.
17 Letter written on behalf of Shoghi Effendi, in *Lights of Guidance*, no. 923, p. 276.
18 *'Abdu'l-Bahá in London*, p. 95.
19 'Abdu'l-Bahá, in *Bahá'í World Faith*, p. 344–5.
20 *The Importance of Obligatory Prayer and Fasting*, no. 15 (1:XV).
21 ibid. no. 47 (2:XXVI).
22 'Abdu'l-Bahá, quoted in Esslemont, *Bahá'u'lláh and the New Era*, p. 184.
23 'Abdu'l-Bahá, *Some Answered Questions*, no. 19, p. 91.

Chapter 5: Fasting for the Body

1 'Abdu'l-Bahá, *Promulgation of Universal Peace*, p. 416.
2 'Abdu'l-Bahá, *Abdul Baha on Divine Philosophy*, p. 127.
3 Letter on behalf of Shoghi Effendi to an individual believer, 24 November 1947, in *Health and Healing*.
4 The Báb, Persian Bayán V:12, in *Selections*, p. 95.
5 The Báb, 'Tafsír-i-Kullu't-Ta'ám' Collection, pp. 221–2, quoted in Saiedi, *Gate of the Heart*, p. 79.
6 ibid. p. 224, quoted in Saiedi, *Gate of the Heart*, p. 62.
7 Maxwell, *Haifa Notes*, vol. 1, p. 5.
8 'Abdu'l-Bahá, *Some Answered Questions*, no. 69, pp. 245–6.
9 Bahá'u'lláh writes in the Tablet to a Physician : 'Jealousy consumeth the body and anger doth burn the liver; avoid these two as you would a lion" (Esslemont, *Bahá'u'lláh and the New Era*, p. 106; also in *Compilation of Compilations*, vol. 1, no. 1020, p. 460).
10 'Abdu'l-Bahá, *Some Answered Questions*. no. 73, pp. 257–9.
11 Hahnemann, *Organon of the Medical Art*, p. 70.
12 'Abdu'l-Bahá, *'Abdu'l-Bahá in London*, p. 95.
13 Bahá'u'lláh, Tablet to a Physician, in *Star of the West*, vol. XXI, no. 5 (August 1930), p. 160.
14 'Abdu'l-Bahá, *Selections*, no. 134, p. 156.

Chapter 6: Preparing the Body for the Fast

1 Letter from the Universal House of Justice to an individual, 24 January 1977, in *The Compilation of Compilations*, vol. 1, no. 1095, p. 486.
2 'Abdu'l-Bahá, *Selections*, no. 134, pp. 154.
3 'Abdu'l-Bahá, as reported in Esslemont, *Bahá'u'lláh and the New Era*, p. 184.
4 Dan Eden, 'Are human really beings of light?', available at .http://viewzone2.com/dnax.html.
5 For instance, 'The American carbon footprint', available at http://brighterplanet.com/research.

6 Such as Benjamin Libet, whose research has given rise to the various attacks on the notion of free will by Wegner and Carpenter.
7 Bahá'u'lláh, Tablet to a Physician, in *Star of the West*, vol. XXI, no. 5 (August 1930), p. 160.
8 'Abdu'l-Bahá, *Selections*, no. 134, pp. 152–3.
9 Bahá'u'lláh, Tablet to a Physician, in *Star of the West*, vol. XXI, no. 5 (August 1930), p. 160.
10 Reported in 'Abdu'l-Bahá, *'Abdu'l-Bahá in London*, p. 81.
11 'Abdu'l-Bahá, *Selections* no. 134, p. 157.
12 See Bahá'u'lláh, *The Kitáb-i-Aqdas*, para. 10; also Questions and Answers no. 51, and notes 16 and 34.
13 Bahá'u'lláh, Tablet to a Physician, in *Star of the West*, vol. XXI, no. 5 (August 1930), p. 160.
14 Bahá'u'lláh, *The Kitáb-i-Aqdas*, note 167, p. 236.
15 'Abdu'l-Bahá, *Selections*, no. 110, p. 135.
16 'Abdu'l-Bahá, *Tablets*, p. 673.

Chapter 7: Recommendations for Fasting
1 Bahá'u'lláh, Tablet to a Physican, in *Star of the West*, vol. XXI, no. 5 (August 1930), p. 160.
2 Tara Packer-Pope, *Wall Street Journal*, 20 March 2006.

Chapter 8: Fasting for the Mind
1 'Abdu'l-Bahá, *Abdul Baha on Divine Philosophy*, p. 121.
2 'Abdu'l-Bahá, *Some Answered Questions*, no. 67, p. 242.
3 Bahá'u'lláh, *Gleanings* XC, para. 1, p. 178.
4 ibid. LXXXIII, para. 4, pp. 165–6.
5 Vithoulkas, *The Science of Homeopathy*, pp. 39–40.
6 Bahá'u'lláh, *Hidden Words*, Persian no. 32.
7 'Abdu'l-Bahá, in *Star of the West*, vol. 17, no. 2, p. 348; also in *Lights of Guidance*, p. 114, no. 390.
8 'Abdu'l-Bahá, Tablet to August Forel, in *The Bahá'í World*, Vol. XV, p. 38.
9 Letter on behalf of Shoghi Effendi to an individual believer, in *Lights of Guidance*, no. 1732, p. 509.
10 Bahá'u'lláh, *Gleanings*, LXXXIII, para. 1, p. 164.
11 'Abdu'l-Bahá, *Abdul Baha on Divine Philosophy*, p. 134.
12 Quoted in a letter from the Universal House of Justice to an individual believer, 8 March 1981, in *Lights of Guidance*, no. 1220, p. 364.
13 As quoted in Esslemont, *Bahá'u'lláh and the New Era*, p. 106; also in *Compilation of Compilations*, vol. 2, no. 1020, p. 460.
14 Sheldon Lewis, in *Spirituality and Health* magazine, March/April 2006.
15 As in Benjamin Libet's experiments, which have had such an influence on recent neuroscience (Wegner, Carpenter) and have led to various attacks on the concept of free will (see Hofman, *The Case for Free Will*, for a discussion, particularly pp. 174–5).
16 Bahá'u'lláh, *Gleanings*, LXXXII, para. 10, p. 162.
17 See Arthur Zajonc, *Catching the Light: The Entwined History of Light and Mind*.
18 'Abdu'l-Bahá, *Selections*, no. 73, p. 111.

19 Bahá'u'lláh, Words of Wisdom, in *Tablets*, p. 156.
20 Letter on behalf of Shoghi Effendi to an individual believer, 10 December 1947, in *Lights of Guidance*, no. 386, p. 113; also in *Compilation of Compilations*, vol. 2, no. 1318, p. 18.
21 Bahá'u'lláh, *Hidden Words*, Persian no. 72.
22 Bahá'u'lláh, *Gleanings*, XLIII, para. 3, p. 93.
23 Bahá'u'lláh, *Hidden Words*, Persian no. 45.
24 Letter on behalf of Shoghi Effendi to an individual believer, 17 December 1943, in *Compilation of Compilations*, vol. 2, no. 1297, p. 12.
25 Letter on behalf of Shoghi Effendi to an individual believer, 8 January 1949, in *Unfolding Destiny*, p. 454.
26 Bahá'u'lláh, *Hidden Words*, Arabic no. 13 and Persian no. 44.
27 'Abdu'l-Bahá, in *Bahá'í Readings*, p. 305.
28 Ahang Rabbani, ''Abdu'l-Baha in Abu-Sinan: September 1914–May 1915', in *Bahá'í Studies Review*, no. 13 (2005), pp. 75–103; available at: <http://www.docstoc.com/docs/1263504/Rabbani_AbdulBaha_in_AbuSinan>.
29 *'Abdu'l-Bahá in London*, p. 65.
30 Letter written on behalf of the Universal House of Justice to an individual, 15 June 1982, in *Lights of Guidance*, no. 955, p. 284.
31 'Abdu'l-Bahá, *Selections*, no. 130, pp. 150–51.
32 Anderson et al., 'The visual impact of gossip', in *Science*, 19 May 2011.
33 Quoted in Robin Nixon, 'Spirituality spot found in brain', Special to *LiveScience*, posted 24 December 2008.
34 See http://www.npr.org/templates/story/story.php?storyId=110997741.
35 ibid.
36 'Abdu'l-Bahá, *Some Answered Questions*, no. 67, p. 242.
37 'Abdu'l-Bahá, *Tablets*, p. 169; also in *Lights of Guidance*, no. 976, p. 288.

Chapter 9: Preparing the Mind for the Fast

1 Letter written on behalf of the Universal House of Justice to an individual, 23 July 1984, in *Lights of Guidance*, p. 282.
2 Bahá'u'lláh, in *The Importance of Obligatory Prayer and Fasting*, no. 17 (1:XVII).
3 See Thich Nhat Hanh, *Anger*.
4 Bahá'u'lláh, Bishárát, in *Tablets of Bahá'u'lláh*, p. 27.
5 Whitman, 'There Was a Child Went Forth', in *Leaves of Grass*, p. 372.
6 Letter on behalf of Shoghi Effendi to an individual believer, 17 February 1933, in *Compilation of Compilations*, vol. 1, p. 84.
7 'Abdu'l-Bahá, *Some Answered Questions*, no. 57, p. 214.
8 Bahá'u'lláh, Tajallíyát, in *Tablets of Bahá'u'lláh*, p. 51.
9 'Abdu'l-Bahá, in *Compilation of Compilations*, vol.1, no. 22, p. 6.
10 'Abdu'l-Bahá, *The Promulgation of Universal Peace*, p. 244.
11 See, for example, Jane Collingwood, 'Writing about trauma can produce health benefits', available at: http://psychcentral.com/lib/2006/writing-about-trauma-can-produce-health-benefits/all/1/.
12 Letter on behalf of Shoghi Effendi to an individual believer, 22 October 1949, in *The Unfolding Destiny of the British Bahá'í Community*, p. 456.
13 Bahá'u'lláh, Ṭarázát, in *Tablets of Bahá'u'lláh*, p. 35.

14 See www.second-opinions.co.uk.
15 See www.themoreyouknow.com.
16 See www.orange-papers.org.
17 Letter on behalf of Shoghi Effendi, 8 May 1947, in *Unfolding Destiny*, p. 199.
18 Bahá'u'lláh, Ṭarázát, in *Tablets of Bahá'u'lláh*, p. 35.
19 Bahá'u'lláh, *Hidden Words*, Arabic no. 2.
20 'Abdu'l-Bahá, *Paris Talks*, no. 2, p. 4.
21 Letter on behalf of Shoghi Effendi to an individual believer, 14 December 1941, in *Compilation of Compilations*, vol. 2, p. 11.
22 'Abdu'l-Bahá, in *Star of the West*, vol. IV, no. 6 (24 June 1913), p. 104.
23 'Abdu'l-Bahá, *Some Answered Questions*, no. 70, p. 248.
24 Bahá'u'lláh, *Gleanings*, LXXVII, p. 149.
25 'Abdu'l-Bahá, *The Promulgation of Universal Peace*, p. 121.
26 Bahá'u'lláh, *Gleanings*, CLX, para. 2, pp. 337–8.
27 'Abdu'l-Bahá, quoted in Grundy, *Ten Days in the Light of Acca*, pp. 30–31.
28 Bahá'u'lláh, *Gleanings*, XLIII, para. 5, p. 94.
29 ibid. LXXXV, para, 2, p. 168.
30 Abdu'l-Bahá, as reported in *'Abdu'l-Bahá in London*, p. 120.
31 Letter on behalf of Shoghi Effendi, no date given, in *Lights of Guidance*, no. 701, p. 237.
32 *Biology Letters*, 2007, no. 3, pp. 435–8.
33 'Abdu'l-Bahá, *The Promulgation of Universal Peace*, p. 453.
34 Letter from the Universal House of Justice to the Bahá'ís of Iran, 23 June 2009.
35 'Abdu'l-Bahá, *Abdul Baha on Divine Philosophy*, pp. 41–2.
36 Bahá'u'lláh, *Gleanings*, XV, para. 1, p. 36.
37 'Abdu'l-Bahá, *Will and Testament*, pp. 18–19.
38 'Abdu'l-Bahá, *The Promulgation of Universal Peace*, p. 453.
39 Marjory Morten, 'Bahíyyih Khánum', in *Bahá'í World*, vol. 5 (1932–1934), pp. 182, 185.
40 Bahá'u'lláh, *Kitáb-i-Íqán*, para. 213, pp. 192–3; also in *Gleanings*, CXXV, para. 2, p. 264.
41 Bahá'u'lláh, Lawḥ-i-Maqṣúd, in *Tablets*, p. 172.
42 'Abdu'l-Bahá, as reported in *Star of the West*, vol. VIII, no. 2 (25 July 1914), pp. 24–5.
43 Bahá'u'lláh, *Gems of Divine Mysteries*, p. 61.
44 Bahá'u'lláh, *Kitáb-i-Íqán*, para. 213, pp. 192–3; also in *Gleanings*, CXXV, para. 2, p. 264.
45 Vithoulkas, *The Science of Homeopathy*, p. 40.
46 Joe Keohane, 'How facts backfire. Researchers discover a surprising threat to democracy: Our brains', in *Boston Globe*, 11 July 2010.
47 'Abdu'l-Bahá, *The Promulgation of Universal Peace*, p. 454.
48 Bahá'u'lláh, *Gleanings*, LXXVII, p. 150.
49 'Abdu'l-Bahá, as reported in *Star of the West*, vol. 13, no. 9 (December 1922); passage reprinted in *Foundations of World Unity*, p. 38.
50 Bahá'u'lláh, *Hidden Words*, Persian no. 56.
51 Letter from Shoghi Effendi to an individual believer in India, 27 March 1938, in *Dawn of a New Day*, p. 200.
52 Taherzadeh, *The Revelation of Bahá'u'lláh*, vol. 3, pp. 35–6.

53 'Abdu'l-Bahá, in Thompson, *Diary*, p. 50.
54 ibid. p. 321.
55 Bahá'u'lláh, *Prayers and Meditations*, XVI, p. 19.
56 ibid. CXLIV, p. 233.
57 ibid. CXXIV p. 210.
58 Bahá'u'lláh, Kalimát-i-Firdawsíyyih, in *Tablets of Bahá'u'lláh*, p. 69.
59 Bahá'u'lláh, *Kitáb-i-Aqdas*, para. 43, p. 35.
60 Bahá'u'lláh, *Kitáb-i-Íqán*, paras. 213–18, pp. 192–8.
61 Rabbani, *The Guardian of the Bahá'í Faith*, p. 180.
62 Beinfield and Korngold, *Between Heaven and Earth: A Guide to Chinese Medicine*.
63 'Abdu'l-Bahá, *Tablets*, p. 309.
64 Shoghi Effendi, as reported in Maxwell, *Haifa Notes*, vol. 1, p. 35.
65 'Abdu'l-Bahá, *The Secret of Divine Civilization*, pp. 108–9, quoting Qur'án 17:31, 110.
66 Bahá'u'lláh, Lawḥ-i-Maqṣúd, in *Tablets of Bahá'u'lláh*, p. 173.
67 Bahá'u'lláh, *Hidden Words*, Arabic no. 35.
68 Letter on behalf of Shoghi Effendi to an individual, 29 April 1933, in *Arohanui*, no. 23, p. 33.
69 Letter on behalf of Shoghi Effendi to an individual, 30 June 1936, in *Lights of Guidance*, no. 2108, p. 624.
70 Taherzadeh, *The Revelation of Bahá'u'lláh*, vol. 3, pp. 290–92.
71 Letter from the Universal House of Justice to all National Spiritual Assemblies, 6 February 1973, in *Messages from the Universal House of Justice 1968–1973*, p. 106.
72 Bahá'u'lláh, *Gleanings*, LXXXV, pp. 167–8.

Chapter 10: Recommendations for the Fast

1 Letter on behalf of Shoghi Effendi to an individual believer, 12 March 1946, in *Compilation of Compilations*, vol. 2, no. 1309, p. 15.
2 Bahá'u'lláh, Ṭarázát, in *Tablets of Bahá'u'lláh*, p. 38.
3 Bahá'u'lláh, *Gleanings*, CLXIII, para. 2, p. 342.
4 'Abdu'l-Bahá, *Selections*, no. 13, p. 28.
5 Bahá'u'lláh, *Hidden Words*, Arabic no. 13.
6 ibid. Persian no. 44.
7 'Abdu'l-Bahá, *Paris Talks*, no. 9, p. 29.
8 Letter written on behalf of Shoghi Effendi to an individual believer, 13 October 1947, in *Unfolding Destiny*, p. 446.
9 Bahá'u'lláh, *Gleanings*, XCVI, para. 2, p. 196.
10 Bahá'u'lláh, quoted by Shoghi Effendi, 'The Dispensation of Bahá'u'lláh', in *The World Order of Bahá'u'lláh*, p. 108.
11 See, for instance, the film *The Power of Forgiveness*, available at www.powerofforgiveness.com.

Chapter 11: Fasting for Spiritual Purposes

1 Taherzadeh, *Revelation of Baha'u'llah*, vol. 1, p. 73.
2 Bahá'u'lláh, *Gleanings*, LXXXII, para. 8, p. 161–2.
3 ibid. LXXX, para. 2, p. 154.
4 ibid. LXXXII, para. 1, p. 158.
5 'Abdu'l-Bahá, *Some Answered Questions*, no. 66, p. 239.

6   ibid. no. 70, pp. 249–50.
7   'Abdu'l-Bahá, *Promulgation of Universal Peace*, p. 416.
8   'Abdu'l-Bahá, *Some Answered Questions*, no. 56, p. 211.
9   'Abdu'l-Bahá, quoted in *Star of the West*, vol. XIII, no. 6 (September 1922), p. 153.
10 'Abdu'l-Bahá, *Some Answered Questions*, no. 67, pp. 242.
11 Bahá'u'lláh, *Gleanings*, LXXVII, p. 149.
12 . 'Abdu'l-Bahá, *'Abdu'l-Bahá on Divine Philosophy*, pp. 130–33.
13 Bahá'u'lláh, *Gleanings*, XCV, para. 1, p. 194.
14 ibid. LXXXI, pp. 156–7.
15 'Abdu'l-Bahá, *Paris Talks*, no. 55, p. 189.
16 'Abdu'l-Bahá, *Selections*, no. 150, p. 178.
17 Bahá'u'lláh, *Hidden Words*, Persian no. 29.
18 Bahá'u'lláh, *Gleanings*, LXXVII, p. 149.
19 ibid. XXIV, para. 8, pp. 81; and CXXIV, para. 2, p. 262.
20 'Abdu'l-Bahá, *Promulgation of Universal Peace*, p. 195.
21 'Abdu'l-Bahá, *Some Answered Questions*, no. 32, pp. 130–31.
22 Bahá'u'lláh, *Gleanings*, LII, para. 4, pp. 106–7.
23 'Abdu'l-Bahá, *Paris Talks*, no. 57, p. 191.
24 Letter on behalf of Shoghi Effendi to an individual believer, 14 December 1941, in *Compilation of Compilations*, vol. 2, no. 1294, p. 11; also in *Lights of Guidance*, no. 2039, p. 601.
25 'Abdu'l-Bahá, *Paris Talks*, no. 14, pp. 42–3.
26 Letter on behalf of Shoghi Effendi to an individual believer, 29 May 1935, in *Unfolding Destiny*, p. 434.
27 'Abdu'l-Bahá, quoted in *Star of the West*, vol. VI, no. 6 (24 June 1915), p. 45.
28 'Abdu'l-Bahá, *Paris Talks*, no. 20, p. 61.
29 Bahá'u'lláh, *Gleanings*, LXXXI, pp. 155–6.
30 ibid. LXXXII, p. 161.
31 ibid. LXXXI, p. 156.
32 'Abdu'l-Bahá, *'Abdu'l-Bahá in London*, p. 96.
33 ibid. p. 74.
34 'Abdu'l-Bahá, quoted in Esslemont, *Bahá'u'lláh and the New Era*, p. 175, quoting from 'Abdu'l-Bahá, *Tablets*, p. 204.
35 Bahá'u'lláh, *Gleanings*, LXXXI, p. 157.
36 'Abdu'l-Bahá, *Some Answered Questions*, no. 67, p. 241.
37 ibid. no. 60, p. 223.
38 Bahá'u'lláh, *Gleanings*, LXXXIX, pp. 151–2.
39 'Abdu'l-Bahá, *Promulgation of Universal Peace*, p. 421.
40 Saiedi, *Gate of the Heart*, pp. 50.
41 Bahá'u'lláh, *Gleanings*, CXXXXIV, para. 3, p. 291.
42 Bahá'u'lláh, *Hidden Words*, Arabic no. 59.
43 Bahá'u'lláh, *Gleanings*, XCIII, para. 5, p. 186.
44 Bahá'u'lláh, *Hidden Words*, Persian no. 27.
45 Bahá'u'lláh, *Kitáb-i-Íqán*, para. 61, pp. 57–8.
46 http://www.heartmath.org/research/featured-research/featured-research-home.html.
47 Rollin McCraty et al., 'The coherent heart: Heart–brain interactions,

     psychophysiological coherence, and the emergence of system-wide order', in *Integral Review*, vol. 5, no. 2 (December 2009).
48   Stephen Harrod Buhner, 'The heart as an organ of perception', in *Spirituality and Health* (March/April 2006).
49   'Abdu'l-Bahá, *Promulgation of Universal Peace*, p. 22.
50   Bahá'u'lláh, *Hidden Words*, Persian no. 26.
51   ibid. Persian no. 6.
52   ibid. Parsian no. 31.
53   Quoted by Bahá'u'lláh in *The Four Valleys*, p. 58.
54   'Abdu'l-Bahá, *Paris Talks*, no. 34, p. 108.
55   'Abdu'l-Bahá, *Selections*, no. 178, p. 205.
56   Bahá'u'lláh, *Hidden Words*, Arabic no. 5.
57   'Abdu'l-Bahá, *Selections*, no. 12, p. 27.

Chapter 12: Preparing the Soul for the Fast
1   Letter on behalf of the Universal House of Justice to a National Spiritual Assembly, 1 September 1983, in *Lights of Guidance*, p. 541.
2   'Abdu'l-Bahá, *Selections*, no. 35, p. 70.
3   'Abdu'l-Bahá , quoted in Esslemont, *Bahá'u'lláh and the New Era*, p. 106.
4   'Abdu'l-Bahá , *Paris Talks*, no. 16, p. 50.
5   'Abdu'l-Bahá, *Tablets*, Epigraph, also p. 524.
6   Bahá'u'lláh, *Kitáb-i-Aqdas*, para. 116, p. 61.
7   'Abdu'l-Bahá, *Selections*, no. 161, p. 192.
8   ibid. no. 68, p. 106.
9   Taherzadeh, *The Revelation of Bahá'u'lláh*, vol. 1, p. 102.
10   Bahá'u'lláh, Súriy-i-Ra'ís, para. 32, in *Summons of the Lord of Hosts*, p. 153.
11   Bahá'u'lláh, *Kitáb-i-Íqán*, para. 270, p. 240.
12   ibid. para. 109, p. 102.
13   Bahá'u'lláh, *Gleanings*, XLIII, pp. 92–3.
14   ibid. CLIII, para. 5, p. 326.
15   Bahá'u'lláh, Kitab-i-Aqdas, para. 149, pp. 73–4.
16   ibid.
17   Bahá'u'lláh, Lawḥ-i-Ḥikmat, in *Tablets of Bahá'u'lláh*, p. 143.
18   Bahá'u'lláh, Tablet of Riḍván, in *Gleanings*, para. 16, p. 33.
19   Bahá'u'lláh, *Hidden Words*, Arabic no. 16.
20   Bahá'u'lláh, *Gleanings*, CXXXVI, para. 2, p. 295.
21   The Báb, Tafsír-i-Súriy-i-Kawthár, quoted in Saiedi, *Gate of the Heart*, p. 73.
22   Letter on behalf of Shoghi Effendi to an individual, 8 December 1935, in *Compilation of Compilations*, vol. 2, no. 1762, p. 238.
23   Bahá'u'lláh, *Kitáb-i-Aqdas*, para. 6, p. 21.
24   'Abdu'l-Bahá, quoted in Baker, *The Path to God* (1937), quoted in Honnold, *Vignettes*, pp. 148–9, no. 27.
25   Letter on behalf of Shoghi Effendi to an individual believer, 26 October 1938, in *Compilation of Compilations*, vol. 2, no. 1768, p. 240.
26   'Abdu'l-Bahá, in *Star of the West*, vol.VIII, no. 4 (17 May 1917), p. 42.
27   'Abdu'l-Bahá, from the diary of Shoghi Effendi, 10 August 1919, quoted in Khadem, *Shoghi Effendi in Oxford*, p. 50.
28   'Abdu'l-Bahá, in *Star of the West*, Vol. VIII, no. 4 (17 May 1917), p. 46.

29 Grundy, *Ten Days in the Light of Acca*, p. 15.
30 'Abdu'l-Bahá, *The Promulgation of Universal Peace*, pp. 246–7.
31 'Abdu'l-Bahá, *Selections*, no. 74, p. 112.
32 Bahá'u'lláh, *Kitáb-i-Aqdas*, para. 51, p. 38.
33 Amen, *Change Your Brain, Change Your Life*, p. 205.
34 Bahá'u'lláh, *Gleanings*, CXXXVI, para. 2, p. 295.
35 'Abdu'l-Bahá, *Selections*, no. 199, p. 241.
36 Weiss, *Through Time into Healing*, p 26.
37 'Abdu'l-Bahá, *Paris Talks*, no. 54, pp. 186–7.
38 Muslim tradition, quoted by Bahá'u'lláh in the *Kitáb-i-Íqan*, para. 267, p. 238.
39 Bahá'u'lláh, Kalimát-i-Firdawsíyyih, in *Tablets of Bahá'u'lláh*, p. 72.
40 'Abdu'l-Bahá, *Paris Talks*, no. 54, pp. 187–8.
41 Shoghi Effendi, quoted in *The Kitáb-i-Aqdas*, note 25, p. 176.
42 'Abdu'l-Bahá, *Some Answered Questions*, no. 73, p. 257.
43 'Abdu'l-Bahá, *Selections*, no. 133, p. 152.
44 'Abdu'l-Bahá, *Abdu'l-Bahá in London*, p. 65.
45 See Wallace et al., 'The effects of the Transcendental Meditation and TM-Sidhi program on the aging process', in *International Journal of Neuroscience*, no. 16, pp. 53–8.
46 Letter on behalf of Shoghi Effendi to an individual believer, 25 January 1943, in *Prayer, Meditation and the Devotional Attitude*, no 50, p. 17.
47 Bhagavad-Gita 6.19, p. 329.
48 Bahá'u'lláh, *Kitáb-i-Aqdas*, para. 134, pp. 66–7.
49 ibid. para. 18, p. 26.
50 Bahá'u'lláh, *Hidden Words*, Arabic no. 31.
51 Bahá'u'lláh, Lawh-i-Hikmat, in *Tablets of Bahá'u'lláh*, pp. 140–41.
52 ibid. p. 140.
53 Saiedi, *Gate of the Heart*, p. 59.
54 Bahá'u'lláh, *Kitáb-i-Íqán*, para. 283, p. 255.
55 'Abdu'l-Bahá, *Tablets*, p. 706.
56 Bahá'u'lláh, *Kitáb-i-Íqán*, para. 213, p. 192.
57 Letter from the Universal House of Justice to an individual believer, 7 December 1969, in *Messages from the Universal House of Justice, 1968–1973*, p. 37; also in *Compilation of Compilations*, vol. 1, no. 765, p. 360.
58 The Báb, Tablet to Mírzá Sa'íd, quoted in Saiedi, *Gate of the Heart*, p. 177.
59 Bahá'u'lláh, Lawh-i-Maqṣúd, in *Tablets of Bahá'u'lláh*, p. 171.
60 Bahá'u'lláh, *Kitáb-i-Íqán*, para. 201, p. 184.
61 Bahá'u'lláh, *Seven Valleys*, p. 8.
62 Bahá'u'lláh, *Kitáb-i-Íqán*, para. 1, p. 3.
63 ibid. para. 213, p. 192.
64 Taherzadeh, *The Revelation of Bahá'u'lláh*, vol. 4, pp. 212–13.
65 'Abdu'l-Bahá, *Abdul Baha on Divine Philosophy*, pp. 136–7.
66 Taherzadeh, *The Revelation of Bahá'u'lláh*, vol. 2, p. 36.
67 ibid. pp. 39-40.
68 'Abdu'l-Bahá, quoted in Blomfield, *The Chosen Highway*, p. 166.
69 'Abdu'l-Bahá, *Abdu'l-Bahá in London*, p. 121.
70 Bahá'u'lláh, quoted in Shoghi Effendi, 'The Dispensation of Bahá'u'lláh', in *The World Order of Bahá'u'lláh*, p. 135.

71 Bahá'u'lláh, *Kitáb-i-Aqdas*, para. 120, p. 62.
72 Bahá'u'lláh, Kalimát-i-Firdawsíyyih, in *Tablets of Bahá'u'lláh*, p. 63.
73 Bahá'u'lláh, *Gleanings*, CXXVI, para. 4, p. 272.
74 ibid. LXVI, para. 2, p. 126.
75 Words attributed to 'Abdu'l-Bahá, from the diary of Ahmad Sohrab, in *Star of the West*, vol. VIII, no 2 (April 1917), p. 17.
76 Bahá'u'lláh, Tablet to a Physician, in *Compilation of Compilations*, vol.. 1, no. 1020, p. 460, from Esslemont, *Bahá'u'lláh and the New Era*, p. 106.
77 See Taherzadeh, *The Revelation of Bahá'u'lláh*, vol. 1, pp. 108–9 for a description.
78 'Abdu'l-Bahá, as reported in *Star of the West*, vol. 13 (March 1922), pp. 24–5.
79 'Abdu'l-Bahá, quoted in Grundy, *Ten Days in the Light of Acca*, p. 29.
80 Bahá'u'lláh, *Prayers and Meditations*, no. VIII, p. 11.
81 Bahá'u'lláh, *Gleanings*, CXVII, p. 250.
82 'Abdu'l-Bahá, *Paris Talks*, no. 55, p. 189.
83 Letter on behalf of Shoghi Effendi to an individual believer, 26 December 1935, in *Lights of Guidance*, no. 1870, pp. 550.
84 Words attributed to 'Abdu'l-Bahá, from the diary of Ahmad Sohrab, *Star of the West*, vol. VIII, no. 1 (9 April 1917), p. 21.
85 Bahá'u'lláh, *Gleanings*, CXXXIX, para. 5, p. 304.
86 'Abdu'l-Bahá, Tablet of Visitation, in most Bahá'í prayer books.
87 Words attributed to 'Abdu'l-Bahá, quotes in Maxwell, *Early Pilgrimage*, p. 40.
88 Words attributed to 'Abdu'l-Bahá, quoted in Gail, *Summon Up Remembrance*, p. 255.
89 Bahá'u'lláh, *Prayers and Meditations*, CLVI, p. 250.
90 Bahá'u'lláh, *Gleanings*, CLIII, para. 5, p. 326.
91 Bahá'u'lláh, *Kitáb-i-Íqán*, para. 216, pp. 195–6.
92 'Abdu'l-Bahá, *Selections*, no. 36, p. 76.
93 Letter on behalf of Shoghi Effendi to an individual, 10 December 1947, in *Compilation of Compilations*, vol. II, p. 18.
94 'Abdu'l-Bahá, new translation provided by the Bahá'í World Centre from *Tablets of Abdul Baha*, pp. 354–5, in *The Wisdom of the Master*, p. 44.
95 Letter on behalf of Shoghi Effendi, 30 June 1923, in *Lights of Guidance*, no. 2048, p. 603.
96 'Abdu'l-Bahá, *The Promulgation of Universal Peace*, pp. 147–8.
97 Bahá'u'lláh, *Gleanings*, CV, para. 2, p. 210.
98 ibid. CLX, para. 3, p. 338.
99 'Abdu'l-Bahá, *Tablets*, p. 709.
100 'Abdu'l-Bahá, *The Promulgation of Universal Peace*, p. 244.
101 Bahá'u'lláh, *Gleanings*, XXXIV, para. 1, pp. 77–8.
102 The Báb, Tafsír-i-Súriy-i-Kawthár, quoted in Saiedi, *Gate of the Heart*, p. 72.
103 Bahá'u'lláh, *Prayers and Meditations*, XIX, p. 22.
104 Bahá'u'lláh, *Kitáb-i-Íqán*, para. 160, p. 151.
105 Bahá'u'lláh, quoted in Shoghi Effendi, *The Promised Day is Come*, para. 204, p. 135 in 1996 ed. (p. 82 in original edition)
106 'Abdu'l-Bahá, *Tablets*, p. 318.
107 Bahá'u'lláh, *Gleanings*, LXVI, para. 13, p. 130.
108 Taherzadeh, *The Revelation of Bahá'u'lláh*, vol. 4, p. 35.
109 'Abdu'l-Bahá, *Selections*, no. 155, p. 182.